Biopharmaceutics and Pharmacokinetics

FV Manvi M Pharm, PhD
Dean of Pharmacy Faculty
KLE University, Belgaum 590010
Karnataka, India

Basavaraj K Nanjwade M Pharm, PhD
Department of Pharmaceutics
KLE University's College of Pharmacy, Belgaum

Mahesh K Patel M Pharm
Department of Pharmaceutics
KLE University's College of Pharmacy, Belgaum

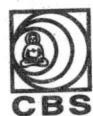

CBS Publishers & Distributors Pvt Ltd

New Delhi • Bengaluru • Chennai • Kochi • Kolkata • Mumbai
Bhopal • Bhubaneswar • Hyderabad • Jharkhand • Nagpur • Patna
• Pune • Uttarakhand • Dhaka (Bangladesh) • Kathmandu (Nepal)

Biopharmaceutics and Pharmacokinetics

ISBN: 978-93-89941-90-6

Copyright © Publisher

First Edition: 2011

CBS Reprint: 2020, 2023

Published by Satish Kumar Jain and produced by Varun Jain for
CBS Publishers & Distributors Pvt Ltd
4819/XI Prahlad Street, 24 Ansari Road, Daryaganj, New Delhi 110 002, India
Ph: 011-23289259, 23266861, 23266867   Website: www.cbspd.com
Fax: 011-23243014   e-mail: delhi@cbspd.com
Corporate Office: 204 FIE, Industrial Area, Patparganj, Delhi 110 092
Ph: 011-4934 4934   Fax: 011-4934 4935   e-mail: publishing@cbspd.com; publicity@cbspd.com

Branches

- **Bengaluru:** Seema House 2975, 17th Cross, KR Road, Banasankari 2nd Stage, Bengaluru 560 070, Karnataka, India
  Ph: +91-80-26771678/79   Fax: +91-80-26771680   e-mail: bangalore@cbspd.com
- **Chennai:** 7, Subbaraya Street, Shenoy Nagar, Chennai 600 030, Tamil Nadu, India
  Ph: +91-44-26680620, 26681266   Fax: +91-44-42032115   e-mail: chennai@cbspd.com
- **Kochi:** 42/1325, 1326, Power House Road, Opp KSEB, Power House, Ernakulam, Kochi 682 018, Kerala, India
  Ph: +91-484-4059061-65   Fax: +91-484-4059065   e-mail: kochi@cbspd.com
- **Kolkata:** 147, Hind Ceramics Compound, 1st Floor, Nilgunj Road, Belghoria, Kolkata 700 056, West Bengal, India
  Ph: +91-33-25633055-56   e-mail: kolkata@cbspd.com
- **Lucknow:** Basement, Khushnuma Complex, 7-Meerabai Marg (behind Jawahar Bhawan), Lucknow 226 001, UP, India
  Ph: +91-522-4000032
                                                          e-mail: tiwari.lucknow@cbspd.com
- **Mumbai:** PWD Shed. Gala no. 25/26, Ramchandra Bhatt Marg, Next to JJ Hospital Gate no. 2, Opp. Union Bank of India, Noorbaug, Mumbai 400 009, Maharashtra, India
  Ph: +91-22-66661880/89
                                                          e-mail: mumbai@cbspd.com

Representatives

- **Hyderabad** 0-9885175004 **Jharkhand** 0-9811541605 **Nagpur** 0-9421945513
- **Patna** 0-9334159340 **Pune** 0-9623451994 **Uttarakhand** 0-9716462459

Printed at Mudrak, Noida, UP, India

PREFACE

Biopharmaceutics basically refers to what happens to the drug inside the body i.e. the various processes of absorption, distribution, metabolism and elimination whereas pharmacokinetics deals with the rate or kinetic of these processes. This book explains each process in detail. In absorption, it explains the key factors affecting absorption-biological, physiological, physicochemical and pharmaceutical. The concept of bioavailability, measurement of bioavailability by different methods, determination of absorption rate constant, the importance of bioequivalence have been discussed. The in-vitro dissolution testing models in-vitro–in-vivo correlation, and bioavailability and bioequivalence including evaluation testing protocols has been covered.

In distribution, the various drug distribution patterns, factors affecting drug distribution have been explained. In protein binding, drug binding to tissues and plasma proteins have been explained. Also, the process of elimination and the concept of renal and organ (hepatic) clearance have been dealt with.

Pharmacokinetics deals with the pharmacokinetic model such as pharmacokinetic model, significance of plasma drug concentration measurement, one compartment and two compartment models. Non-linear pharmacokinetics is the other topics of discussion.

Clinical pharmacokinetics, being an important chapter, discusses the adjustment of drug dosage in various situations such as with and without renal and hepatic failure. This chapter also discusses the pharmacokinetic drug interactions and its significance in combination therapy.

Each chapter is explained with the help of graphical illustrations wherever necessary and examples are worked out in case of mathematical concepts to make them clear to the students.

The objective of writing this book is to present this subject in a simple way and make it as informative as possible. Although this book is targeted to the undergraduate and postgraduate students, it caters to anyone who is interested or working in the R&D department of an industry, clinician, and research scholars.

Although, several books of foreign authors are available in the market, all the chapters are not covered in a single book or they are not simple enough to follow from the student's point of view. Very few books are available from the Indian authors. The growing importance of this subject and my love for this wonderful subject has inspired me to write this book. I hope to inspire students and other readers through this book to understand and appreciate the application of biopharmaceutics and pharmacokinetics in various pharmaceutical fields such as product development, R&D, hospitals etc.

The authors express their sincere thanks and appreciation to Prof. Ashok D.Taranahalli, Principal, KLE University College of Pharmacy, Belgaum, Prof. Dr. Chandrakant K. Kokate, Vice-Chancellor and Prof. Dr. P.F. Kotur, Registrar, KLE University, Belgaum, Karnataka, India for rendering useful suggestions and inputs, apart from being intensely persuasive to complete the project.

We are grateful to Mr. Gowrishetty Madhusudhan, IKON BOOKS who has taken keen interest and spared no pains for the fine getup of the book.

CONTENTS

Chapter—1

INTRODUCTION

Biopharmaceutics

A drug can be obtained from different sources such as, plant source, animal source, mineral source or it can be synthetic. A drug is usually administered in different dosage forms (drug +excipients/additives) by a suitable route. The therapeutic response produced by the drug depends on 2 main factors – intrinsic pharmacological activity of the drug and the route by which the drug is administered. The drug-response relationships obtained by the drug administered by oral and that administered by parentral route are different. Variations are observed when the same drug is administered in different dosage forms or similar dosage forms produced by different manufacturers, this depends upon the physicochemical properties of the drug, the excipients present in the formulation, the method of formulation and the manner of administration. Thus biopharmaceutics was developed to study the dose-response relationship of the drug and the factors affecting it.

All pharmaceuticals, from the generic analgesic tablet in the community pharmacy to the state-of-the-art immunotherapy in specialized hospitals, undergo extensive research and development prior to approval by the U.S. Food and Drug Administration (FDA). The physicochemical characteristics of the active pharmaceutical ingredient (API, or drug substance), the dosage form or the drug, and the route of administration are critical determinants of the *in-vivo* performance, safety and efficacy of the drug product. The properties of the drug and its dosage form are carefully engineered and tested to produce a stable drug product that upon administration provides the desired therapeutic response in the patient. Both the pharmacist and the pharmaceutical scientist must understand these complex relationships to comprehend the proper use and development of pharmaceuticals.

To illustrate the importance of the drug substance and the drug formulation on absorption, and distribution of the drug to the site of action, one must first consider the sequence of events that precede elicitation of a drug's therapeutic effect. First, the drug in its dosage form is taken by the patient either by an oral, intravenous, subcutaneous, transdermal, etc., route of administration. Next, the drug is released from the dosage form in a predictable and characterizable manner. Then, some fraction of the drug is absorbed from the site of administration into either the surrounding tissue, into the body (as with oral dosage forms), or both. Finally, the drug reaches the site of action. If the drug concentration at the site of action exceeds the minimum effective concentration (MEC), a pharmacologic response results. The actual dosing regimen (dose, dosage form, dosing interval) was carefully determined in clinical trials to provide the correct drug concentrations at the site of action. This sequence of events is profoundly affected—in fact, sometimes orchestrated—by the design of the dosage form, the drug itself, or both.

Historically, pharmaceutical scientists have evaluated the relative drug availability to the body *in vivo* after giving a drug product to an animal or human, and then comparing specific pharmacologic, clinical, or possible toxic responses. For example, a drug such as isoproterenol causes an increase in heart rate when given intravenously but has no observable effect on the heart when given orally at the same dose level. In addition, the bioavailability (a measure of systemic availability of a drug) may differ from one drug product to another containing the same drug, even for the same route of administration. This difference in drug bioavailability may be manifested by observing the difference in the therapeutic effectiveness of the drug products. In other words, the nature of the drug molecule, the route of delivery, and the formulation of the dosage form can determine whether an administered drug is therapeutically effective, toxic, or has no apparent effect at all.

Many factors have been found to influence the time course of a drug in the plasma and thereby its concentration at the site(s) of action. These include the foods eaten by the patient, the effect of the disease state on drug absorption, the age of the patient, the site(s) of absorption of the administered drug, co-administration of other drugs, the physical and chemical properties of the administered drug, the type of dosage form, the composition and method of manufacture of the dosage form and the size of dose and frequency of administration of the dosage form. Thus, a given drug may exhibit differences in its bioavailability if-

(1) It is administered in the same type of dosage form by different route, e.g., an aqueous solution of a given drug administered by the intramuscular and oral routes of administration.

(2) It is given by the same route of administration and in the same dosage form, but formulation and methods of manufacture of the dosage form are different, e.g. different formulations of an aqueous suspension of a given drug administered by the peroral route.

(3) It is given by same route of administration but in different dosage forms, e.g., an emulsion, suspension and tablet administered by peroral route.

The variability by a drug in bioavailability from different formulations of the same type of dosage form or from different types of dosage forms etc., can cause the patient to be under or over medicated. The result may be a therapeutic failure or serious adverse effects, particularly in the case of drugs that have narrow therapeutic indices.

The entry of a drug into the systemic circulation following its administration usually involves:

(1) The release of the drug from its dosage form into a solution in the biological fluids at the absorption site, and

(2) The movement of the dissolved drug across the biological membranes into the systemic circulation.

Biopharmaceutics may be defined as the study of factor influencing the rate and amount of drug that reaches the systemic circulation and the use of this information to optimize the therapeutic efficacy of the drug products.

Biopharmaceutics is the science that examines this interrelationship of the physicochemical properties of the drug, the dosage form in which the drug is given, and the route of administration on the rate and extent of systemic drug absorption. Thus, biopharmaceutics involves factors that influences are as follows:

(1) The stability of the drug within the drug product,

(2) The release of the drug from the drug product,

(3) The rate of dissolution/release of the drug at the absorption site, and

(4) The systemic absorption of the drug.

The study of biopharmaceutics is based on fundamental scientific principles and experimental methodology. Studies in biopharmaceutics use both *in-vitro* and *in-vivo* methods. *In-vitro* methods are procedures employing test apparatus and equipment without involving laboratory animals or humans. *In-vivo* methods are more complex studies involving human subjects or laboratory animals. These methods must be able to

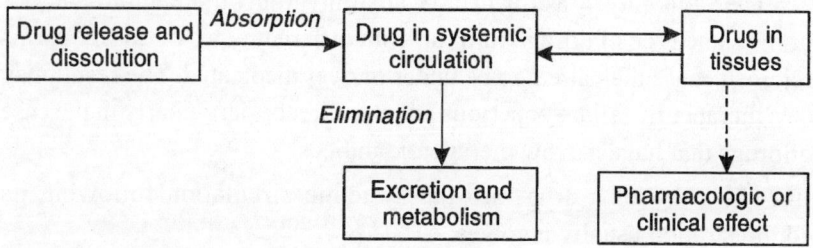

Fig.1.1: Scheme demonstrating the dynamic relationship between the drug, the drug product, and the pharmacologic effect.

assess the impact of the physical and chemical properties of the drug, drug stability, and large-scale production of the drug and drug product on the biologic performance of the drug. Moreover, biopharmaceutics considers the properties of the drug and dosage form in a physiologic environment, the drug's intended therapeutic use, and the route of administration. The dynamic relationship between the drug, the drug product, and the pharmacologic effect is given in fig. 1.1.

Absorption may be defined as the process of movement of drug from its site of administration to the systemic circulation.

Bioavailability may be defined as the rate and extent (amount) of drug absorption. If there occurs any alteration in drug's bioavailability, it is reflected in its pharmacological response. The bioavailability may differ from one drug product to another containing the same drug. The difference in drug bioavailability may be manifested by observing the difference in the therapeutic effectiveness of the drug products.

If a change is made in the drug's bioavailability, it is reflected in its pharmacological effects. The bioavailability of a drug depends upon the following aspects:

(1) The rate at which the drug is released from its dosage form,

(2) The extent to which the drug is released from its dosage form,

(3) The extent of subsequent absorptions from the dissolved (solution) state, and

(4) The biotransformation occurring during the process of absorption.

Drug distribution is the movement of drug between one compartment and the other. Generally the site of drug administration and site of drug action are different, thus drug distribution play a vital role in determining the onset, intensity and duration of action of the drug. The intensity of action also depends on the effective concentration of the drug and the duration for which the concentration is maintained at the site of action. The maintenance of drug concentration at the site of action depends upon elimination processes.

Elimination is process of removal of the drug from the body and thus terminates its action. Elimination takes place by involving the following two processes:

(1) **Biotransformation:** The metabolism of drug in the body is known as biotransformation. This process usually inactivates the drug.

(2) **Excretion:** The exit of drug/metabolites from the body is known as excretion.

Pharmacokinetics

After a drug is released from its dosage form, the drug is absorbed into the surrounding tissue, the body, or both. The distribution through and elimination of the drug in the body varies for each patient but can be characterized using mathematical models and statistics. **Pharmacokinetics** is the science of the kinetics of drug absorption, distribution, and elimination (i.e. excretion and metabolism). The description of drug distribution and elimination is often termed **drug disposition.** Characterization of drug disposition is an important prerequisite for determination or modification of dosing regimens for individuals and groups of patients.

The study of pharmacokinetics involves both experimental and theoretical approaches. The experimental aspect of pharmacokinetics involves the development of biologic sampling techniques, analytical methods for the measurement of drugs and metabolites, and procedures that facilitate data collection and manipulation. The theoretical aspect of pharmacokinetics involves the development of pharmacokinetic models that predict drug disposition after drug administration. The application of statistics is an integral part of pharmacokinetic studies. Statistical methods are used for pharmacokinetic parameter estimation and data interpretation ultimately for the purpose of designing and predicting optimal dosing regimens for individuals or groups of patients. Statistical methods are applied to pharmacokinetic models to determine data error and structural model deviations. Mathematics and computer techniques form the theoretical basis of many pharmacokinetic methods. Classical pharmacokinetics is a study of theoretical models focusing mostly on model development and parameterization.

Clinical pharmacokinetics may be defined as the application of pharmacokinetic methods in drug therapy. This is useful in optimizing the drug dose to suit individual patient needs and achieving maximum utility. The study of clinical pharmacokinetics of drugs in disease state requires input from medical and pharmaceutical research.

Pharmacodynamics refers to the relationship between the drug concentration at the site of action (receptor) and pharmacologic response, including biochemical and physiologic effects that influence the interaction of drug with the receptor. The interaction of a drug molecule with a receptor causes the initiation of a sequence of molecular events resulting in a pharmacologic or toxic response. Pharmacokinetic-pharmacodynamic models are constructed to relate plasma drug level to drug concentration in the site of action and establish the intensity and time course of the drug.

Toxicokinetics is the application of pharmacokinetic principles to the design, conduct, and interpretation of drug safety evaluation studies and in validating dose-related exposure in animals. Toxicokinetic data aids in the interpretation of toxicologic findings in animals and extrapolation of the resulting data to humans. Toxicokinetic studies are performed in animals during preclinical drug development and may continue after the drug has been tested in clinical trials.

Clinical toxicology is the study of adverse effects of drugs and toxic substances (poisons) in the body. The pharmacokinetics of a drug in an overmedicated (intoxicated) patient may be very different from the pharmacokinetics of the same drug given in lower therapeutic doses. At very high doses, the drug concentration in the body may saturate enzymes involved in the absorption, biotransformation, or active renal secretion mechanisms, thereby changing the pharmacokinetics from linear to nonlinear pharmacokinetics. Drugs frequently involved in toxicity cases include acetaminophen, salicylates, morphine, and the tricylic antidepressants (TCAs). Many of these drugs can be assayed conveniently by fluorescence immunoassay (FIA) kits.

Basic Pharmacokinetics

Drugs are in a dynamic state within the body as they move between tissues and fluids, bind with plasma or cellular components, or are metabolized. The biologic nature of drug distribution and disposition is complex, and drug events often happen simultaneously. Yet such factors must be considered when designing drug therapy regimens. The inherent and infinite complexity of these events requires the use of mathematical models and statistics to estimate drug dosing and to predict the time course of drug efficacy for a given dose.

A model is a hypothesis using mathematical terms to describe quantitative relationships concisely. The predictive capability of a model lies in the proper selection and development of mathematical function(s) that parameterize the essential factors governing the kinetic process. The key parameters in a process are commonly estimated by fitting the model to the experimental data, known as variables. A pharmacokinetic parameter is a constant for the drug that is estimated from the experimental data. For example, estimated pharmacokinetic parameters such as k depend on the method of tissue sampling, the timing of the sample, drug analysis, and the predictive model selected.

A pharmacokinetic function relates an independent variable to a dependent variable, often through the use of parameters. For example, a pharmacokinetic model may predict the drug concentration in the liver 1 hour after an oral administration of a 20-mg dose. The independent variable is time and the dependent variable is the drug concentration in the liver. Based on a set of time-versus-drug concentration data, a model equation is derived to predict the liver drug concentration with respect to time. In this case, the drug concentration depends on the time after the administration of the dose, where the time: concentration relationship is defined by a pharmacokinetic parameter, k, the elimination rate constant.

Such mathematical models can be devised to simulate the rate processes of drug absorption, distribution, and elimination to describe and predict drug concentrations in the body as a function of time. Pharmacokinetic models are used to:

1. Predict plasma, tissue, and urine drug levels with any dosage regimen
2. Calculate the optimum dosage regimen for each patient individually
3. Estimate the possible accumulation of drugs and/or metabolites
4. Correlate drug concentrations with pharmacologic or toxicologic activity
5. Evaluate differences in the rate or extent of availability between formulations (bioequivalence)
6. Describe how changes in physiology or disease affect the absorption, distribution, or elimination of the drug
7. Explain drug interactions

Simplifying assumptions are made in pharmacokinetic models to describe a complex biologic system concerning the movement of drugs within the body. For example, most pharmacokinetic models assume that the plasma drug concentration reflects drug concentrations globally within the body. A model may be empirically, physiologically, or compartmentally based. The model that simply interpolates the data and allows an empirical formula to estimate drug level over time is justified when limited information is available. Empirical models are practical but not very useful in explaining the mechanism of the actual process by which the drug is absorbed, distributed, and eliminated in the body.

Physiologically based models also have limitations. Using the example above, and apart from the necessity to sample tissue and monitor blood flow to the liver *in vivo*, the investigator needs to understand the following questions. What does liver drug concentration mean? Should the drug concentration in the blood within the tissue be determined and subtracted from the drug in the liver tissue? What type of cell is representative of the liver if a selective biopsy liver tissue sample can be collected without contamination from its surroundings? Indeed, depending on the spatial location of the liver tissue from the hepatic blood vessels, tissue drug concentrations can differ depending on distance to the blood vessel or even on the type of cell in the liver. Moreover, changes in the liver blood perfusion will alter the tissue drug concentration. If heterogeneous liver tissue is homogenized and assayed, the homogenized tissue represents only a hypothetical concentration that is an average of all the cells and blood in the liver at the time of collection. Since tissue homogenization is not practical for human subjects, the drug concentration in the liver may be estimated by knowing the liver extraction ratio for the drug based on knowledge of the physiologic and biochemical composition of the body organs.

A very simple and useful tool in pharmacokinetics is compartmentally based models. For example, assume a drug is given by intravenous injection and that the drug dissolves (distributes) rapidly in the body fluids. One pharmacokinetic model that can describe this situation is a tank containing a volume of fluid that is rapidly equilibrated with the drug. The concentration of the drug in the tank after a given dose is governed by two parameters: (1) the fluid volume of the tank that will dilute the drug, and (2) the elimination rate of drug per unit of time. Though this model is perhaps an overly simplistic view of drug disposition in the human body, a drug's pharmacokinetic properties can frequently be described using a fluid-filled tank model called the one-compartment open model (see below). In both the tank and the one-compartment body model, a fraction of the drug would be continually eliminated as a function of time. In pharmacokinetics, these parameters are assumed to be constant for a given drug. If drug concentrations in the tank are determined at various time intervals following administration of a known dose, then the volume of fluid in the tank or compartment (V_D, volume of distribution) and the rate of drug elimination can be estimated.

In practice, pharmacokinetic parameters such as k and V_D are determined experimentally from a set of drug concentrations collected over various times and known as data. The number of parameters needed to describe the model depends on the complexity of the process and on the route of drug administration. In general, as the number of parameters required to model the data increases, accurate estimation of these parameters becomes increasingly more difficult. With complex

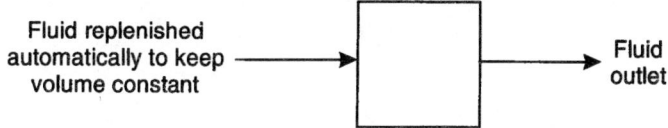

Fig. 1.2: Tank with a constant volume of fluid equilibrated with drug. The volume of the fluid is 1.0 L. The fluid outlet is 10 mL/min. The fraction of drug removed per unit of time is 10/1000, or 0.01 min^{-1}

pharmacokinetic models, computer programs are used to facilitate parameter estimation. However, for the parameters to be valid, the number of data points should always exceed the number of parameters in the model.

Because a model is based on a hypothesis and simplifying assumptions, a certain degree of caution is necessary when relying totally on the pharmacokinetic model to predict drug action. For some drugs, plasma drug concentrations are not useful in predicting drug activity. For other drugs, an individual's genetic differences, disease state, and the compensatory response of the body may modify the response of a drug. If a simple model does not fit all the experimental observations accurately, a new, more elaborate model may be proposed and subsequently tested. Since limited data are generally available in most clinical situations, pharmacokinetic data should be interpreted along with clinical observations rather than replacing sound judgment by the clinician. Development of pharmacometric statistical models may help to improve prediction of drug levels among patients in the population. However, it will be some time before these methods become generally accepted.

Measurement of Drug Concentration

Because drug concentrations are an important element in determining individual or population pharmacokinetics, drug concentrations are measured in biologic samples, such as milk, saliva, plasma, and urine.

Sensitive, accurate, and precise analytical methods are available for the direct measurement of drugs in biologic matrices. Such measurements are generally validated so that accurate information is generated for pharmacokinetic and clinical monitoring. In general, chromatographic methods are most frequently employed for drug concentration measurement, because chromatography separates the drug from other related materials that may cause assay interference.

Drug concentration in Blood, plasma, or serum

Measurement of drug concentration (levels) in the blood, serum, or plasma is the most direct approach to assessing the pharmacokinetics of the drug in the body. Whole blood contains cellular elements including red blood cells, white blood cells, platelets, and various other proteins, such as albumin and globulins. In general, serum or plasma is most commonly used for drug measurement. To obtain serum, whole blood is allowed to clot and the serum is collected from the supernatant after centrifugation. Plasma is obtained from the supernatant of centrifuged whole blood to which an anticoagulant, such as heparin, has been added. Therefore, the protein content of serum and plasma is not the same. Plasma perfuses all the tissues of the body, including the cellular elements in the blood. Assuming that a drug in the plasma is in dynamic equilibrium with the tissues, then changes in the drug concentration in plasma will reflect changes in tissue drug concentrations.

Sampling of biologic specimens

Only a few biologic specimens may be obtained safely from the patient to gain information as to the drug concentration in the body. Invasive methods include sampling blood, spinal fluid, synovial fluid, tissue biopsy, or any biologic material that requires parenteral or surgical intervention in the patient. In contrast, noninvasive methods include sampling of urine, saliva, feces, expired air, or any biologic material that can be obtained without parenteral or surgical intervention. The measurement of drug and metabolite concentration in each of these biologic materials yields important information, such as the amount of drug retained in, or transported into, that region of the tissue or fluid, the likely pharmacologic or toxicologic outcome of drug dosing, and drug metabolite formation or transport.

Plasma Level–Time Curve

The plasma level–time curve is generated by obtaining the drug concentration in plasma samples taken at various time intervals after a drug product is administered. The concentration of drug in each plasma sample is plotted on rectangular-coordinate graph paper against the corresponding time at which the plasma sample was removed. As the drug reaches the general (systemic) circulation, plasma drug concentrations will rise up to a maximum. Usually, absorption of a drug is more rapid than elimination. As the drug is being absorbed into the systemic circulation, the drug is distributed to all the tissues in the body and is also simultaneously being eliminated. Elimination of a drug can proceed by excretion, biotransformation, or a combination of both.

The relationship of the drug level–time curve and various pharmacologic parameters for the drug is shown in. MEC and MTC represent the minimum effective concentration and minimum toxic concentration of drug, respectively. For some drugs, such as those acting on the autonomic nervous system, it is useful to know the concentration of drug that will just barely produce a pharmacologic effect (i.e., MEC). Assuming the drug concentration in the plasma is in equilibrium with the tissues, the MEC reflects the minimum concentration of drug needed at the receptors to produce the desired pharmacologic effect. Similarly, the MTC represents the drug concentration needed to just barely produce a toxic effect. The onset time corresponds to the time required for the drug to reach the MEC. The intensity of the pharmacologic effect is proportional to the number of drug receptors occupied, which is reflected in the observation that higher plasma drug concentrations produce a greater pharmacologic response, up to a maximum. The duration of drug action is the difference between the onset time and the time for the drug to decline back to the MEC.

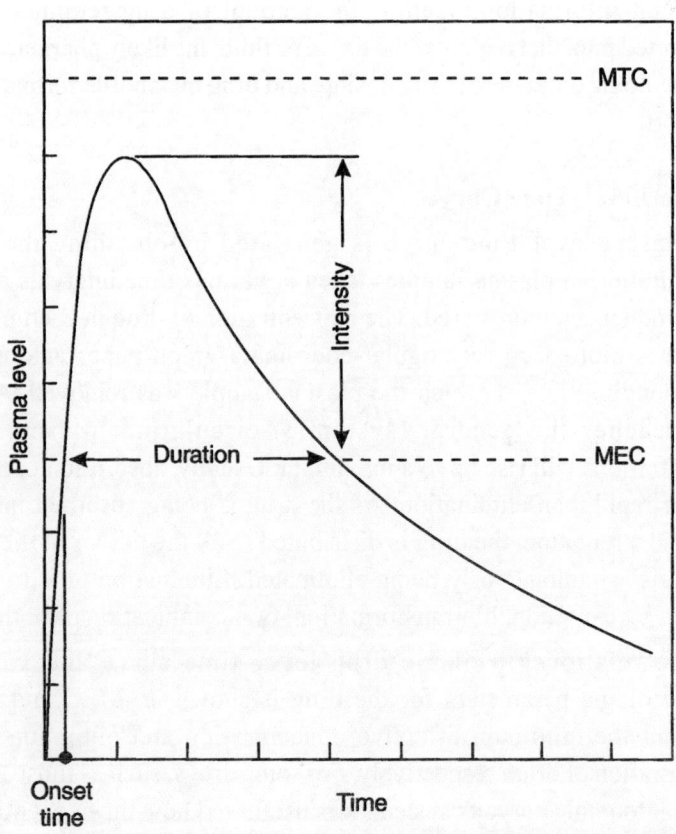

Fig. 1.3:   Generalized plasma level–time curve after oral administration of a drug.

In contrast, the pharmacokineticist can also describe the plasma level–time curve in terms of such pharmacokinetic terms as peak plasma level, time for peak plasma level, and area under the curve, or AUC. The time of peak plasma level is the time of maximum drug concentration in the plasma and is a rough marker of average rate of drug absorption. The peak plasma level or maximum drug concentration is related to the dose, the rate constant for absorption, and the elimination constant of the drug. The AUC is related to the amount of drug absorbed systemically.

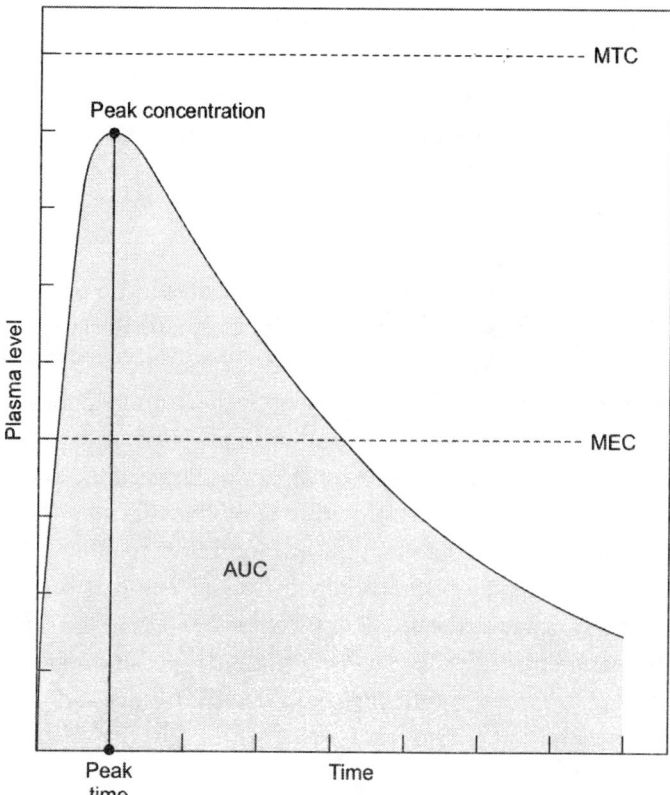

Fig.1.4: Plasma level–time curve showing peak time and concentration. The shaded portion represents the AUC (area under the curve).

Drug concentrations in urine and feces

Measurement of drug in urine is an indirect method to ascertain the bioavailability of a drug. The rate and extent of drug excreted in the urine reflects the rate and extent of systemic drug absorption. Measurement of drug in feces may reflect drug that has not been absorbed after an oral dose or may reflect drug that has been expelled by biliary secretion after systemic absorption. Fecal drug excretion is often performed in mass balance studies, in which the investigator attempts to account for the entire dose given to the patient. For a mass balance study, both urine and feces are collected and their drug content measured. For certain solid oral dosage forms that do not dissolve in the gastrointestinal tract but slowly leach out drug, fecal collection is performed to recover the dosage form. The undissolved dosage form is then assayed for residual drug.

Drug concentrations in tissues

Tissue biopsies are occasionally removed for diagnostic purposes, such as the verification of a malignancy. Usually, only a small sample of tissue is removed, making drug concentration measurement difficult. Drug concentrations in tissue biopsies may not reflect drug concentration in other tissues nor the drug concentration in all parts of the tissue from which the biopsy material was removed. For example, if the tissue biopsy was for the diagnosis of a tumor within the tissue, the blood flow to the tumor cells may not be the same as the blood flow to other cells in this tissue. In fact, for many tissues, blood flow to one part of the tissues need not be the same as the blood flow to another part of the same tissue. The measurement of the drug concentration in tissue biopsy material may be used to ascertain if the drug reached the tissues and reached the proper concentration within the tissue.

Drug concentrations in saliva

Saliva drug concentrations have been reviewed for many drugs for therapeutic drug monitoring. Because only free drug diffuses into the saliva, saliva drug levels tend to approximate free drug rather than total plasma drug concentration. The saliva/plasma drug concentration ratio is less than 1 for many drugs. The saliva/plasma drug concentration ratio is mostly influenced by the pKa of the drug and the pH of the saliva. Weak acid drugs and weak base drugs with pKa significantly different than pH 7.4 (plasma pH) generally have better correlation to plasma drug levels. The saliva drug concentrations taken after equilibrium with the plasma drug concentration generally provide more stable indication of drug levels in the body. The use of salivary drug concentrations as a therapeutic indicator should be used with caution and preferably as a secondary indicator.

Forensic drug measurements

Forensic science is the application of science to personal injury, murder, and other legal proceedings. Drug measurements in tissues obtained at autopsy or in other bodily fluids such as saliva, urine, and blood may be useful if a suspect or victim has taken an overdose of a legal medication, has been poisoned, or has been using drugs of abuse such as opiates (eg., heroin), cocaine, or marijuana. The appearance of social drugs in blood, urine, and saliva drug analysis shows short-term drug abuse. These drugs may be eliminated rapidly, making it more difficult to prove that the subject has been using drugs of abuse. The analysis for drugs of abuse in hair samples by very sensitive assay methods, such as gas chromatography coupled with mass spectrometry, provides information regarding past drug exposure. A study by showed that the hair samples from subjects who were known drug abusers contained cocaine and 6-acetylmorphine, a metabolite of heroine (diacetylmorphine).

Significance of measuring plasma drug concentrations

The intensity of the pharmacologic or toxic effect of a drug is often related to the concentration of the drug at the receptor site, usually located in the tissue cells. Because most of the tissue cells are richly perfused with tissue fluids or plasma, measuring the plasma drug level is a responsive method of monitoring the course of therapy. Clinically, individual variations in the pharmacokinetics of drugs are quite common. Monitoring the concentration of drugs in the blood or plasma ascertains that the calculated dose actually delivers the plasma level required for therapeutic effect. With some drugs, receptor expression and/or sensitivity in individuals varies, so monitoring of plasma levels is needed to distinguish the patient who is receiving too much of a drug from the patient who is supersensitive to the drug. Moreover, the patient's physiologic functions may be affected by disease, nutrition, environment, concurrent drug therapy, and other factors. Pharmacokinetic models allow more accurate interpretation of the relationship between plasma drug levels and pharmacologic response.

In the absence of pharmacokinetic information, plasma drug levels are relatively useless for dosage adjustment. For example, suppose a single blood sample from a patient was assayed and found to contain 10 mg/mL. According to the literature, the maximum safe concentration of this drug is 15 mg/mL. In order to apply this information properly, it is important to know when the blood sample was drawn, what dose of the drug was given, and the route of administration. If the proper information is available, the use of pharmacokinetic equations and models may describe the blood level–time curve accurately. Monitoring of plasma drug concentrations allows for the adjustment of the drug dosage in order to individualize and optimize therapeutic drug regimens. In the presence of alteration in physiologic functions due to disease, monitoring plasma drug concentrations may provide a guide to the progress of the disease state and enable the investigator to modify the drug dosage accordingly. Clinically, sound medical judgment and observation are most important. Therapeutic decisions should not be based solely on plasma drug concentrations.

In many cases, the pharmacodynamic response to the drug may be more important to measure than just the plasma drug concentration. For example, the electrophysiology of the heart, including an electrocardiogram (ECG), is important to assess in patients medicated with cardiotonic drugs such as digoxin. For an anticoagulant drug, such as dicumarol, prothrombin clotting time may indicate whether proper dosage was achieved. Most diabetic patients taking insulin will monitor their own blood or urine glucose levels. For drugs that act irreversibly at the receptor site, plasma drug concentrations may not accurately predict pharmacodynamic response. Drugs used in cancer chemotherapy often interfere with nucleic acid or protein biosynthesis to destroy tumor cells. For these drugs, the plasma drug concentration does not relate directly to the pharmacodynamic response. In this case, other pathophysiologic parameters and side effects are monitored in the patient to prevent adverse toxicity.

Drug administration and therapy can now be conveniently divided into four processes or phases:

(1) **The pharmaceutics process:** It is concerned with the formulation of an effective dosage form of the drug for administration by a suitable route.

(2) **The pharmacokinetic process:** It is concerned with the ADME of drugs as elicited by the plasma drug concentration- time profile and its relationship with the dose, dosage form and frequency and route of administration. In shortly, it is the sum of all the processes inflicted by the body on the drug.

(3) **The pharmacodynamic process:** it is concerned with the physiologic and biochemical effects of the drug and its mechanism of action. It is characterized by the concentration of drug at the site of action and its relation to the magnitude of effects observed. Simply, pharma-codynamics deals with what the drug does to the body in contrast to pharmacokinetics which is a study of what the body does to drug.

(4) **The therapeutic process:** it is concerned with the translation of pharmacologic effect into clinical benefit.

To achieve optimal therapy with a drug, the drug product must be designed to deliver the active principle at an optimal rate and amount, depending upon the patient's needs. A knowledge of the factors affecting the bioavailability of drug helps in designing such an optimum formulation and saves many drugs that may be discarded as useless. On the other hand, rational use of drug or the therapeutic objective can only be achieved through a better understanding of pharmacokinetics (in addition to pharmacodynamics of the drug), which helps in designing a proper **dosage regimen** (the manner in which the drug should be taken). This avoids the use of the empirical where a considerable experimentation is needed to arrive at the balance between the desired therapeutic and the undesired toxic effects in order to define an appropriate dosage regimen.

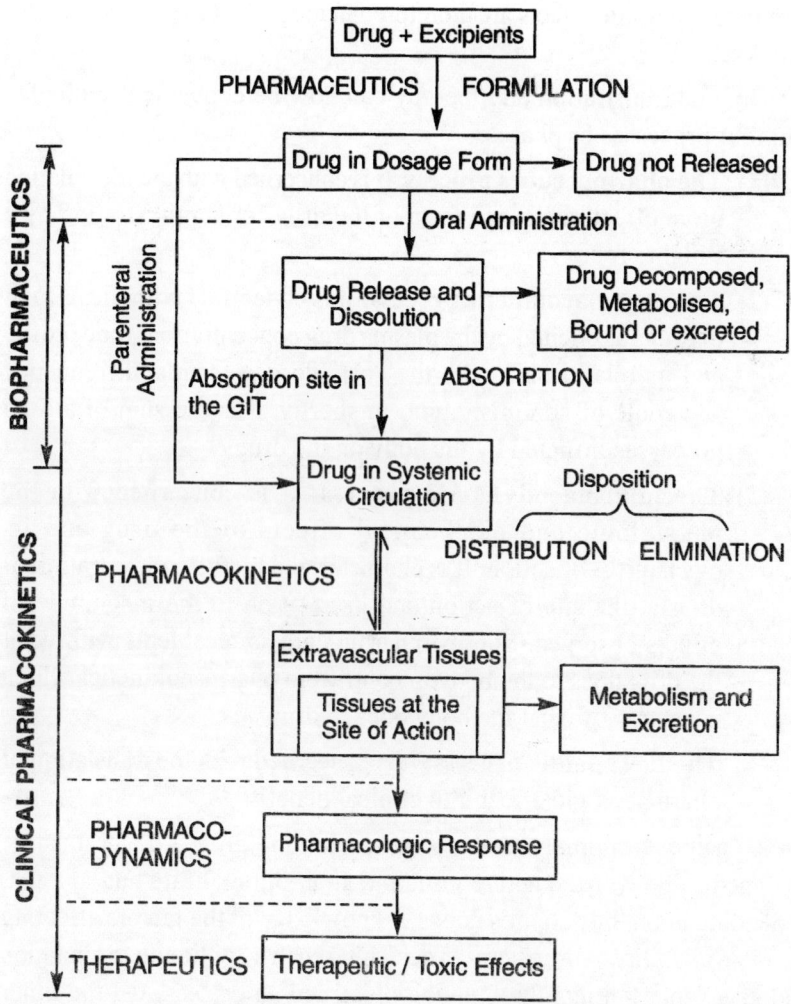

Fig. 1.5: Schematic representation of the processes involved in drug therapeutics

Application of Biopharmaceutics and Pharmacokinetics

(1) In the design and development of new drugs and their appropriate dosage regimen.

(2) In the safe and effective therapeutic management of the patients by improving drug therapy.

(3) In the design and utilization of *in vitro* model systems that can evaluate the dissolution characteristics of new compounds formulated as solid dosage forms and establish meaningful *in vitro - in vivo* correlations.

(4) To understand the processes of absorption, distribution and elimination after the administration of a drug/dosage form, which affect the onset and intensity of a biologic response.

(5) To assess a drug moiety in terms of plasma drug concentration response this is now considered as a more appropriate parameter than the intrinsic pharmacological activity.

(6) To understand the concept of bioavailability which has been used successfully by regulatory authorities, to evaluate and monitor the in vivo performance of new drugs, new dosage forms and generic formulations.

(7) To carry out bioavailability and bioequivalence studies which have now been accepted as an integral part of the drug product approval process across the world.

A schematic representation of the various processes involved in the therapy with a drug is given in Fig.1.5.

The knowledge and concepts of biopharmaceutics and pharmacokinetics thus have an integral role in the formulation and development of new drugs and their dosage forms and clinical setting.

Questions

Essay questions

1. What is biopharmaceutics? Write their role in formulation development and clinical setting.

2. What is pharmacokinetics? Write their role in formulation development and clinical setting.

Short question

1. Write application of biopharmaceutics and pharmacokinetics.
2. What is basic pharmacokinetics? Write uses of pharmacokinetic models.
3. Give two reasons for the measurement of the plasma drug concentration, C_p assuming (a) the C_p relates directly to the pharmacodynamic activity of the drug and (b) the C_p does not relate to the pharmacodynamic activity of the drug.
4. Explain various processes for drug administration and therapy.
5. Write a note on measurement of drug concentration.

Chapter—2

ABSORPTION OF DRUGS

Drug absorption may be defined as the process of movement of unchanged drug from the site of administration to systemic circulation. Following absorption, the effectiveness of a drug can only be assessed by its concentration at the site of action. However, it is difficult to measure the drug concentration at such a site. Instead, the concentration can be measured more accurately in plasma There always exist a correlation between the plasma concentration of a drug and the therapeutic response

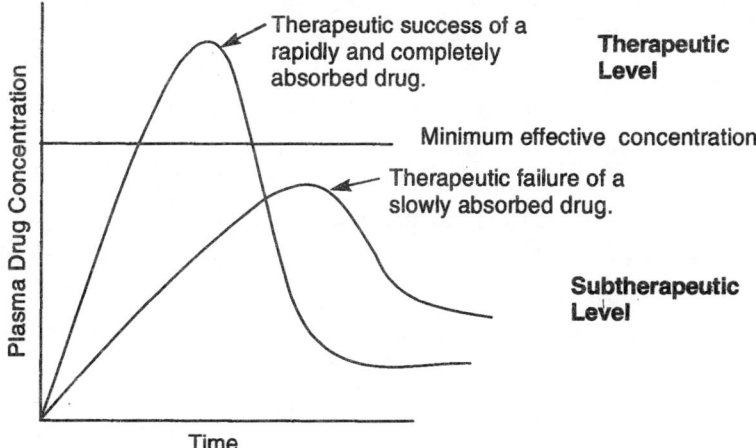

Fig. 2.1: Plots showing significance of rate and extent of absorption in drug therapy

and thus, **absorption** can also be defined as the process of movement of unchanged drug from the site of administration to the site of measurement. i.e. plasma. This definition takes into account the loss of drug that occurs after oral administration due to first- pass effect or presystemic metabolism. Not only the magnitude of drug that comes into the systemic circulation but also the rate at which it is absorbed is important. This is clear from Fig. 2.1.

A drug that is completely but slowly absorbed may fail to show therapeutic response as the plasma concentration for desired effect is never achieved. On the contrary, a rapidly absorbed drug attains the therapeutic level easily to elicit pharmacologic effect. Thus, both the rate and the extent of drug absorption are important.

Structure of Cell Membrane

It is also called the plasma membrane, plasmalemma or phospholipid bilayer. The cell membrane is a flexible yet sturdy barrier that surrounds and contains the cytoplasm of a cell. For a drug to be absorbed and distributed into organs and tissues and eliminated from the body, it must pass through one or more barrier/membrane at various locations. Such a movement of drug across the membrane is called as **drug transport**. The barriers are mainly biological membranes such as gastrointestinal epithelium, lungs, blood and brain. A drug substance must pass through one or more than one of these membranes before reaching its site of action. Though the chemistry of body membranes differ from one another, they are made up of basic structure of cell membrane. The structure of cell membrane is shown in Fig. 2.2. Cell membrane mainly consists of:

    (1) Lipid bilayer: (a) phospholipid

                           (b) Cholesterol

                           (c) Glycolipids.

    (2) Proteins: (a) Integral membrane proteins

                           (b) Lipid anchored proteins

                           (c) Peripheral Proteins

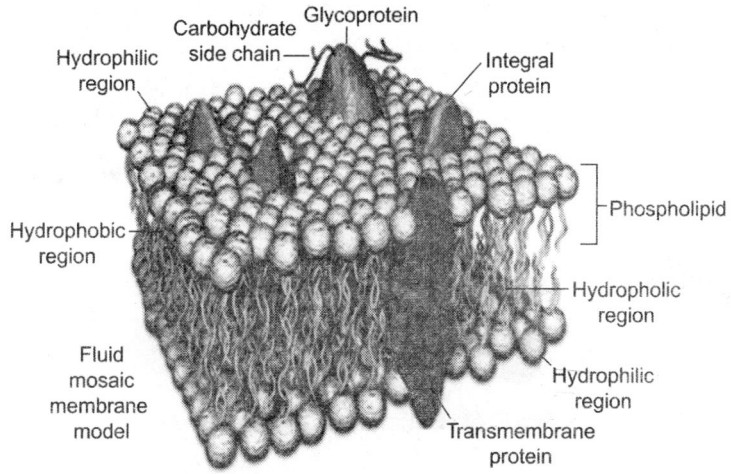

Fig. 2.2: Structure of cell membrane

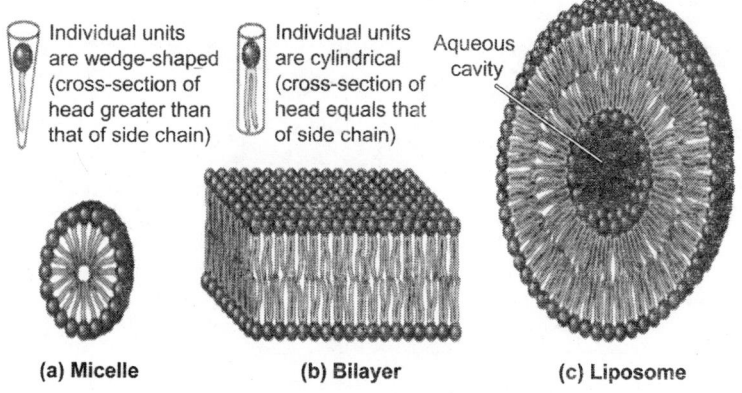

(a) Micelle　　　　**(b) Bilayer**　　　　**(c) Liposome**

Fig. 2.3: Structure of lipid bilayer

(1) Lipid bilayer: The basic structural framework of the cell membrane is the lipid bilayer. It consists primarily of a thin layer of amphipathic phospholipids which spontaneously arrange so that the hydrophobic "tail" regions are shielded from the the resulting bilayer. This forms a continuous, spherical lipid bilayer (7nm thick). The structure of lipid bilayer is shown in Fig. 2.3.

(a) **Phospholipid:** Phospholipid is a pair of fatty acid chains and a phosphate group attached to a glycerol backbone. Polar (water-soluble) heads face out and the non-polar fatty acids hang inside. The structure of phospholipid is shown in Fig. 2.4.

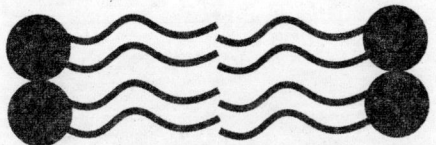

Fig 2.4: Structure of phospholipid

(b) **Cholesterol:** Cholesterol amount in membrane is 20 %. Cholesterol inserts in membrane with same orientation as

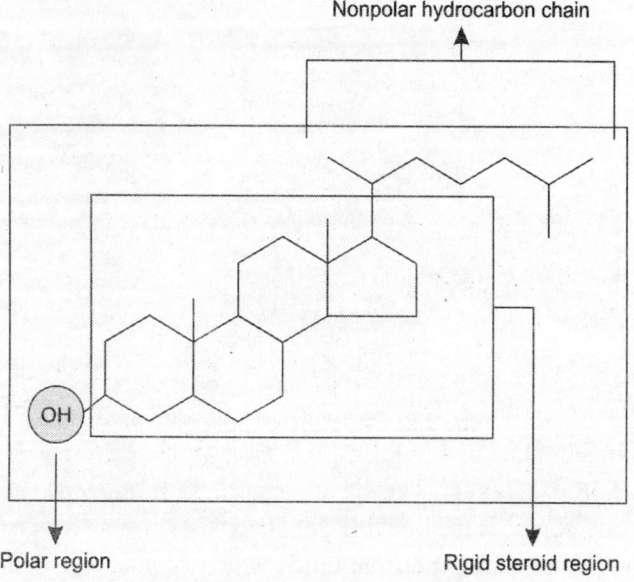

Fig. 2.5: Structure of cholesterol.

phospholipids molecules. Polar head of cholesterol is aligned with polar head of phospholipids. Structure of cholesterol is shown in Fig.2.5. Functions of cholesterol are as follows:

(1) Immobilize first few hydrocarbons groups' phospholipids molecules.

(2) Prevents crystallization of hydrocarbons and phase shift in membrane.

(c) **Glycolipids:** Glycolipids amount in membrane is about 5 %. Carbohydrate groups form polar "head". Fatty acids "tails" are non polar. Glycolipids present in membrane layer that faces the extracellular fluid (Shown in Fig. 2.6). This is one reason due to which bilayer is asymmetric. Glycolipids functions are as follows:

(1) Protective

(2) Insulator

(3) Site of receptor binding

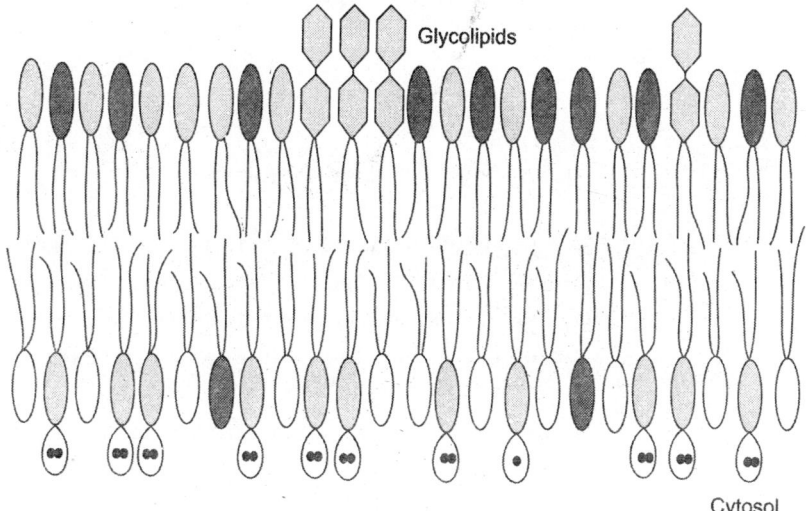

Fig. 2.6: Glycolipids present in cell membrane layer

(2) **Proteins:** Proteins determine membrane's specific functions. Cell membrane and organelle membranes each have unique collections of proteins. Many functions of proteins are shown in Fig. 2.7.

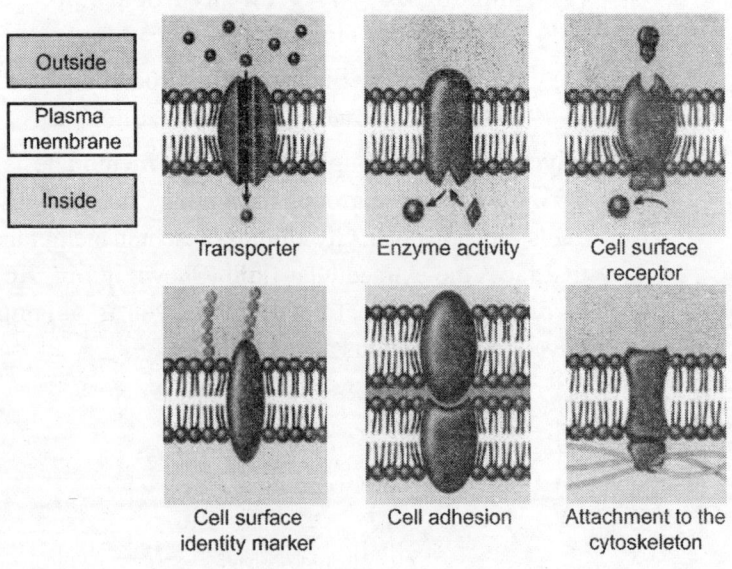

Fig. 2.7: Many functions of proteins

(a) **Integral proteins:** It is also known as transmembrane protein. It have hydrophilic and hydrophobic domain. Hydrophobic domain anchor within the cell membrane and hydrophilic domain interacts with external molecules. Hydrophobic domain consists of one, multiple or combination of α – helices and β – sheets protein motifs. Example of integral proteins are ion channels, proton pump etc.

(b) **Lipid anchored proteins:** Covalently bound to single or multiple lipid molecules. Hydrophobically inert into cell membrane and anchors the protein. The protein itself is not in contact with membrane. Example of lipid anchored proteins is G Proteins.

(c) **Peripheral proteins:** Attached to integral membrane proteins or associated with peripheral regions of lipid bilayer. It has only temporary interaction with biological membrane. Once reacted with molecule, dissociates to carry on its work in cytoplasm. Examples of peripheral proteins are some enzyme, some hormones etc.

Gastrointestinal Absorption of Drugs

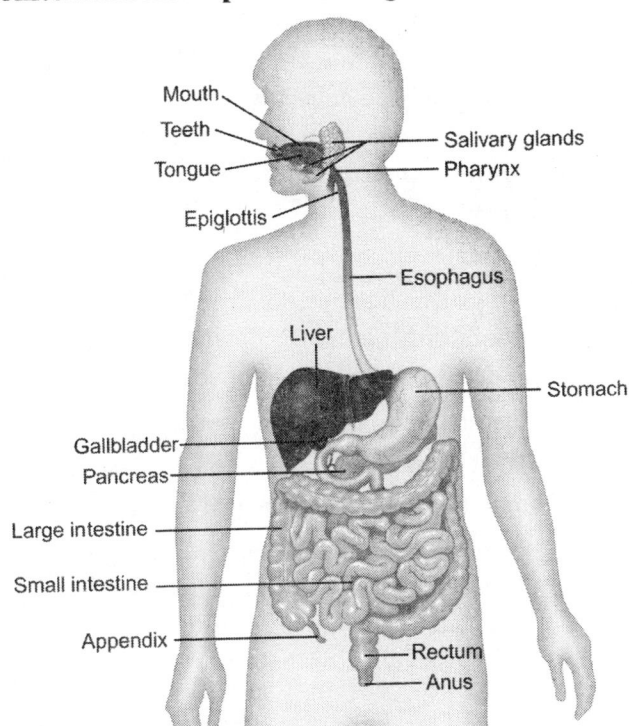

Fig. 2.8: Gastrointestinal absorption of drugs

(1) Stomach

(a) The surface area for absorption of drugs is relatively small in the stomach due to the absence of macrovilli and microvilli.

(b) Extent of drug absorption is affected by variation in the time it takes the stomach to empty, i.e., how long the dosage form is able to reside in stomach.

(c) Drugs which are acid labile must not be in contact with the acidic environment of the stomach.

(d) Stomach emptying applies more to the solid dosage forms because the drug has to dissolve in the GI fluid before it is available for absorption.

(e) Since solubility and dissolution rate of most drugs is a function of pH, it follows that, a delivery system carrying a drug that is predominantly absorbed from the stomach, must stay in the stomach for an extended period of time in order to assure maximum dissolution and therefore to extent of absorption.

(2) Small intestine:

(a) The drugs which are predominantly absorbed through the small intestine, the transit time of a dosage form are the major determinant of extent of absorption.

(b) Various studies to determine transit time:

- Early studies using indirect methods placed the average normal transit time through the small intestine at about 7 hours.

- These studies were based on the detection of hydrogen after an oral dose of lactulose. (Fermentation of lactulose by colon bacteria yields hydrogen in the breath).

- Newer studies suggest the transit time to be about 3 to 4 hours.

- Use gamma scintigraphy.

- Thus, if the transit time in small intestine for most healthy adults is between 3 to 4 hours, a drug may take about 4 to 8 hours to pass through the stomach and small intestine during fasting state.

- During the fed state, the small intestine transit time may take about 8 to 12 hours.

(3) Large intestine:

(a) The major function of large intestine is to absorb water from ingestible food residues which are delivered to the large intestine in a fluid state, and eliminate them from the body as semi solid feces.

(b) Only a few drugs are absorbed in this region.

Mechanisms of Drug Absorption

(1) Passive diffusion

(2) Pore transport

(3) Carrier- mediated transport

    (a) Facilitated diffusion

    (b) Active transport

(4) Ionic or Electrochemical diffusion

(5) Ion-pair transport

(6) Endocytosis

(1) Passive diffusion: It is also known as non-ionic diffusion. It is defined as the difference in the drug concentration on either side of the membrane. It is major process for absorption of more than 90% of the drugs. The driving force for this process is the concentration or electrochemical gradient. Drug movement is a result of the kinetic energy of molecules. Since no energy source is required, the process is called as **passive diffusion.** During passive diffusion, the drug present in the aqueous solution at the absorption site partitions and dissolves in the lipid material of the membrane and finally leaves it by dissolving again in an aqueous medium, this time at the inside of the membrane. Passive diffusion of water and water soluble substances are shown in Fig. 2.9.

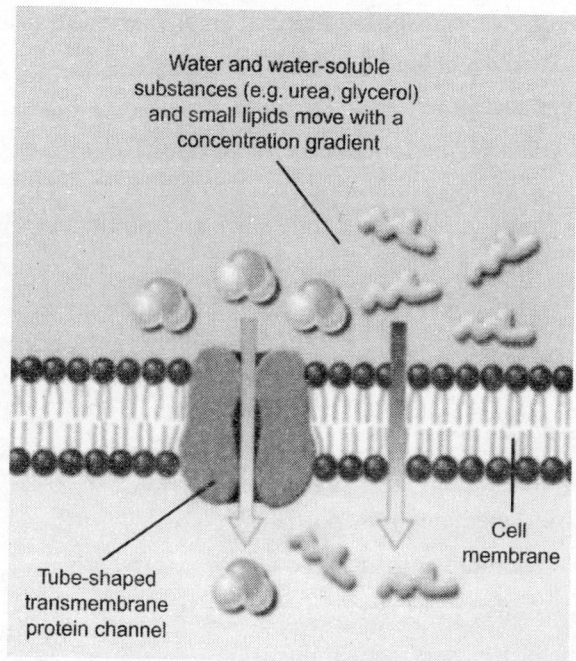

Fig. 2.9: Passive diffusion of water and water soluble arug

Passive diffusion is best expressed by Fick's first law of diffusion which states that the drug molecules diffuse from a region of higher concentration to one of lower concentration until equilibrium is attained and the rate of diffusion is directly proportional to the concentration gradient across the membrane. It can be mathematically expressed by the following equation:

$$\frac{dQ}{dt} = \frac{DAK_{\frac{m}{w}}}{h}(C_{GIT} - C) \qquad \dots (2.1)$$

Where,

dQ/dt	=	rate of drug diffusion (amount/time). It also represents the rate of appearance of drug in blood
D	=	diffusion coefficient of the drug through the membrane (area/time)
A	=	surface area of the absorbing membrane for drug diffusion (area)
$K_{m/w}$	=	partition coefficient of the drug between the lipoidal membrane and the aqueous GI fluids
$(C_{GIT} - C)$	=	difference in the concentration of drug in the GI fluids and the plasma, called as the concentration gradient (amount/volume)
h	=	thickness of the membrane (length)

Certain characteristics of passive diffusion can be generalized, based on the above equation:

(1) The drug moves down the concentration gradient indicating downhill transport.

(2) The rate of drug transfer is directly proportional to the concentration gradient between GI fluids and the blood compartment.

(3) Greater the area and lesser the thickness of the membrane, faster the diffusion; thus, more rapid is the rate of drug absorption from the intestine than from the stomach.

(4) When the concentration on either side of the membrane becomes equal, equilibrium is attained.

(5) The drug diffuses rapidly when the volume of GI fluid is low; conversely, dilution of GI fluids (C_{GIT}) and lower the concentration gradient ($C_{GIT} - c$). This phenomena is, however, made use of in treating cases of oral overdose or poisoning.

(6) Drug which can exist in both ionized and unionized forms approach equilibrium primarily by the transfer of the unionized

species; the rate of transfer of unionized species is 3 to 4 times the rate for ionized drugs.

(7) Greater the membrane/water partition coefficient of drug, faster the absorption; since the membrane is lipoidal in nature, a lipophilic drug diffuses at a faster rate by solubilizing in the lipid layer of the membrane.

Passive diffusion process is energy independent but depends more or less on the square root of the molecular size of the drugs. The molecular weight of the most drugs lie between 100 to 400 daltons which can be effectively absorbed passively. The diffusion decreases with increase in the molecular weight of compound. However, there are exceptions- for example, cyclosporine A, a peptide of molecular weight 1200, is absorbed orally much better than any other peptide. When the drug is ingested, $C_{GIT} >> C$ and a large concentration gradient exists thereby acting as the driving force for absorption. The drug diffusion should stop and consequently a large fraction of drug may remain unabsorbed, as the equilibrium approaches. But this is not the case; once the passively absorbed drug enters blood, it is rapidly swept away and distributed into a much larger volume of body fluids and hence, the concentration of drug at the absorption site, C_{GIT} is maintained greater than the concentration of drug in plasma. Such condition is called as **sink condition** for drug absorption. Hence under usual conditions of absorption, D, A, $K_{m/w}$ and h are constants, $DAK_{m/w} / h$ can be replaced by a combined constant P called as **permeability coefficient**. Permeability may be defined as the ease with which a drug can penetrate or diffuse through a membrane. In addition, due to sink conditions, the concentration of drug in plasma C is very small in comparison to C_{GIT} As a result, equation 2.1 may be simplified to:

$$dQ/dt = P C_{GIT} \qquad \qquad ... (2.2)$$

Equation 2.2 is an expression for a first order process. Thus, passive diffusion follows first order kinetics. A large concentration gradient exist at the absorption site for passive diffusion, the rate of drug absorption is usually more rapid than the rate of elimination. Besides, dilution and distribution of the absorbed drug into a large pool of body fluids and its subsequent binding to various tissues are other reasons for elimination being slower than absorption.

(2) **Pore transport:** It is also known as convective transport, bulk flow or filtration. It is important in the absorption of low molecular weight (less than 100), Low molecular size (smaller than the diameter of the pore) and generally water-soluble drugs through narrow, aqueous filled channels or pores in the membrane structure for example, urea, water and sugars. The driving force for the passage of the drugs is the hydrostatic or the osmotic pressure difference across the membrane. The rate of absorption via pore transport depends on the number and size of the pores, and given as follows:

$$dQ/dt = P\ C_{GIT}$$
$$dc/dt = N.R^2.A.\Delta C/(\eta)(h) \qquad \qquad ... (2.3)$$

Where,

dc/dt	=	rate of absorption
N	=	number of pores
R	=	radius of pores
Δ_c	=	concentration gradient
η	=	viscosity of fluid in the pores

(3) **Carrier mediated transport:** It involves a carrier (a component of the membrane) which binds reversibly with the solute molecules to be transported to yield the carrier solute complex which transverses across the membrane to the other side where it dissociates to yield the solute molecule. The carrier then returns to its original site to accept a fresh molecule of solute. There are two types of carrier mediated transport system:

(a) **Facilitated diffusion:** This mechanism involves the driving force is concentration gradient. In this system, no expenditure of energy is involved (down-hill transport), therefore the process is not inhibited by metabolic poisons that interfere with energy production. Facilitated diffusion of some nutrients is shown in Fig. 2.10.

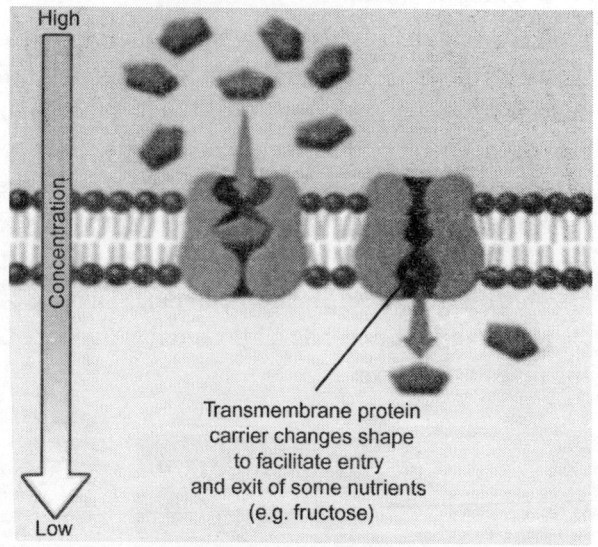

High

Concentration

Low

Transmembrane protein
carrier changes shape
to facilitate entry
and exit of some nutrients
(e.g. fructose)

Fig. 2.10: Facilitated diffusion of some nutrients

Facilitated diffusion is of limited importance in the absorption of drugs - for example, such a transport system includes entry of glucose into RBCs and intestinal absorption of vitamins B_1 and B_2. A classical example of passive facilitated diffusion is the gastro-intestinal absorption of vitamin B_{12}. An intrinsic factor (IF), a glycoprotein produced by the gastric parietal cells, forms a complex with vitamin B_{12} which is then transported across the intestinal membrane by a carrier system.

(b) **Active transport:** It is more important process than facilitated diffusion. The driving force is against the concentration gradient or uphill transport. Since the process is uphill, energy is required in the work done by the barrier. As the process requires expenditure of energy, it can be inhibited by metabolic poisons that interfere with energy production. If drugs (especially used in cancer) have structural similarities to such agents, they are absorbed actively. A good example of competitive inhibition of drug absorption via active transport is the impaired absorption of levodopa when ingested with meals rich in proteins. The rate of absorption by active transport can be determined by applying the equation used for Michalies-menten kinetics:

$$dc/dt = [C].(dc/dt)_{max}/K_m + [C] \qquad ...(2.4)$$

Where,

$(dc/dt)_{max}$ = maximal rate of drug absorption at high drug concentration.

$[C]$ = concentration of drug available for absorption

K_m = affinity constant of drug for the barrier.

(4) **Ionic or Electrochemical diffusion:** This charge influences the permeation of drugs. Molecular forms of solutes are unaffected by the membrane charge and permeate faster than ionic forms. The permeation of anions and cations is also influenced by pH. Thus, at a given pH, the rate of permeation may be as follows:

Unionized molecule > anions > cations

The permeation of ionized drugs, particularly the cationic drugs, depends on the potential difference or electrical gradient as the driving force across the membrane. Once inside the membrane, the cations are attached to negatively charge intracellular membrane, thus giving rise to an electrical gradient. If the same drug is moving from a higher to lower concentration, i.e., moving down the electrical gradient, the phenomenon is known as electrochemical diffusion.

(5) **Ion-pair transport:** It is another mechanism is able to

explain the absorption of such drugs which ionize at all pH condition. Transport of charged molecules due to the formation of a neutral complex with another charged molecule carrying an opposite charge. Drugs have low o/w partition coefficient values, yet these penetrate the membrane by forming reversible neutral complexes with endogenous ions – for example, mucin of GIT. Such neutral complexes have both the required lipophilicity as well as aqueous solubility for passive diffusion. This phenomenon is known as ion-pair transport (Fig. 2.11).

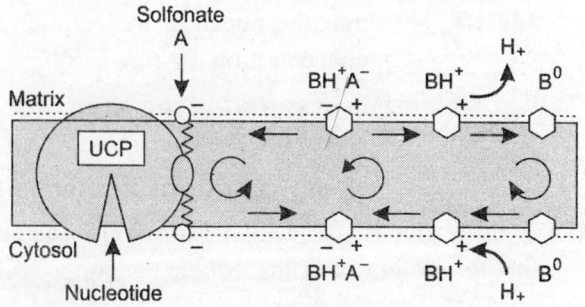

Fig. 2.11: Ion-pair transport of a cationic drug

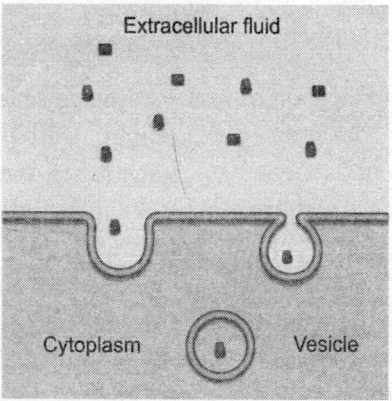

Fig. 2.12: Endocytic uptake of macromolecules

(6) Endocytosis: It involves engulfing extracellular materials within a segment of the cell membrane to form a saccule or a vesicle (hence also called as corpuscular or vesicular transport) which is then pinched off intracellularly (Fig. 2.12).

In endocytosis, there are three processes:

(a) Phagocytosis (cell eating): adsorptive uptake of solid particulates. Phases of Phagocytosis are shown in fig.2.13.

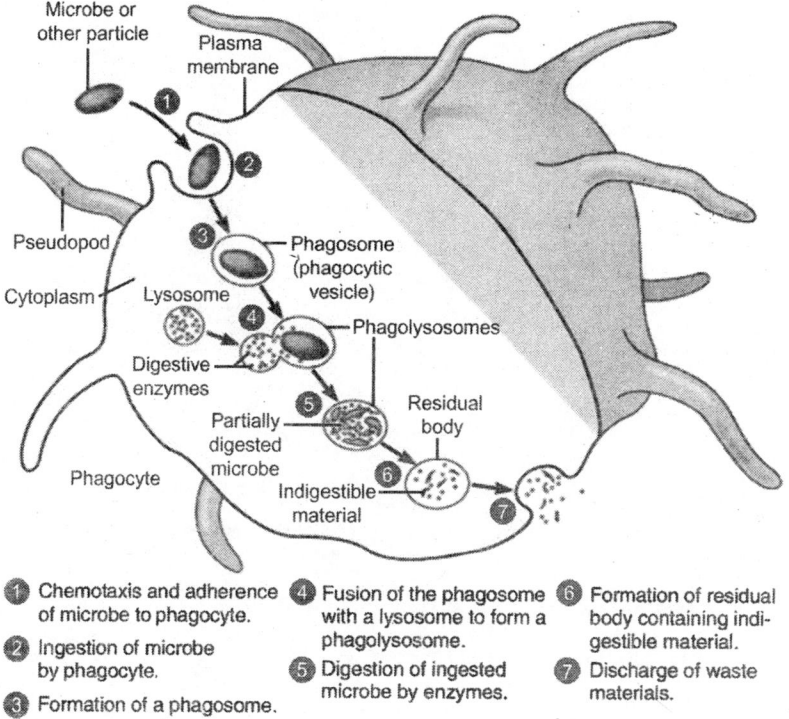

① Chemotaxis and adherence of microbe to phagocyte.

② Ingestion of microbe by phagocyte.

③ Formation of a phagosome.

④ Fusion of the phagosome with a lysosome to form a phagolysosome.

⑤ Digestion of ingested microbe by enzymes.

⑥ Formation of residual body containing indigestible material.

⑦ Discharge of waste materials.

Fig. 2.13: Phases of phagocytosis

(b) Pinocytosis (cell drinking): uptake of fluid solute (Fig.2.14). Orally administered Sabin polio vaccine and large protein molecules are thought to be absorbed by pinocytosis.

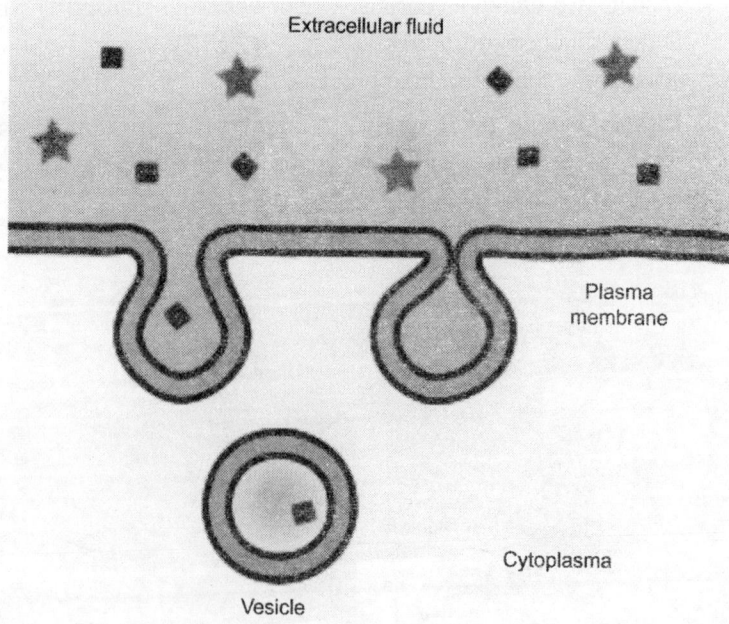

Fig. 2.14: Uptake of fluid solute

(c) **Transcytosis:** It is a phenomenon in which endocytic vesicle is transferred from one extracellular compartment to another.

Factors Affecting Absorption

1. Physico- chemical Factors
2. Pharmaceutical Factors
3. Physiological Factors

1. **Physico-chemical Factors:** The physicochemical factors that affect the rate of drug absorption are:

   (a) **Drug solubility and dissolution rate:** The absorption of drug requires that molecules be in solution at the absorption site. The dissolution of solid dosage forms in gastrointestinal fluid is an important step for the delivery of drug to systemic circulation after oral administration. Dissolution depends on the solubility of the drug substances in the surrounding medium. Polar molecules are more soluble in water than in organic phases. Ionized molecules are also easily soluble than unionized molecules. The solubility of acids or base in the aqueous medium is dependent on pH. The drugs having high solubility in aqueous medium are absorbed faster by passive diffusion than that of drugs with low aqueous solubility.

(b) **Particle size and effective surface area of the drugs:** Smaller the particle size, greater the effective surface area and higher will be the dissolution rate. Particle size reduction results in increased bioavailability provided that absorption of the drug is dissolution rate limited. For examples:

(1) By using the micronized form of the drug, spironolactone, the therapeutic dose has been reduced from 500 mg to 25 mg.

(2) Reduction in the particle size of the digoxin from 20 to 30 microns to 3.7 microns leads to an increase in rate and extent of absorption of drug.

In case of few drugs, the inclusion of small sized particles gave an increased incidence of undesirable side effects. For example, Nitrofurantoin

(c) **Polymorphism and amorphism:** Depending upon the internal structure, a solid can exist either in crystalline or amorphous form. When a substance exists in more than one crystalline form, the different forms are designated as polymorphs and the phenomenon is called as polymorphism. Polymorphs are of the two types:

(1) **Enantiotropic polymorph:** In this one form can be

reversibly changed into another form by altering the temperature or pressure. For example, sulfur.

(2) **Monotropic polymorph:** It is the form which is unstable at all temperatures and pressures. For example, glyceryl stearates.

The polymorphs differ from each other with respect to their physical properties such as solubility, melting point, density, hardness and compression characteristics. The existence of polymorphs can be determined by using techniques such as optical crystallography, x-ray diffraction, differential scanning calorimetry etc. one of the several polymorphic forms is more stable than others. Such stable polymorphs have low energy state and high melting point and least aqueous solubility. The remaining polymorphs are called as metastable forms which have high energy state, low melting points and higher aqueous solubilities. Since, the metastable forms have greater aqueous solubility; they have better absorption characteristics and better bioavailability. About 40% of all organic compounds exhibit polymorphism. For example, barbiturates, sulfonamide etc.

Some drugs exist in amorphous forms which have no internal crystal structure. Such drugs have high energy states and can be considered as super cooled liquids. Hence, they have greater aqueous solubility than crystalline forms. For example, novobiocin, chloramphenicol- palmitate, cortisone acetate etc. The order of dissolution of different solid forms is amorphous > metastable > stable.

(d) **Solvates and Hydrates (Pseudo polymorphism):** Many drugs can associate with solvents to produce crystalline forms called solvates. When the solvent is water then, the crystal is termed as hydrate. For example:

(1) Anhydrous form of caffeine, theophylline and glutethimide.

(2) The anhydrous form of ampicillin.

Solvate forms of drug with organic solvents may dissolve in water much faster than the non-solvated forms. For example:

(1) N-pentanol and ethyl acetate solvates of Fluoro-cortisone.

(2) N-pentanol solvate of Succinyl sulphathiazole.

(3) Chloroform solvate of Griseofulvin.

(e) **Complexation:** Complexation influence the effective drug concentration in GI fluids, alter the rate and extent of drug absorption. The complexing agent may be,

— Substance normal to the GIT.

— A dietary component.

— A component of the dosage form.

For example:

(1) Polysaccharide mucin of the intestinal mucosa forms a complex with Streptomycin and Dihydro streptomycin leading to the poor absorption of the drugs.

(2) Calcium ion complexes with Tetracycline and thus its absorption are substantially reduced if taken with milk or other source of calcium.

(3) Amphetamine interacts with carboxymethyl cellullose to form a poorly soluble complex that leads to reduced absorption of the drug.

Drugs which are poorly water soluble and thus incompletely absorbed can be administered as water soluble complexes.

For example:

(1) Hydroquinones form a water soluble, rapidly dissolving complex with digoxin.

(2) Caffeine forms a complex with Benzocaine in the ratio 1:1 resulting in the faster dissolution rate and absorption.

(f) **Adsorption:** It is a physical and surface phenomenon where the drug molecules are held on the surface of certain substances (adsorbents) by Vanderwaal's forces. For example,

(1) When charcoal is co-administered with Promazine, it significantly reduced both the rate and extent of drug absorption as it adsorbs Promazine.

(g) **Drug stability and Hydrolysis in GIT:** The wide pH spectrum and enzymatic activity of GI fluids lead to the acid and enzymatic hydrolysis of the drugs in GIT. For example,

(1) The half life of degradation of Penicillin G is less than 1 minute at pH 1. The drug is stable in the less acidic fluids of the duodenum.

(2) The antibiotic Erythromycin and its various esters are very unstable in the gastric fluids, having a degradation half life of less than 2 minutes.

In certain cases, ester hydrolysis in the GIT is very beneficial, since it is a prerequisite for the absorption of the parent drug. For example,

(1) Chloramphenicol is administered as Chloramphenicol Stearate or Palmitate Ester. The ester must undergo hydrolysis in the GIT to form the parent compound in order for absorption to occur.

(2) Erythromycin Stearate, Erythromycin estolate, the prodrugs of Erythromycin, after hydrolysis in the intestinal fluid yield Erythromycin, which is absorbed.

(h) **Salt form of the drug:** Sodium or potassium salts of weak acids dissolve more rapidly than the free acid. Same is observed for the HCl or other strong acid salts of weak bases. For example,

(1) Novobiocin is a weak acid. The administration of sodium salt shows improved bioavailability 50 times that of free acid.

(2) Potassium salt of penicillin V gives higher peak concentration of the antibiotic than the free acid.

(3) The dissolution rate of sodium salt of Phenobarbital

is 820 times greater in pH 6.8 phosphate buffer compared to Phenobarbital.

Certain salts have low solubility and dissolution rate compared to the parent drug. For example,

(1) Aluminium aspirin is more slowly absorbed and less available than aspirin after oral administration.

(i) **Viscosity:** Changes in viscosity of a solution affects the drug absorption by several possible mechanisms including modification of gastric emptying rate or intestinal transit rate. If a high viscosity is produced around a drug due to the excipients, it would limit the diffusion of drug to the GI fluids to attain dissolution and thus limits its absorption.

(j) **Lipophilicity of the drug:** The P^{ka} of a drug determines the degree of ionization at a particular P^H. The unionized drug is absorbed into systemic circulation if it is sufficiently lipid soluble. Thus for optimum absorption a drug should have sufficient aqueous solubility to dissolve in the fluids at absorption site and enough lipid solubility to facilitate partition into the lipoidal membrane and into systemic circulation.

(k) **P^{ka} of the drug:** The amount of drug that exists in unionized form is a function of dissociation constant (P^{ka}) of the drug. The absorption of the drug is faster if it remains in unionized form. The ionization of acidic and basic drugs is hence dependent on the dissociation constants.

2. **Pharmaceutical Factors:** The pharmaceutical factors that affect the rate of absorption are:

(a) **Disintegration and Dissolution times:** the disintegration and dissolution times have particular importance in case of solid dosage forms like tablets and capsules. The *in-vitro* disintegration test does not guarantee drugs bioavailability because if the drug particle does not dissolve, absorption is not possible. The disintegration time of a tablet is influenced by the amount of binder present and the compression force of a tablet. After disintegration, the particles must be deaggregate into fine particles for dissolution.

(b) Manufacturing variables: the manufacturing variables that influence drug dissolution and hence absorption from dosage forms are:

(1) Method of granulation, and

(2) Compression force

(1) Method of granulation: The wet granulation technique which is a conventional technique for manufacture of tablets has many limitations such as:

    (a) Formation of crystal bridge by the presence of liquid.

    (b) The liquid may act as a medium affecting chemical reactions such as hydrolysis and

    (c) The drying may harm thermolabile drugs

    (d) A number of steps such as duration of blending method, time and temperature of drying which affects dissolution.

The method of dry granulation or dry compression can be used to produce tablets that dissolve at faster rate.

(2) Compression force: The compression force used in manufacture of tablets influence density, hardness, disintegration and dissolution of tablets. Higher compression forces increase hardness of tablet decreasing porosity which effects disintegration.

(c) Pharmaceutical ingredients/excipients: drugs are rarely administered in their original form. A number of additives or excipients are added to the drug to formulate the drug in a desired dosage form. Excipients are added to provide stability, acceptability and to achieve uniformity of dose. Though they are inert they have a major influence on the absorption of drugs. Increase in numbers of excipients may result in multiple problems for its absorption and hence bioavailability.

(d) **Nature and type of dosage form:** The successful achievement of bioavailability of a drug depends to a greater extent on the proper selection of dosage form of that drug. The bioavailability of a drug depends upon the nature and type of the dosage form. The difference in absorption rates of different dosage forms is due to the difference in release of drug from the dosage forms. The more complex a dosage form greater the number of rate-limiting steps and greater the potential for bioavailability problems. The bioavailability of a drug from various dosage forms is in the following order.

Solution > Emulsion > Suspension > Capsules > Tablets > Coated tablets > Enteric coated tablets > Sustained release products.

(e) **Product Age and storage conditions:** The alteration in storage conditions and using of the dosage form can result in the changes in the physicochemical properties of the drug in dosage form. The drug in dosage forms may precipitate due to altered solubility in case of polymorphic forms of drugs. The change in particle size of the drug molecule can be observed in suspension and emulsions on storage which can cause change in drug dissolution and absorption. The disintegration and dissolution rates of tablets can increase due to aging and storage conditions which depend on binder used. The shelf life of a dosage form can be affected by large variations in temperature and humidity.

3. **Physiological factors / patient related factors:** This include the physiologic and pathologic characteristics of patients that affect drug absorption. They are:

(1) **Age:** In infants, the gastric pH is high intestinal surface

and blood flow to GIT is low resulting in altered absorption pattern in comparison to adults. In elderly persons, cause of impaired drug absorption include altered gastric emptying, decreased intestinal surface area and GI blood flow, higher incidents of achlorhydria and bacterial overgrowth in small intestine.

(2) **Gastric emptying:** Apart from dissolution of drug and its penetration through the biomembrane, passage from stomach to small intestine called as gastric emptying, can also be rate-limiting step in the drug absorption because the major site of drug absorption is intestine. Rapid gastric emptying is advisable where,

1) Rapid onset of action is desired. Example, sedatives.

2) Dissolution of drug occurs in the intestine. Example, enteric coated dosage form.

3) The drugs are not stable in gastric fluids. Example, penicillin G and erythromycin

4) The drug is best absorbed from the distal part of the small intestine. Example, vitamin B12

For better absorption and dissolution, the gastric emptying can be promoted by taking the drug in emptying stomach. Such gastric emptying is altered by several factor due to which large intersubject variation are observed, all biopharmaceutics study that require the drug to be taken orally or performed in volunteers on emptying stomach.

Gastric emptying of is delayed by co-administrating food because unless the gastric contents are fluid enough or size of the solid particles is reduced below 2mm, its passage through the pylorus into the intestine is not possible. Delayed in gastric emptying is recommended in particular where,

1) Food promotes drug dissolution and absorption. Example, Griseofulvin.

2) Disintegration and dissolution of dosage form is Promoted by gastric fluids.

3) The drugs dissolve slowly. Example, Griseofulvin.

4) The drug irritating gastric mucosa. Example, aspirin, nitrofurantoin.

5) The drugs are absorbed from the proximal part of the small intestine and prolong drug absorption site contact is desired. Example, vitamin-B2, vitamin-C

Gastric emptying is a first order process. Several parameters are used to quantify gastric emptying.

1) **Gastric emptying rate:** is the speed at which the stomach contents into the intestine.

2) **Gastric emptying time:** is the time required for the gastric content to empty into the intestine. Longer the gastric emptying time, lesser the gastric emptying rate.

3) **Gastric emptying, $t_{1/2}$:** is the time taken for half the stomach to emptying.

A large number of factor influence gastric emptying as discussed below.

1. **Volume of meal:** Larger the bulk of the meals, longer the gastric emptying time. However, an intestinal rapid rate of emptying is observed with a large meal volume and in initial lag phase in emptying of small volume of meal. Since gastric emptying is first order process, a plot of log of volume of contents remaining in the stomach versus time yields a straight line.

2. **Composition of meals:** Predictably the rate of gastric emptying for various food materials is in the following order: carbohydrates > proteins > fats.

3. **Physical state and viscosity of meal:** Liquid meals take less than an hour to empty whereas a solid meal may take as long as 6 to7 hours.

4. **Temperature of the meal:** High or low temperature of the intestinal fluid reduce the gastric emptying rate.

5. **Gastrointestinal pH:** Gastric emptying is retarded at low

stomach pH and promoted at higher or alkaline pH.Chemicals that affects gastrointestinal pH also alters gastric emptying.

6. **Electrolytes and osmotic pressure:** Water, isotonic solutions and solutions of low salt concentration empty the stomach rapidly whereas a high electrolyte concentration decreases.

7. **Body posture:** Gastric emptying is favored while standing and by lying on the right side since the normal curvature of the stomach provides the downhill path whereas lying on the left side or in supine position retards it.

8. **Emotional state:** Stress and anxiety promote gastric motility whereas depression retards it.

9. **Drugs:** Drugs that retards gastric emptying includes poorly soluble antacids, anticholinergics, and narcotic analgesic, tricyclic antidepressants. Metachlopramide, domperidone and cisapride stimulate gastric emptying.

(3) **Intestinal transit:** Small intestine is the major site for absorption of drugs. The residence time depends on the intestinal contractions which promote drug absorption,

(a) By increasing the drug intestinal membrane contact.

(b) By enhancing the drug dissolution through induced agitation.

Delayed intestinal transit is desirable for,

(a) Drug that dissolve or release slowly from their dosage form. Example, sustained release products.

(b) Drug that dissolve only in intestine. Example, enteric coated formulations.

(c) Drug absorbed from specific sites in the intestine. Example, vitamin-B

Intestinal transit time is relatively short in comparison to the gastric emptying time and as the contents moves down the intestine into the colon, viscosity gradually increase due to the absorption of the water and electrolytes which limits the designed of sustained release product of drug having small biological half lives.

(4) **Gastrointestinal pH:** A tremendous 107 fold difference in the hydrogen ion concentration is observed between the gastric and colon fluids. The GI fluid pH influence drug absorption in a several ways:

(a) **Disintegration:** Disintegration of some dosage forms is depends on pH. With enteric coated formulations, the coat dissolves in the intestine followed by disintegration of the tablet.

(b) **Dissolution:** A large number of drugs are either week acids or bases, whose solubility is greatly affected by pH. A pH that favors formation of salts of the drug enhances the dissolution, since dissolution is the important rate limiting step in absorption.

(c) **Absorption:** Depending upon the drug pKa and whether it is an acidic or basic drug the GI pH influence drug absorption by determining the amount of drug that would exist in unionized form at the site of absorption.

(d) **Stability:** GI pH also influences the chemical stability of drugs. The acidic stomach pH is known to effect degradation of penicillin G and erythromycin. This can be overcome by preparing prodrug of such drug that do not degrade or dissolve in acidic pH e.g. carindacillin and erythromycin estolate. With basic drug, formation of insoluble drug hydroxide in the alkaline pH of the intestine has been observed.

(5) **Disease states**: Several disease states can influence the rate and extent of drug absorption is as follows:

(a) **Gastrointestinal disease and infection:** The influence of achlorhydria (decreased gastric acid secretion and increase stomach pH) on gastric emptying and drug absorption especially that of acidic drug (decreased absorption, e.g. aspirin). Two of the intestinal disorders are related with malabsorption syndrome, (Celiac disease, and Crohn's disease).

- Abnormalities associated with celiac disease include,
  — Gastric emptying rate increases.
  — GI permeability increases.
  — Altered intestinal drug metabolism.
  — Steatorrhea.
- Abnormalities associated with Crohn's disease include,
  — Altered absorption pattern by altered gut wall microbial flora.
  — Decreased gut surface area and intestinal transit rate.
- GI infections,
  — Shigellosis, gastroenteritis, cholera and food poisoning.
- Colonic diseases,
  — Colitis, amebiasis, constipation.
- Gastrointestinal surgery: Gastrectomy can result in drug dumping in the intestine, osmotic diarrhea and reduced intestinal transit time. Intestinal surgery also influences drug absorption for predictable reason.

(b) **Cardiovascular diseases:** Several changes associated with congestive cardiac failure influence bioavailability of a drug viz. edema of the intestine, decreased blood flow to the GIT and gastric emptying rate and altered GI pH, secretion and microbial flora.

(c) **Hepatic disease:** Disorder such as hepatic cirrhosis influence bioavailability mainly of drug that undergo considerable first-pass hepatic metabolism e.g. propranolol.

(6) **Blood flow to GIT:** The GIT is extensively supplied by blood capillary network and lymphatic system. The absorbed drug can thus be taken up by blood or the lymph. The high perfusion rate of GIT ensure that once the drug crossed the membrane it is rapidly removed from the absorption site, thus maintaining the sink condition. For highly lipid soluble drug GI perfusion rate could be rate limiting step in absorption. Blood flow is important for actively absorbed drugs, since oxygen and energy is required for transportation.

(7) **Gastrointestinal contents:** The contents present in the GIT influence the drug absorption as discussed below:

(1) **Food-drug interaction:** The contents in the stomach may decrease or increase the absorption of the drug by interacting with it.

(2) **Fluid volume:** When drugs are administered with large fluid volume, it helps in better dissolution, rapid gastric emptying and better absorption.

(3) **Interaction of drug with normal GI constituents:** The contents of GIT such as mucin, bile salts and enzymes influence the drug absorption. These may retard the absorption by acting as a barrier and forming or insoluble complexes enhance absorption by solubilization.

(4) **Drug-Drug interactions in the GIT:** when two or more drugs are co-administered, the absorption of the drugs may be increased, decreased or unaltered due to the drug-drug interactions that take place between them.

(8) **Presystemic metabolism/First-pass effects:** For a drug

administered orally, the two main reasons for its decreased bioavailability are,

(a) Decreased absorption.

(b) First pass/ pre-systemic metabolism.

The loss of drug through biotransformation by such eliminating organs during its passage to systemic circulation is called as first pass or pre-systemic metabolism. The four primary systems which affect pre- systemic metabolism of the drug are,

(a) Luminal enzymes.

(b) Gut wall enzymes/mucosal enzymes.

(c) Bacterial enzymes.

(d) Hepatic enzymes.

(a) **Luminal enzymes:** These are the enzymes present in the gut fluids and include enzyme from intestinal and pancreatic secretions. The latter contains hydrolases which hydrolyse ester drug like chloramphenicol palmitate into active chloramphenicol.

(b) **Gut wall enzymes/mucosal enzymes:** They are present in stomach, intestine and colon. Alcohol dehydrogenase is an enzyme of stomach that inactivates ethanol. Intestinal mucosa contains both phase I and phase II enzyme, e.g. sulfation of ethinyl estradiol and isoprenaline.

(c) **Bacterial enzymes:** The GI microflora is scantily present in stomach and small intestine and is reach in colon. Hence most orally administered drug remains unaffected by them. The colonic microbes generally render the drug more active or toxic on biotransformation for example sulfosalazine, a drug use in ulcerative colitis, is hydrolyse to sulfa pyridine and 5-amino salicylic acid by the microbial enzyme of the colon.

(d) **Hepatic enzymes:** Several drugs undergo first-pass hepatic metabolism, the highly extracted ones being isoprenaline, propranolol, atenolol, deltiazem, nifedipine, morphine etc.

Questions

Essay questions

1. What is drug absorption? Explain various mechanisms of drug absorption.

2. Classify and enumerate the biopharmaceutics factors influencing bioavailability of a drug from its dosage form.

Short questions

1. What is presystemic metabolism? Write factor affecting presystemic metabolism.

2. List characteristics of passive diffusion of drugs.

3. Discuss the similarities and differences between passive and facilitated diffusion.

4. Define polymorphism, amorphism, and Pseudopolymorphism.

5. Discuss briefly the influence of pharmaceutical excipients on drug bioavailability.

Chapter—3

DISTRIBUTION OF DRUGS

Once a drug has gained excess to the blood stream, the drug is subjected to a number of processes called as **Disposition Processes** that tend to lower the plasma concentration. The two major drug disposition processes are:

1. **Distribution** which involves reversible transfer of a drug between compartments.

2. **Elimination** which involves irreversible loss of drug from the body. It comprises of **biotransformation** and **excretion**.

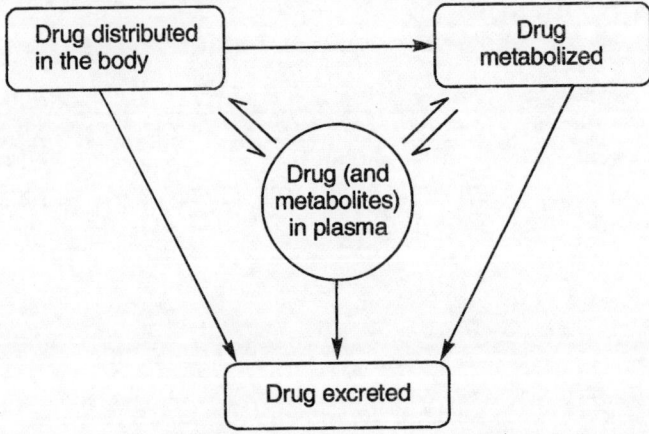

Fig. 3.1: Interrelationship between different processes of drug disposition

The interrelationship between drug distribution, biotransformation and excretion and the drug in plasma is shown in Fig. 3.1.

Distribution is defined as the reversible transfer of a drug between one compartment and another. Since the process is carried out but the circulation of blood, one of the compartments is always the blood or the plasma and the other represents extra vascular fluids and other body tissues. In other words, **distribution** is reversible transfer of a drug between the blood and the extra vascular fluids and tissues. Distribution is a passives process, for which, the driving force is concentration gradient a passive process, for which, the driving force is concentration gradient between the blood and the extra vascular tissues. The process occurs by diffusion of free drug only until equilibrium is achieved. As the pharmacologic action of a drug depends upon its concentration at the site of action, distribution plays a significant role in the onset, intensity and sometimes duration of drug action.

Physiologic Factors of Distribution

After a drug is absorbed into plasma, the drug molecules are distributed throughout the body by the systemic circulation. The drug molecules are carried by the blood to the target site (receptor) for drug action and to other (nonreceptor) tissues as well, where side effects or adverse reactions may occur. Drug molecules are distributed to eliminating organs, such as the liver and kidney, and to noneliminating tissues, such as the brain, skin, and muscle. In pregnancy, drugs cross the placenta and may affect the developing fetus. Drugs can also be secreted in milk via the mammillary glands. A substantial portion of the drug may be bound to proteins in the plasma and/or tissues. Lipophilic drugs deposit in fat, from which the drug may be slowly released.

The circulatory system consists of a series of blood vessels; these include the arteries that carry blood to tissues, and the veins that return the blood back to the heart. An average subject (70 kg) has about 5 L of blood, which is equivalent to 3 L of plasma. About 50% of the blood is in the large veins or venous sinuses. The volume of blood pumped by the heart per minute—the cardiac output—is the product of the stroke volume of the heart and the number of heart beats per minute. An average cardiac output is 0.08 L/left ventricle contraction x 69 contractions (heart beats)/ min, or about 5.5 L/min in subjects at rest. The cardiac output may be five to six times higher during exercise. Left ventricular contraction may produce a systolic blood pressure of 120 mm Hg, and moves blood at a linear speed of 300 mm/sec through the aorta. Mixing of a drug solution in the blood occurs rapidly at this flow rate.

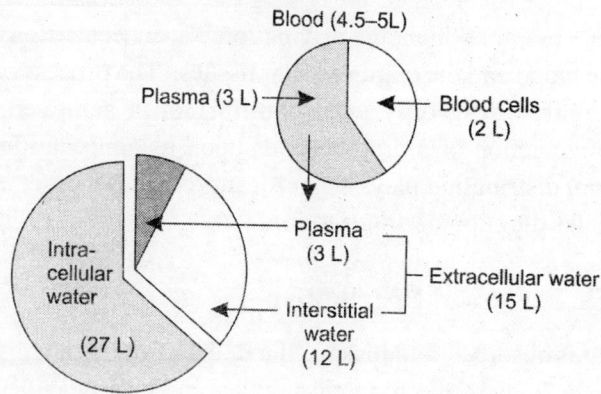

Fig. 3.2: Major water volumes (L) in average 70–kg human.

Drug molecules rapidly diffuse through a network of fine capillaries to the tissue spaces filled with interstitial fluid. The interstitial fluid plus the plasma water is termed extracellular water, because these fluids reside outside the cells. Drug molecules may further diffuse from the interstitial fluid across the cell membrane into the cell cytoplasm.

Drug distribution is generally rapid, and most small drug molecules permeate capillary membranes easily. The passage of drug molecules across a cell membrane depends on the physicochemical nature of both the drug and the cell membrane. Cell membranes are composed of protein and a bilayer of phospholipid, which act as a lipid barrier to drug uptake. Thus, lipid-soluble drugs generally diffuse across cell membranes more

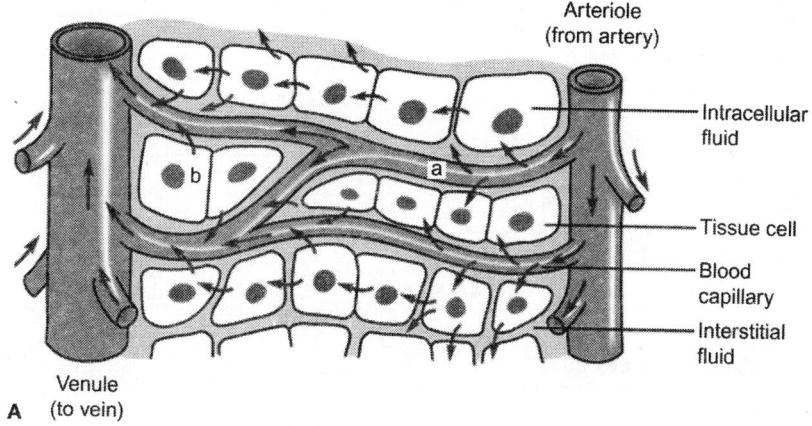

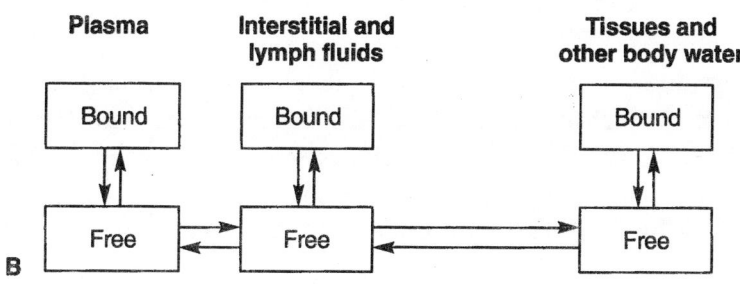

Fig. 3.3 Diffusion of drug from capillaries to interstitial spaces

easily than highly polar or water-soluble drugs. Small drug molecules generally diffuse more rapidly across cell membranes than large drug molecules. If the drug is bound to a plasma protein such as albumin, the drug–protein complex becomes too large for easy diffusion across the cell or even capillary membranes. A comparison of diffusion rates for water-soluble molecules is given in:

Table. 3.1 Permeability of molecules of various sizes to capillaries

	Mole-cular Weight	Radlus of Equi-valent Sphere A (0.1 mm)	Diffusion coefficient	
			In water (cm²/sec) × 10⁵	Across capillary (cm²/sec × 100 g)
Water	18		3.20	3.7
Urea	60	1.6	1.95	1.83
Glucose	180	3.6	0.91	0.64
Sucrose	342	4.4	0.74	0.35
Raffinose	594	5.6	0.56	0.24
Inulin	5,500	15.2	0.21	0.036
Myoglobin	17,000	19	0.15	0.005
Hemoglobin	68,000	31	0.094	0.001
Serum albumin	69,000		0.085	<0.001

(a) Diffusion and Hydrostatic Pressure

The processes by which drugs transverse capillary membranes include passive diffusion and hydrostatic pressure. Passive diffusion is the main process by which most drugs cross cell membranes. **Passive diffusion** is the process by which drug molecules move from an area of high concentration to an area of low concentration. Passive diffusion is described by Fick's law of diffusion:

$$\text{Rate of drug diffusion} = \frac{dQ}{dt} = -DKA(C_P - C_t)/h \quad ...(3.1)$$

Where,

$C_p - C_t$ = the difference between the drug concentration in the plasma (C_p) and in the tissue (C_t), respectively.

A = the surface area of the membrane

h = the thickness of the membrane

K = the lipid–water partition coefficient, and

D = the diffusion constant

The negative sign denotes net transfer of drug from inside the capillary lumen into the tissue and extracellular spaces. Diffusion is spontaneous and temperature dependent. Diffusion is distinguished from blood flow-initiated mixing, which involves hydrostatic pressure.

Hydrostatic pressure represents the pressure gradient between the arterial end of the capillaries entering the tissue and the venous capillaries leaving the tissue. Hydrostatic pressure is responsible for penetration of water-soluble drugs into spaces between endothelial cells and possibly into lymph. In the kidneys, high arterial pressure creates a filtration pressure that allows small drug molecules to be filtered in the glomerulus of the renal nephron. Blood flow-induced drug distribution is rapid and efficient, but requires pressure. As blood pressure gradually decreases when arteries branch into the small arterioles, the speed of flow slows and diffusion into the interstitial space becomes diffusion or concentration driven and facilitated by the large surface area of the capillary network. The average pressure of the blood capillary is higher (+18 mm Hg) than the mean tissue pressure (–6 mm Hg), resulting in a net total pressure of 24 mm Hg higher in the capillary over the tissue. This pressure difference is offset by an average osmotic pressure in the blood of 24 mm Hg, pulling the plasma fluid back into the capillary. Thus, on average, the pressures in the tissue and most parts of the capillary are equal, with no net flow of water.

At the arterial end, as the blood newly enters the capillary, however, the pressure of the capillary blood is slightly higher (about 8 mm Hg) than that of the tissue, causing fluid to leave the capillary and enter the tissues. This pressure is called **hydrostatic** or **filtration pressure**. This filtered fluid (filtrate) is later returned to the venous capillary due to a lower venous pressure of about the same magnitude. The lower pressure of the venous blood compared with the tissue fluid is termed **absorptive pressure**. A small amount of fluid returns to the circulation through the lymphatic system.

(b) Distribution half-life, blood flow, and drug uptake by organs
Because the process of drug transfer from the capillary into the tissue

fluid is mainly diffusional, the membrane thickness, diffusion coefficient of the drug, and concentration gradient across the capillary membrane are important factors in determining the rate of drug diffusion. Kinetically, if a drug diffuses rapidly across the membrane in such a way that blood flow is the rate-limiting step in the distribution of drug, then the process is **perfusion** or **flow limited**. A person with congestive heart failure has decreased cardiac output, resulting in impaired blood flow, which may reduce renal clearance through reduced filtration pressure and blood flow. In contrast, if drug distribution is limited by the slow diffusion of drug across the membrane in the tissue, then the process is termed **diffusion** or **permeability limited**. Drugs that are permeability limited may have an increased distribution volume in disease conditions that cause inflammation and increased capillary membrane permeability. The delicate osmotic pressure balance may be altered due to albumin and/or blood loss or due to changes in electrolyte levels in renal and hepatic disease, resulting in net flow of plasma water into the interstitial space

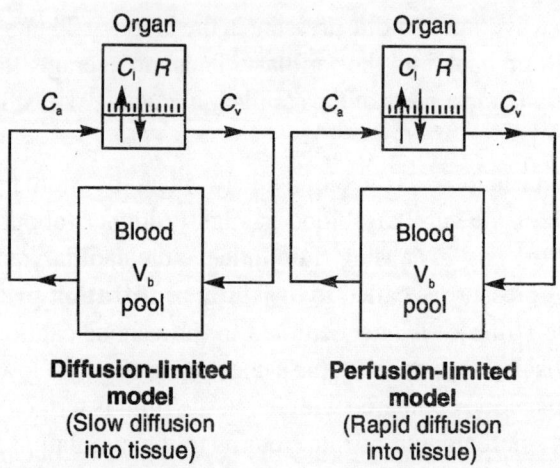

Diffusion-limited model
(Slow diffusion into tissue)

Perfusion-limited model
(Rapid diffusion into tissue)

Fig. 3.4: Drug distribution to body organs by blood flow (perfusion). **Right.** Tissue with rapid permeability; **Left.** Tissue with slow permeability.

(edema). This change in fluid distribution may partially explain the increased extravascular drug distribution during some disease states. Blood flow, tissue size, and tissue storage are also important in determining the time it takes the drug to become fully distributed. List the blood flow and tissue mass for many tissues in the human body. Drug affinity for a tissue or organ refers to the partitioning and accumulation of the drug in the tissue. The time for drug distribution is generally measured by the distribution half-life or the time for 50% distribution. The factors that determine the distribution constant of a drug into an organ are related to the blood flow to the organ, the volume of the organ, and the partitioning of the drug into the organ tissue, as shown in Equation 3.2.

$$K_d = \frac{Q}{VR} \qquad \qquad ... (3.2)$$

Where,

K_d = first-order distribution constant

Q = blood flow to the organ

V = volume of the organ

R = ratio of drug concentration in the organ tissue to drug concentration in the blood (venous).

The distribution half-life of the drug to the tissue, $t_{d1/2}$ may easily be determined from the distribution constant, $t_{d1/2} = 0.693/k_d$. The ratio R must be determined experimentally from tissue samples. With many drugs, however, only animal tissue data are available. Pharmacokineticists have estimated the ratio R based on knowledge of the partition coefficient of the drug. The partition coefficient is a physical property that measures the ratio of the solubility of the drug in the oil phase and in aqueous phase. The **partition coefficient ($P_{o/w}$)** is defined as a ratio of the drug concentration in the oil phase (usually represented by octanol) divided by the drug concentration in the aqueous phase measured at equilibrium under specified temperature *in vitro* in an oil/water two-layer system. The partition coefficient is one of the most important factors that determine the tissue distribution of a drug.

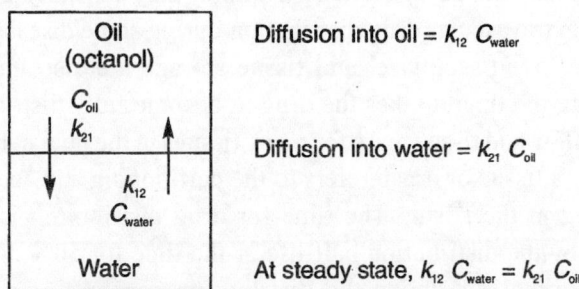

Fig. 3.5: Diagram showing equilibration of drug between oil and water layer *in vitro.*

Table 3.2 Blood flow to human tissues

Tissue	Percent Body Weight	Percent Cardiac Output	Blood Flow (mL/100g tissue/min)
Adrenals	0.02	1	550
Kidneys	0.4	24	450
Thyroid	0.04		400
Liver			
Hepatic	2.0	5	20
Portal		20	75
Portal-drained viscera	2.0	20	75
Heart (basal)	0.4	4	70
Brain	2.0	15	55
Skin	7.0	5	5
Muscle (basal)	40.0	15	3
Connective tissue	7.0	1	1
Fat	15.0	2	1

If each tissue has the same ability to store the drug, then the distribution half-life is governed by the blood flow, Q, and volume (size), V, of the organ. A large blood flow, Q, to the organ decreases the distribution time, whereas a large organ size or volume, V, increases the distribution time because a longer time is needed to fill a large organ volume with drug. illustrates the distribution time (for 0, 50, 90, and 95% distribution) for the adrenal gland, kidney, muscle (basal), skin, and fat tissue in an average human subject (ideal body weight, IBW =70kg). In this illustration, the blood drug concentration is equally maintained at 100 g/mL, and the drug is assumed to have equal distribution between all the tissues and blood, i.e. when fully equilibrated, the partition or drug concentration ratio (R) between the tissue and the plasma will equal 1. Vascular tissues such as the kidneys and adrenal glands achieve 95% distribution in less than 2 minutes. In contrast, drug distribution time in fat tissues takes 4 hours, while less vascular tissue, such as the skin and muscles, take between 2 and 4 hours. When drug partition of the tissues is the same, the distribution time is dependent only on the tissue volume and its blood flow:

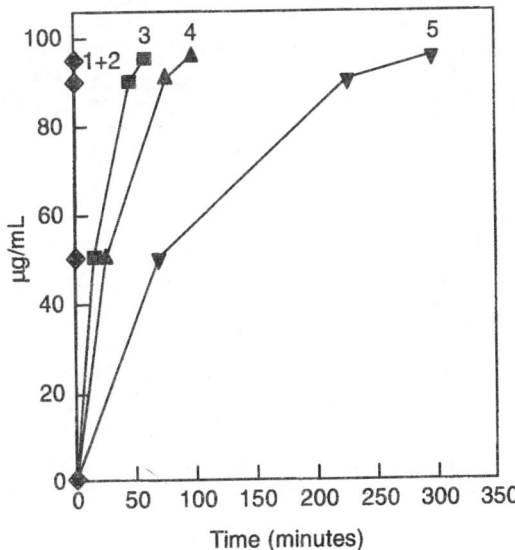

Fig. 3.6: Drug distribution in five groups of tissues at various rate of equilibration. (1 = adrenal, 2 = kidney, 3 = skin, 4 = muscle [basal], 5 = fat).

Blood flow is an important consideration in determining how rapid and how much drug reaches the receptor site. Under normal conditions, limited blood flow reaches the muscles. During exercise, the increase in blood flow may change the fraction of drug reaching the muscle tissues. Diabetic patients receiving intramuscular injection of insulin may experience the effects of changing onset of drug action during exercise. Normally, the blood reserve of the body stays mostly in the large veins and sinuses in the abdomen. During injury or when blood is lost, constrictions of the large veins redirect more blood to needed areas and, therefore, affect drug distribution. Accumulation of carbon dioxide may lower the pH of certain tissues and may affect the level of drugs reaching those tissues. Illustrate the distribution of a drug to three different tissues when the partition of the drug for each tissue varies. For example, the adrenal glands have five times the concentration of the plasma (R = 5), while for drug partition for the kidney, R = 3, and for basal muscle,

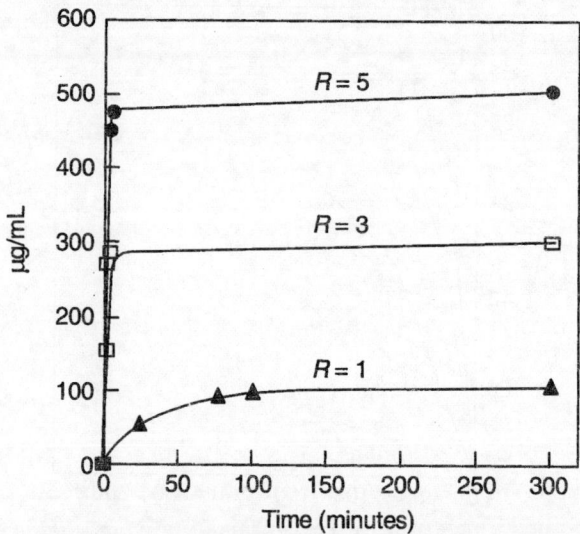

Fig. 3.7: Drug distribution in three groups of tissues with various ability to store drug (R) (**top** = adrenal; **middle** = kidney; **bottom** = muscle).

R = 1. In this illustration, the adrenal gland and kidney take 5 and 3 times as long to be equilibrated with drug. Thus, it can be seen that, even for vascular tissues, high drug partition can take much more time for the tissue to become fully equilibrated. In the example in, drug administration is continuous (as in IV infusion), since tissue drug levels remain constant after equilibrium.

Some tissues have great ability to store and accumulate drug, as shown by large R values. For example, the antiandrogen drug flutamide and its active metabolite are highly concentrated in the prostate. The prostate drug concentration is 20 times that of the plasma drug concentration; thus, the antiandrogen effect of the drug is not fully achieved until distribution to this receptor site is complete. Digoxin is highly bound to myocardial membranes. Digoxin has a high tissue/plasma concentration ratio (R = 60 – 130) in the myocardium. This high R ratio for digoxin leads to a long distributional phase despite abundant blood flow to the heart. It is important to note that if a tissue has a long distribution half-life, a long time is needed for the drug to leave the tissue when blood level decreases. Understanding drug distribution is important because the activities of many drugs are not well correlated with plasma drug level. Kinetically, both protein binding or favorable solubility in the tissue site lead to longer distribution times. Chemical knowledge in molecular structure often helps to estimate the lipid solubility of a drug, and a drug with large oil/water partition coefficient tends to have high R values *in vivo*. A reduction in the partition coefficient of a drug often reduces the rate of drug uptake into the brain. This may decrease drug distribution to the central nervous system and decrease undesirable central nervous system side effects. Extensive tissue distribution is kinetically evidenced by an increase in the volume of distribution, while a secondary effect is a prolonged elimination half-life of the drug distributed over a larger volume (thus, more diluted) and, therefore, less efficiently removed by the kidney or the liver. For example, etretinate (a retinoate derivative) for acne treatment has an unusually long elimination half-life of about 100 days, due to its extensive distribution to body fats. Newly synthesized agents have been designed to reduce lipophilicity and distribution. These new agents have less accumulation and less potential for teratogenicity.

(c) Drug accumulation

The deposition or uptake of the drug into the tissue is generally controlled by the diffusional barrier of the capillary membrane and other cell membranes. For example, the brain is well perfused with blood, but many drugs with good aqueous solubility have high kidney, liver, and lung concentrations and yet little or negligible brain drug concentration. The brain capillaries are surrounded by a layer of tightly joined glial cells that act as a lipid barrier to impede the diffusion of polar or highly ionized drugs. A diffusion-limited model may be necessary to describe the pharmacokinetics of these drugs that are not adequately described by perfusion models. Tissues receiving high blood flow equilibrate quickly with the drug in the plasma. However, at steady state, the drug may or may not accumulate (concentrate) within the tissue. The accumulation of drug into tissues is dependent on both the blood flow and the affinity of the drug for the tissue. Drug uptake into a tissue is generally reversible. The drug concentration in a tissue with low capacity equilibrates rapidly with the plasma drug concentration and then declines rapidly as the drug is eliminated from the body.

In contrast, drugs with high tissue affinity tend to accumulate or concentrate in the tissue. Drugs with a high lipid/water partition coefficient are very fat soluble and tend to accumulate in lipid or adipose (fat) tissue. In this case, the lipid-soluble drug partitions from the aqueous environment of the plasma into the fat. This process is reversible, but the extraction of drug out of the tissue is so slow that the drug may remain for days or even longer in adipose tissues, long after the drug is depleted from the blood. Because the adipose tissue is poorly perfused with blood, drug accumulation is slow. However, once the drug is concentrated in fat tissue, drug removal from fat may also be slow. For example, the chlorinated hydrocarbon DDT (dichlorodiphenyltrichloroethane) is highly lipid soluble and remains in fat tissue for years. Drugs may accumulate in tissues by other processes. For example, drugs may accumulate by binding to proteins or other macromolecules in a tissue. Digoxin is highly bound to proteins in cardiac tissue, leading in a large volume of distribution (440 L/70 kg) and long elimination $t_{1/2}$ (approximately 40 hours). Some drugs may complex with melanin in the skin and eye, as observed after long-term administration of high doses of phenothiazine to chronic schizophrenic patients. The antibiotic tetracycline forms an insoluble chelate with calcium. In growing teeth and bones, tetracycline will complex with the calcium and remain in these tissues.

Some tissues have enzyme systems that actively transport natural biochemical substances into the tissues. For example, various adrenergic tissues have a specific uptake system for catecholamines, such as norepinephrine. Thus, amphetamine, which has a phenylethylamine structure similar to norepinephrine, is actively transported into adrenergic tissue. Other examples of drug accumulation are well documented. For some drugs, the actual mechanism for drug accumulation may not be clearly understood. In a few cases, the drug is irreversibly bound into a particular tissue. Irreversible binding of drug may occur when the drug or a reactive intermediate metabolite becomes covalently bound to a macromolecule within the cell, such as to a tissue protein. Many purine and pyrimidine drugs used in cancer chemotherapy are incorporated into nucleic acids, causing destruction of the cell.

(d) Permeability of cell and capillary membranes

Cell membranes vary in their permeability characteristics, depending on the tissue. For example, capillary membranes in the liver and kidneys are more permeable to transmembrane drug movement than capillaries in the brain. The sinusoidal capillaries of the liver are very permeable and allow the passage of large-molecular-weight molecules. In the brain and spinal cord, the capillary endothelial cells are surrounded by a layer of glial cells, which have tight intercellular junctions. This added layer of cells around the capillary membranes acts effectively to slow the rate of drug diffusion into the brain by acting as a thicker lipid barrier. This lipid barrier, which slows the diffusion and penetration of water-soluble and polar drugs into the brain and spinal cord, is called the **blood–brain barrier.**

Under certain pathophysiologic conditions, the permeability of cell membranes, including capillary cell membranes, may be altered. For example, burns will alter the permeability of skin and allow drugs and larger molecules to permeate inward or outward. In meningitis, which involves inflammation of the membranes of the spinal cord or brain, drug uptake into the brain will be enhanced. The diameters of the capillaries are very small and the capillary membranes are very thin. The high blood flow within a capillary allows for intimate contact of the drug molecules with the cell membrane, providing for rapid drug diffusion. For capillaries that perfuse the brain and spinal cord, the layer of glial cells functions effectively to increase the thickness term h in Equation 3.1, thereby slowing the diffusion and penetration of water-soluble and polar drugs into the brain and spinal cord.

Apparent Volume Distribution

The concentration of drug in the plasma or tissues depends on the amount of drug systemically absorbed and the volume in which the drug is distributed. The apparent volume of distribution, V_D in a model, is used to estimate the extent of drug distribution in the body. Although the apparent volume of distribution does not represent a true anatomical or physical volume, the V_D represents the result of dynamic drug distribution between the plasma and the tissues and accounts for the mass balance of the drug in the body. To illustrate the use of V_D, consider a drug dissolved in a simple solution. A volume term is needed to relate drug concentration in the system (or human body) to the amount of drug present in that system. The volume of the system may be estimated if the amount of drug added to the system and the drug concentration after equilibrium in the system are known.

$$\text{Volume (L)} = \frac{\text{amount (mg) of drug added to system}}{\text{drug concentration (mg/L) in system after equilibrium}}$$

$$...(3.3)$$

Equation 3.3 describes the relationship of concentration, volume, and mass, as shown in Equation 3.4.

Concentration (mg/mL) × volume (L) = mass (mg)   ...(3.4)

Considerations in the Calculation of Volume of Distribution: A Simulated Example

The objective of this exercise is to calculate the fluid volume in each beaker and to compare the calculated volume to the real volume of water in the beaker. Assume that three beakers are each filled with 100 mL of aqueous fluid. Beaker 1 contains water only; beakers 2 and 3 each contain aqueous fluid and a small compartment filled with cultured cells. The cells in beaker 2 can bind the drug, while the cells in beaker 3 can metabolize the drug. The three beakers represent the following, respectively:

Beaker 1. Drug distribution in a fluid (water) compartment only, without drug binding and metabolism

Beaker 2. Drug distribution in a fluid compartment containing cell clusters that reversibly bind drugs

Beaker 3. Drug distribution in a fluid compartment containing cell clusters (similar to tissues *in vivo*) in which the drug may be metabolized and the metabolites bound to cells:

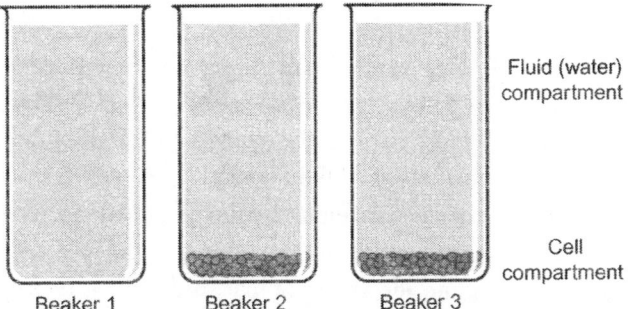

Beaker 1   Beaker 2   Beaker 3

Fluid (water) compartment

Cell compartment

Fig. 3.8: Experiment simulating drug distribution in the body. Three beakers each contain 100 mL of water (fluid compartment) and 100 mg of a water-soluble drug. Beakers 2 and 3 also contain 5 mL of cultured cell clusters.

Suppose 100 mg of drug is then added to each beaker. After the fluid concentration of drug in each beaker is at equilibration, and the concentration of drug in the water (fluid) compartment has been sampled and assayed, the volume of water may be computed.

Case 1

The volume of water in beaker 1 is calculated from the amount of drug added (100 mg) and the equilibrated drug concentration using Equation 3.3. After equilibration, the drug concentration was measured to be 1 mg/mL.

$$\text{Volume} = 100 \text{ mg} / 1 \text{ mg} / \text{mL} = 100 \text{ mL}$$

The calculated volume in beaker 1 confirms that the system is a simple, homogeneous system and, in this case, represents the "true" fluid volume of the beaker.

Case 2

Beaker 2 contains cell clusters stuck to the bottom of the beaker. Binding of drug to the proteins of the cells occurs on the surface and within the cytoplasmic interior. This case represents a heterogeneous system consisting of a well-stirred fluid compartment and a tissue (cell). To determine the volume of this system, more information is needed than in Case 1:

1. The amount of drug dissolved in the fluid compartment must be determined. Because some of the drug will be bound within the cell compartment, the amount of drug in the fluid compartment will be less than the 100 mg placed in the beaker.

2. The amount of drug taken up by the cell cluster must be known to account for the entire amount of drug in the beaker. Therefore, both the cell and the fluid compartments must be sampled and assayed to determine the drug concentration in each compartment.

3. The volume of the cell cluster must be determined.

Assume that the above measurements were made and that the following information was obtained:

❖ Drug concentration in fluid compartment = 0.5 mg/mL
❖ Drug concentration in cell cluster = 10 mg/mL
❖ Volume of cell cluster = 5 mL
❖ Amount of drug added = 100 mg
❖ Amount of drug taken up by the cell cluster = 10 mg/mL × 5 mL
= 50 mg
❖ Amount of drug dissolved in fluid (water) compartment = 100
mg (total) – 50 mg (in cells) = 50 mg (in water)

Using the above information, the true volume of the fluid (water) compartment is calculated using Equation 3.3.

$$\text{Volume of fluid compartment} = \frac{50 \text{ mg}}{0.5 \text{ mg/mL}} = 100 \text{ mL}$$

The value of 100 mL agrees with the volume of fluid we put into the beaker.

If the tissue cells were not accessible for sampling as in the case of *in-vivo* drug administration, the volume of the fluid (water) compartment is calculated using Equation 3.3 assuming the system is homogenous and that 100 mg drug was added to the system

$$\text{Apparent volume} = \frac{100 \text{ mg}}{0.5 \text{ mg/mL}} = 200 \text{ mL}$$

The value of 200 mL is a substantial overestimation of the true volume (100 mL) of the system.

When a heterogeneous system is involved, the real or true volume of the system may not be accurately calculated by monitoring only one compartment. Therefore, an apparent volume of distribution is calculated and the infrastructure of the system is ignored. The term apparent volume of distribution refers to the lack of true volume characteristics. The apparent volume of distribution is used in pharmacokinetics because the tissue (cellular) compartments are not easily sampled and the true volume is not known. When the experiment in beaker 2 is performed with an equal volume of cultured cells that have different binding affinity for the drug, then the apparent volume of distribution is very much affected by the extent of cellular drug binding.

Table 3.3: Relationship of volume of distribution and amount of drug in tissue (cellular) compartment

Total Drug (mg)	Volume of Cells (mL)	Drug in Cells (mg)	Drug in Water (mg)	Drug Concentration in Water (mg/mL)	V_D in Water (mL)
100	15	75	25	0.25	400
100	10	50	50	0.50	200
100	5	25	75	0.75	133
100	1	5	95	0.95	105

For each condition, the true water (fluid) compartment is 100 mL. Apparent volume of distribution (V_D) is calculated according to Equation 3.3.

As shown in, as the amount of drug in the cell compartment increases (column 3), the apparent V_D of the fluid compartment increases (column 6). Extensive cellular drug binding effectively pulls drug molecules out of the fluid compartment, decreases the drug concentration in the fluid compartment, and increases V_D. In biological systems, the quantity of cells, cell compartment volume, and extent of drug binding within the cells affect V_D. A large cell volume and/or extensive drug binding in the cells reduce the drug concentration in the fluid compartment and increase the apparent volume of distribution. In this example, the fluid compartment is comparable to the central compartment and the cell compartment is analogous to the peripheral or tissue compartment. If the drug is distributed widely into the tissues or concentrates unevenly into the tissues, the V_D for a drug may exceed the physical volume of the body (about 70 L of total volume or 42 L of body water for a 70-kg subject). Besides cellular protein binding, partitioning of drug into lipid cellular components may greatly inflate V_D. Many drugs have oil/water partition coefficients above 10,000. These lipophilic drugs are mostly concentrated in the lipid phase of adipose tissue, resulting in a very low drug concentration in the extracellular water. Generally, drugs with very large V_D values have very low drug concentrations in plasma.

A large V_D is often interpreted as broad drug distribution for a drug, even though many other factors also lead to the calculation of a large apparent volume of distribution. A true V_D that exceeds the volume of the body is physically impossible. Only if the drug concentrations in both the tissue and plasma compartments are sampled, and the volumes of each compartment are clearly defined, can a true physical volume be calculated.

Case 3

The drug in the cell compartment in beaker 3 decreases due to undetected metabolism because the metabolite formed is bound to the inside the cells. Thus, the apparent volume of distribution is also greater than 100 mL. Any unknown source that decreases the drug concentration in the fluid compartment will increase the V_D, resulting in an overestimated apparent volume of distribution. This is illustrated with the experiment in beaker 3. In beaker 3, the cell cluster metabolizes the drug and binds the metabolite to the cells. Therefore, the drug is effectively removed from the fluid concentration. The data for this experiment (note that metabolite is expressed as equivalent intact drug) are as follows:

❖ Total drug placed in beaker = 100 mg
❖ Cell compartment:
   Drug concentration = 0.2 mg/mL
   Metabolite-bound concentration = 9.71 mg/mL
   Metabolite-free concentration = 0.29 mg/mL
   Cell volume = 5 mL
❖ Fluid (water) compartment:
   Drug concentration = 0.2 mg/mL

Metabolite concentration = 0.29 mg/mL

To calculate the total amount of drug and metabolite in the cell compartment, Equation 3.3 is rearranged as shown:

Total drug and metabolite in cells = 5 mL × (0.2 + 9.96 + 0.29 mg/mL)

$$= 52.45 \text{ mg}$$

Therefore, the total drug and metabolites in the fluid compartment is

$$100 - 52.45 \text{ mg} = 47.55 \text{ mg}.$$

If only the intact drug is considered, V_D is calculated using Eqn. 3.3.

$$V_D = \frac{50 \text{ mg}}{0.2 \text{ mg/mL}} = 500 \text{mL}$$

Considering that only 100 mL of water was placed into beaker 3, the calculated apparent volume of distribution of 500 mL is an overestimate of the true fluid volume of the system. The following conclusions can be drawn from this beaker exercise:

1. Drug must be at equilibrium in the system before any drug concentration is measured. In nonequilibrium conditions, the sample removed from the system for drug assay does not represent all parts of the system.

2. Drug binding distorts the true physical volume of distribution when all components in the system are not properly sampled and assayed. Extravascular drug binding increases the apparent V_D.

3. Both intravascular and extravascular drug binding must be determined to calculate meaningful volumes of distribution.

4. The apparent V_D is essentially a measure of the relative extent of drug distribution outside the plasma compartment. Greater tissue drug binding and drug accumulation increases V_D, whereas greater plasma protein drug binding decreases the V_D distribution.

5. Undetected cellular drug metabolism increases V_D.

6. An apparent V_D larger than the combined volume of plasma and body water is indicative of (4) and (5), or both, above.

7. Although the V_D is not a true physiologic volume, the V_D is useful to relate the plasma drug concentration to the amount of drug in the body (Eq. 3.3). This relationship of the product of the drug concentration and volume to equal the total mass of drug is important in pharma-cokinetics.

Practice Problem

The amount of drug in the system calculated from V_D and the drug concentration in the fluid compartment is shown in. Calculate the amount of drug in the system using the true volume and the drug concentration in the fluid compartment.

Solution

In each case, the product of the drug concentration (column 5) times the apparent volume of distribution (column 6) yields 100 mg of drug, accurately accounting for the total amount of drug present in the system. For example, 0.25 mg/mL x 400 mL = 100 mg. Notice that the total amount of drug presents cannot be determined using the true volume and the drug concentration (column 5).

The physiologic approach requires detailed information, including (1) cell drug concentration, (2) cell compartment volume, and (3) fluid compartment volume. Using the physiologic approach, the total amount of drug is equal to the amount of drug in the cell compartment and the amount of drug in the fluid compartment.

$$(15 \text{ mg/mL} \times 5 \text{ mL}) + (100 \text{ mL} \times 0.25 \text{ mg/mL}) = 100 \text{ mg}$$

The two approaches shown above each account correctly for the amount of drug present in the system. However, the second approach requires more information than is commonly available. The second approach does, however, make more physiologic sense. Most physiologic compartment spaces are not clearly defined for measuring drug concentrations.

Apparent Volume of Distribution

The apparent volume of distribution, in general relates the plasma drug concentration to the amount of drug present in the body. In classical compartment models, V_{DSS} is the volume of distribution determined at steady state when the drug concentration in the tissue compartment is at equilibrium with the drug concentration in the plasma compartment (, top). In a physiological system involving a drug distributed to a given tissue from the plasma fluid (, bottom), the two-compartment model is not assumed, and drug distribution from the plasma to a tissue is equilibrated by perfusion with arterial blood and returned by venous blood. The model parameter V_{app} is used to represent the apparent distribution volume in this model, which is different from V_{DSS} used in the compartment model. Similar to the apparent volume simulated in the beaker experiment in Equation 3.3, V_{app} is defined by Equation 3.5, and the amount of drug in the body is given by Equation 3.6.

$$V_{app} = D_B / C_P \qquad \qquad \text{... (3.5)}$$

$$D_B = V_P C_P + V_t C_t \qquad \qquad \text{... (3.6)}$$

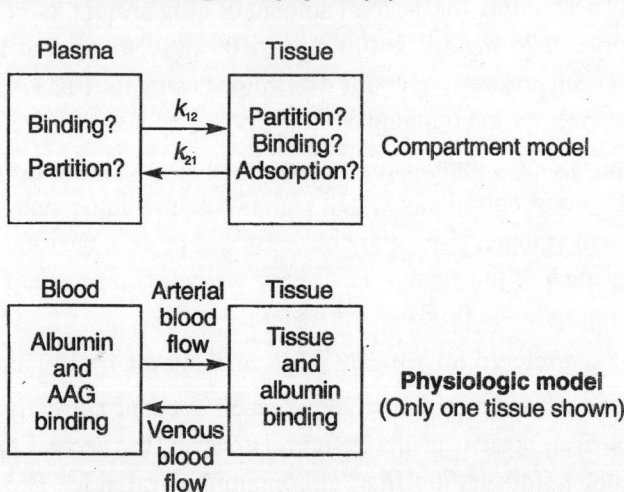

Fig. 3.9: A diagram showing (top) a two-compartment model approach to drug distribution; (bottom) a physiologic approach to drug distribution.

Where,

D_B = the amount of drug in the body

V_p = the plasma fluid volume

V_t = the tissue volume

C_p = the plasma drug concentration, and

C_t = the tissue drug concentration.

For many protein-bound drugs, the ratio of D_B/C_p is not constant over time, and this ratio depends on the nature of dissociation of the protein–drug complex and how the free drug is distributed; the ratio is best determined at steady state. Protein binding to tissue has an apparent effect of increasing the apparent volume of distribution. Several V_D terms were introduced in the classical compartment models. However, protein binding was not introduced in those models.

Equation 3.6 describes the amount of drug in the body at any time point between a tissue and the plasma fluid. Instead of assuming the drug distributes to a hypothetical compartment, it was assumed that, after injection, the drug diffuses from the plasma to the extracellular fluid/water, where it further equilibrates with the given tissue. One or more tissue types may be added to the model if needed. If the drug penetrates inside the cell, distribution into the intracellular water may occur. If the volume of body fluid and the protein level are known, this information may be incorporated into the model. Such a model may be more compatible with the physiology and anatomy of the human body. When using pharmacokinetic parameters from the literature, it is important to note that most calculations of steady-state V_D involve some assumptions on how and where the drug distributes in the body; it could involve a physiologic or a compartmental approach.

For a drug that involves protein binding, some models assume that the drug distributes from the plasma water into extracellular tissue fluids, where the drug binds to extravascular proteins, resulting in a larger V_D due to extravascular protein binding. Unfortunately, drug binding and distribution to lipoid tissues are generally not distinguishable. If the pharmacokineticist suspects' distribution to body lipids because the drug involved is very lipophilic, he or she may want to compare results simulated with different models before making a final conclusion. List the steady-state volume of distribution of 10 common drugs in ascending order. Most of these drugs follow multicompartment kinetics with various tissue distribution phases. The physiologic volumes of an ideal 70-kg subject are also plotted for comparison: (1) the plasma (3 L), (2) the extracellular fluid (15 L), and (3) the intracellular fluid (27 L). Drugs such as penicillin, cephalosporin, valproic acid, and furosemide are polar compounds that stay mostly within the plasma and extracellular fluids and therefore have a relatively low V_D.

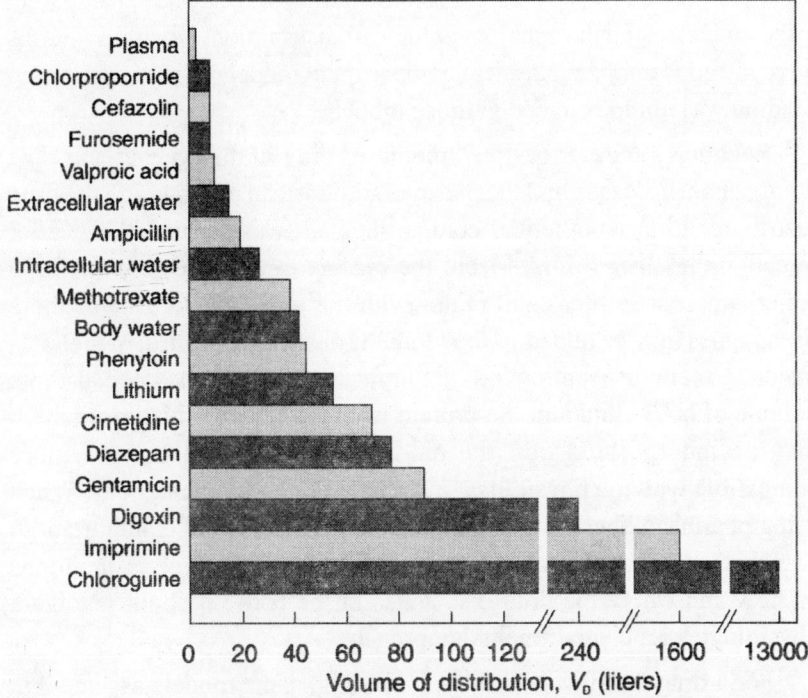

Fig. 3.10: Lists of steady-state volumes of distribution of 10 common drugs in ascending order showing various factors affect V_D. Drugs with high V_D generally has high tissue affinity or low binding to serum albumin. Polar or hydrophilic drugs tend to have V_D similar to the volume of extracellular water.

In contrast, drugs with lower distribution to the extracellular water are more extensively distributed inside the tissues and tend to have a large V_D. An excessively high volume of distribution (greater than the body volume of 70 L) is due mostly to special tissue storage, tissue protein binding, carrier, or efflux system which removes drug from the plasma fluid. Digoxin, for example, is bound to myocardial membrane that has drug levels that are 60 and 130 times the serum drug level in adults and children, respectively. The high tissue binding is responsible for the large steady-state volume of distribution. The greater drug affinity also results in longer distribution half-life in spite of the heart's great vascular blood perfusion. Imipramine is a drug that is highly protein bound and concentrated in the plasma, yet its favorable tissue partition and binding accounts for a large volume of distribution. Several tricyclic antidepressants (TCAs) also have large volumes of distribution due to tissue (CNS) penetration and binding.

Real Volume of Distribution

The **real volume of distribution** has direct physiologic meaning and is related to the body water. The body water is made up of 3 distinct compartments as shown in the Table 3.4.

Table 3.4: Fluid compartments of a 70 kg adult

Body Fluid	Volume (liters)	% of Body Weight	% of TBW
1. Vascular fluid/blood (Plasma)	6(3)	9(4.5)	15(7.5)
2. Extracellular fluid (excluding plasma)	12	17	28
3. Intracellular fluid (excluding blood cells)	24	34	57
Total Body Water (TBW)	42	60	100

The volume of each of these real physiologic compartments can be determined by use of specific tracers or markers (Table 3.5). The plasma volume can be determined by use of substances of high molecular weight or substances that are totally bound to plasma albumin, for e.g. high molecular weight dyes such as Evans blue, indocyanine green and I-131 albumin. When given i.v., these remain confined to the plasma. The total blood volume can also be determined if the hematocrit is known. The extracellular fluid (ECF) volume can be determined by substances that easily penetrates the capillary membrane and rapidly distribute throughout the ECF but do not cross the cell membranes, for e.g. the Na^+, Cl^-, Br^-, SCN^- and So ions and inulin, mannitol and raffinose. However, none of these substances are completely kept out of the cells. The ECF volume, excluding plasma is approximately 15 liters. The total body water (TBW) volume can be determined by use of substances that distribute equally in all water compartments of the body (both intra- and extracellular), for e.g. heavy water ($D2O$), tritiated water (HTO) and lipid soluble substances such as antipyrine. The intracellular fluid volume is determined as the

Table 3.5: Markers used to measure the volume of real physiologic compartments.

Physiologic Fluid Compartment	Markers Used	Approximate Volume (liters)
Plasma	Evans blue, indocyanine green, I-131 albumin	3
Erythrocytes	Cr-51	2
Extracellular fluid	Nonmetabolizable saccharides like raffinose, inulin, mannitol and radioisotopes of selected ions: Na^+, Cl^-, Br^-, SO_4^{2-}	15
Total body water	D_2O, HTO, antipyrine	42

difference between the TBW and ECF volume. The intracellular fluid volume including those of blood cells is approximately 27 liters.

Since the tracers are not bound or negligibly bound to plasma or tissue proteins, their apparent volume of distribution is same as their true volume of distribution. The situation is different with most drugs which bind to plasma proteins or extravascular tissues or both. Certain generalizations can be made regarding the apparent volume of distribution of such drugs:

1. Drugs which bind selectively to plasma proteins or other blood components, e.g. warfarin (i.e. those that are less bound to extravascular tissues), have apparent volume of distribution smaller than their true volume of distribution. The V_d of such drugs lies between blood volume and TBW volume (i.e. between 6 to 42 liters); for example, warfarin has a V_d of about 10 liters.

2. Drugs which bind selectively to extravascular tissues, e.g. chloroquine (i.e. those that are less bound to blood components), have apparent volume of distribution larger than their real volume of distribution. The V_d of such drugs is always greater than 42 liters or TBW volume; for example, chloroquine has a V_d of approximately 15,000 liters. Such drugs leave the body slowly and are generally more toxic than drugs that do not distribute deeply into body tissues.

Thus, factors that produce an alteration in binding of drug to blood components result in an increase in V_d and those that influence drug binding to extravascular components result in a decrease in V_d. Other factors that may influence V_d are changes in tissue perfusion and permeability, changes in the physicochemical characteristics of the drug e.g. ionization, changes in the body weight and age and several disease states.

Apparent volume of distribution is expressed in liters and sometimes in liters / Kg body weight. The V_d of various drugs range from as low as 3 liters (plasma volume) to as high as 40,000 liters (much above the total body size). Many drugs have V_d greater than 30 liters. The V_d is a characteristic of each drug under normal conditions and is altered under conditions that affect distribution pattern of the drug.

Factors Influencing Distribution

1. Tissue permeability of the drug:
   a. Physicochemical properties of the drug like molecular size, pK_a and o/w partition coefficient
   b. Physiological barriers to diffusion of drugs
2. Organ/tissue size and perfusion rate
3. Binding of drugs to tissue components:
   a. Binding of drugs to blood components
   b. Binding of drugs to extravascular tissue proteins
4. Miscellaneous factors:
   c. Age
   d. Pregnancy
   e. Obesity
   f. Diet
   g. Disease states
   h. Drug interactions

Tissue permeability of drugs:

Of the several factors listed above, the two major rate-determining steps in the distribution of drugs are:

1. Rate of tissue permeability, and
2. Rate of blood perfusion.

If the blood flow to the entire body tissues were rapid and uniform, differences in the degree of distribution between tissues will be indicative of differences in the tissue penetrability of the drug and the process will be tissue permeability rate-limited. The tissue permeability of a drug depends upon the physicochemical properties of the drug into tissues.

(a) Physicochemical Properties of the Drug

Important physicochemical properties that influence drug distribution are molecular size, degree of ionization and partition coefficient. Almost all drugs having molecular weight less than 500 to 600 Daltons cagily cross the capillary membrane to diffuse into the extra cellular interstitial fluids. However, penetration of drugs from the extracellular fluid into the cells is a function of molecular size, ionization constant and lipophilicity of the drug. Only small, water-soluble molecules and ions of size below 50 daltons enter the cell through aqueous filled channels whereas those of larger size are restricted unless a specialized transport system exists for them.

The degree of ionization of a drug is an important determinant in its tissue penetrability. The pH of the blood and the extravascular fluid also play a role in the ionization and diffusion of drugs into cells. A drug that remains unionized at these pH values can permeate the cells relatively more rapidly. Since the blood and the ECF pH normally remain constant at 7.4, they do not have much of an influence on drug diffusion unless altered in conditions such as systemic acidosis or alkalosis.

Most drugs are either weak acids or weak bases and their degree of ionization at plasma or ECG pH depends upon their pK_a. All drugs that ionize at plasma pH (i.e. polar, hydrophilic drugs), cannot penetrate the lipoidal cell membrane and tissue permeability is the rate-limiting step in the distribution of such drugs. Only unionized drugs which are generally lipophilic rapidly cross the cell membrane. Among the drugs that have same o/w partition coefficient but differ in the extent of ionization at blood pH the one that ionizes to a lesser extent will have greater penetrability than that which ionizes to a larger extent; for example, pentobarbital and salicylic acid have almost the same $K_{o/w}$ but former is more unionized at blood pH and therefore distributes rapidly. The influence of drug pK_a and $K_{o/w}$ on distribution is illustrated by the example that thiopental, a nonpolar, lipophilic drug, largely unionized at plasma pH do not cross the blood-brain barrier. Since the extent to which a drug exists in unionized form governs the distribution pattern, acidosis (metabolic or respiratory) results in decreased ionization of acidic drugs and thus increased intracellular drug concentration and pharmacologic action. Opposite is the influence of alkalosis. Sodium bicarbonate induced alkalosis is sometimes useful in the treatment of barbiturate (and other acidic drugs) poisoning to drive the drug out and prevent further entry into the CNS and promote their urinary excretion by favoring ionization. Converse is true for basic drugs; acidosis favors extra cellular whereas alkalosis, intracellular distribution.

In case of polar drugs where permeability is the rate-limiting step in the distribution, the driving force is the effective partition coefficient of drug. It is calculated by the following formula:

Effective $K_{o/w}$ = Fraction unionized at pH 7.4 ×

$K_{o/w}$ of unionized drug   ... (3.7)

The extent to which the effective partition coefficient influences rapidity of drug distribution can be seen from the example given in Table 3.6.

Table 3.6: Distribution of acidic drugs in CSF

Drug	Relative acidity	Effective $K_{o/w}$ at pH 7.4	Relative rate of distribution
Thiopental	Weaker acid	2.0	80
Salicylic acid	Stronger acid	0.0005	1

Thus, thiopental distributes in CSF at a rate 80 times faster than salicylic acid.

(b) Physiologic Barriers to Distribution of Drugs

A membrane (or a barrier) with special structural features can be a permeability restriction to distribution of drugs to some tissues. Some of the important simple and specialized physiologic barriers are:

1. Simple capillary endothelial barrier
2. Simple cell membrane barrier
3. Blood-brain barrier
4. Cerebrospinal fluid barrier
5. Placental barrier
6. Blood-testis barrier

1. **The simple capillary endothelial barrier:** The membrane of capillaries that supply blood to most tissues is, practically speaking, not a barrier to moieties which we call drugs. Thus, all drugs, ionized or unionized, with a molecular size less than 600 daltons, diffuse through the capillary endothelium and into the interstitial fluid. Only drugs bound to the blood components are restricted because of the large molecular size of the complex.

2. **The simple cell membrane barrier:** Once a drug diffuses from the capillary wall into the extracellular fluid, its further entry into cells of most tissues is limited by its permeability through the membrane that lines such cells. Such a simple cell membrane is similar to the lipoidal barrier in the GI absorption of drugs.

3. **Blood-Brain Barrier (BBB):** Unlike the capillaries found in other parts of the body, the capillaries in the brain are highly specialized and much less permeable to water-soluble drugs. The brain capillaries consist of endothelial cells which are joined to one another by continuous tight intercellular junctions comprising what is called as the **blood-brain barrier**.

   Moreover, the presence of special cells called as **astrocytes,** which are the elements of the supporting tissue found at the base of endothelial membrane, from a solid envelope around the brain capillaries. As a result, the intercellular passage is blocked and for a drug to gain access from the capillary circulation into the brain, it has to pass through access from the cells rather than between them. (However, there are specific sites in the brain where the BBB does not exist, namely, the trigger area and the median hypothalamic eminence. Moreover, drugs administered intranasally may diffuse directly into the CNS because of the continuity between sub-mucosal areas of the nose and the subarachnoid space of the olfactory lobe).

Since the BBB is a lipoidal barrier, it allows only the drugs having high o/w partition coefficient to diffuse passively whereas moderately lipid soluble and partially ionized molecules penetrate

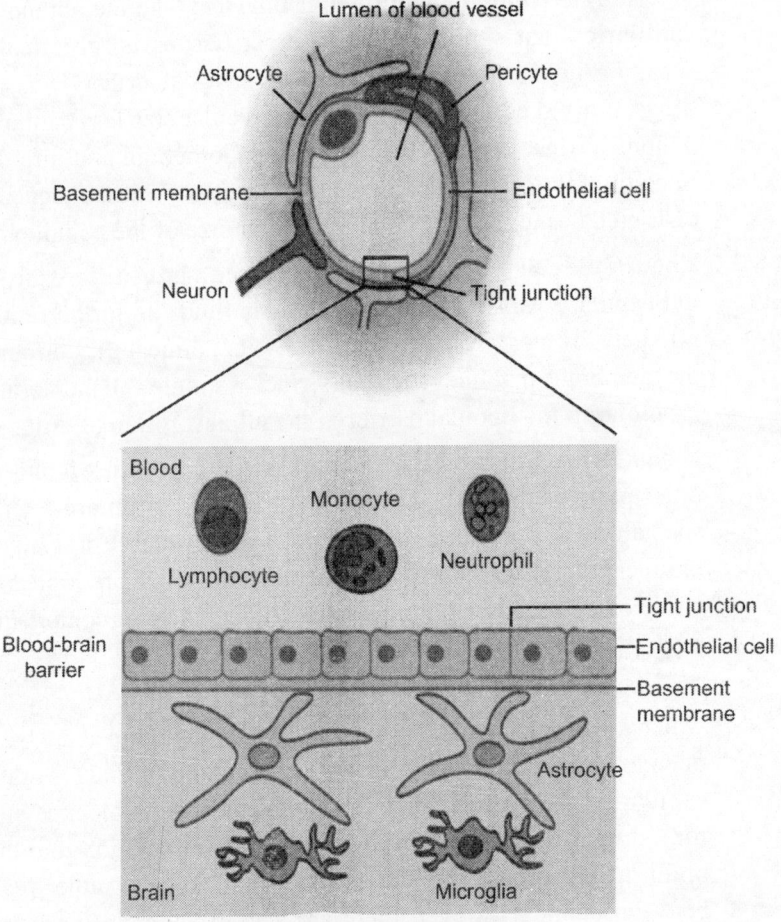

Fig. 3.11: Blood-brain barrier

at a slow rate. The effective partition coefficient of thiopental, a highly lipid soluble drug is 50 times that of pentobarbital and crosses the BBB much more rapidly polar natural substances such as sugars and amino acids are transported to brain actively.

Thus, structurally similar foreign molecules can also penetrate the BBB by the same mechanism. Most antibiotics such as penicillin which are polar, water-soluble and ionized at plasma pH do not cross the BBB under normal circumstances.

The selective permeability of lipid soluble moieties through the BBB makes appropriate choice of a drug to treat CNS disorders an essential part of therapy; for example, Parkinsonism, a disease characterized by depletion of dopamine in the brain, cannot be treated by administration of dopamine as it does not cross the BBB. Hence, levodopa, which can penetrate the CNS where it is metabolized to dopamine, is used in its treatment. Three different approaches have been utilized successfully to promote crossing the BBB by drugs:

i. Use of permeation enhancers such as dimethyl sulfoxide (DNSI)

ii. Osmotic disruption of the BBB by infusing internal carotid artery with mannitol

iii. Use of dihydropyridine redox system as drug carriers to the brain

In the latter case, the lipid soluble dihydropyridine is linked as a carrier to the polar drug to form a prodrug that readily crosses the BBB. In the brain, the CNS enzymes oxidize the dihydropyridine moiety to the polar pyridinium ion form that cannot diffuse back out of the brain. As a result, the drug gets trapped in the CNS. Such a redox system has been used to deliver steroidal drugs to the brain.

4. **Blood-Cerebrospinal Fluid Barrier:** The cerebrospinal fluid (CSF) is formed mainly by the choroids plexus of the lateral,

third and fourth ventricles and is similar in composition to the ECF of brain. The capillary endothelium that lines the choroids plexus has open junctions or gaps and drugs can flow freely into the extracellular space between the capillary wall and the choroidal cells. However, the choroidal cells are joined to each other by tight junctions forming the blood-CSF barrier which has permeability characteristics similar to that of the BBB.

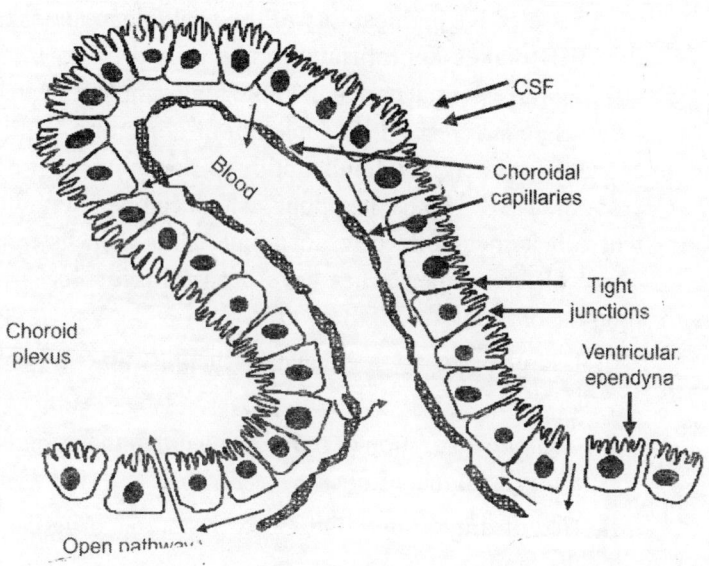

Fig. 3.12 The blood-CSF barrier

As in the case of BBB, only highly lipid soluble drugs can cross the blood-CSF barrier with relative ease whereas moderately lipid soluble and partially ionized drugs permeate slowly. A drug that enters the CSF slowly cannot achieve a high concentration as the bulk flow of CSF continuously removes the drug. For any given drug, its concentration in the brain will always be higher than in the CSF.

Although the mechanisms for diffusion of drugs into the CNS and CSF are similar, the degree of uptake may vary significantly. In some cases, CSF drug concentration may be higher than its cerebral concentration e.g. sulfamethoxazole and trimethoprim, and vice versa in other cases, e.g. certain â-blockers.

5. **Placental Barrier:** The maternal and the fetal blood vessels are separated by a number of tissue layers made of fetal trophoblast basement membrane and the endothelium which together constitute the placental barrier.

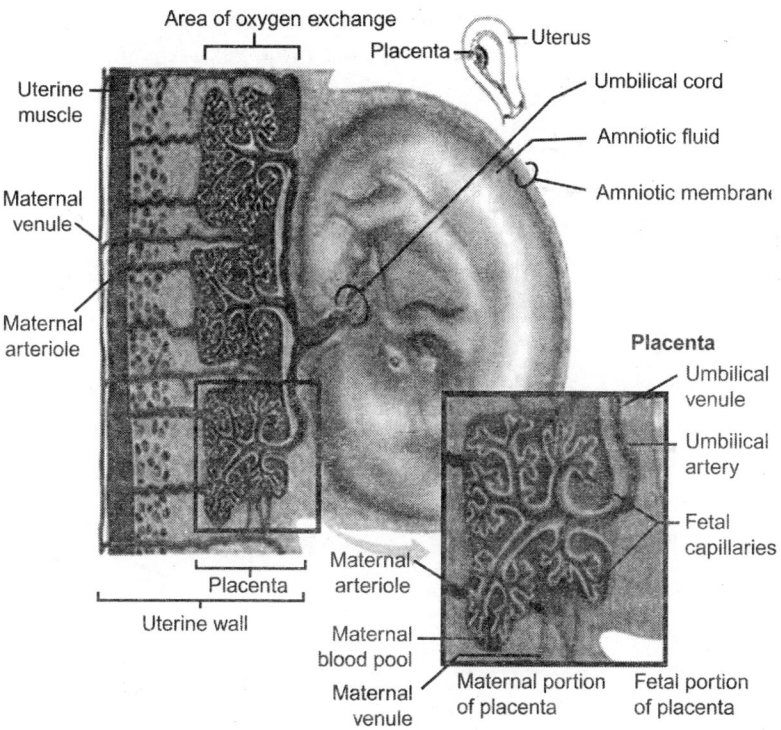

Fig. 3.13: Placental barrier

The human placental barrier has a mean thickness of 25 microns in early pregnancy that reduces to 2 microns at full term which however does not reduce its effectiveness. Many drugs having molecular weight less than 1000 daltons and moderate to high lipid solubility e.g. ethanol, sulfonamides, barbiturates, gaseous anesthetic, steroids, narcotic analgesics, anticonvulsants and some antibiotics, cross the barrier by simple diffusion quite rapidly. This shows that the placental barrier is not as effective a barrier as BBB Nutrients essential for the fetal growth are transported by carrier-mediated processes. Immunoglobulins are transported by endocytosis. Drugs are particularly dangerous to the fetus during 2 stages

i. In the first trimester when the fetal organs develop; it is during this stage that most drugs show their teratogenic effects (congenital defects) e.g. thalidomide, phenytoin, isotretinoin, testosterone, methotrexate, etc.

ii. In the latter stages of pregnancy when drugs are known to affect physiologic functions, e.g. respiratory depression by morphine.

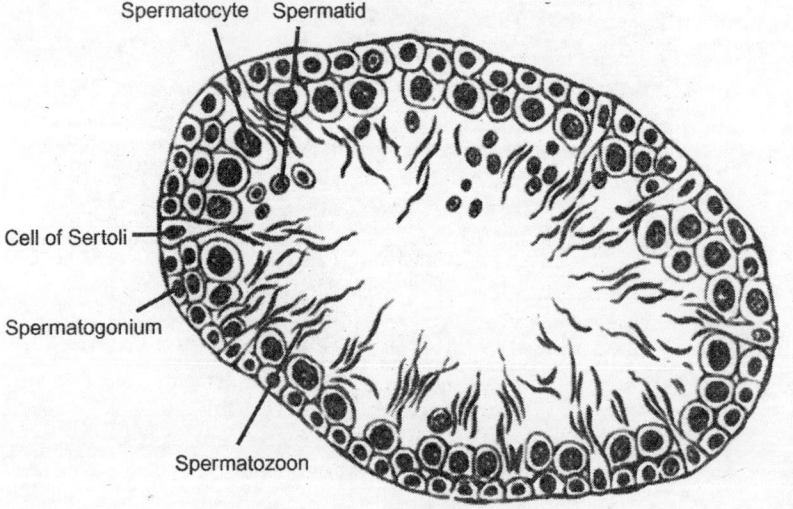

Fig. 3.14: Blood-testis barrier

It is, therefore, always better to restrict all drugs during pregnancy because of the uncertainty of their hazardous effects.

6. **Blood-Testis Barrier:** This barrier is located not at the capillary endothelium level but at sertoli-sertoli cell junction. It is the tight junctions between the neighboring sertoli cells that act as the blood-testis barrier. This barrier restricts the passage of drugs to spermatocytes and spermatids.

Organ/tissue size and perfusion rate

As discussed until now, distribution is permeability rate-limited in the following cases:

   i. When the drug under consideration is ionic, polar or water soluble

  ii. Where the highly selective physiologic barriers restrict the diffusion of such drugs to the inside of the cell

In contrast, distribution will be perfusion rate-limited when:

   i. The drug is highly lipophilic

  ii. The membrane across which the drug is supposed to diffuse is highly permeable such as those of the capillaries and the muscles.

Whereas only highly lipophilic drugs such as thiopental can cross the most selective of the barriers like the BBB, highly permeable capillary wall permits passage of almost all drugs (except those bound to plasma proteins). In both circumstances, the tart-limiting step is the rate of blood flow or perfusion to the tissue. Greater the blood flow, faster the distribution.

Perfusion rate is defined as the volume of blood that flows per unit time per unit volume of the tissue. It is expressed in ml/min/ml of the tissue. The perfusion rates of various tissues are given in Table 3.7.

In Table 3.7 the various tissues are listed in decreasing order of their perfusion rate which indicates the rapidity with which the drug will be distributed to the tissues. Highly perfused tissues such as lungs, kidneys, adrenal, liver, heart and brain are rapidly equilibrated with lipid soluble drugs.

Table 3.7: Relative Volume of Different Organs, Blood Flow and Perfusion Rate under Basal Conditions Assuming the Total Body Volume to be 70 liters

Organ/tissue	% of Body Volume	Blood Flow (ml/min)	% of Cardiac Output	Perfusion Rate (ml/min/ml)
I. Highly Perfused				
1. Lungs	0.7	5000	100.0	10.2
2. Kidneys	0.4	1250	25.0	4.5
3. Adrenals	0.03	25	0.5	1.2
4. Liver	2.3	1350	27.0	0.8
5. Heart	0.5	200	4.0	0.6
6. Brain	2.0	700	14.0	0.5
II. Moderately Perfused				
7. Muscles	42.0	1000	20.0	0.034
8. Skin	15.0	350	7.0	0.033
III. Poorly Perfused				
9. Fat (adipose)	10.0	200	4.0	0.03
10. Bone (skeleton)	16.0	250	5.0	0.02

If $K_{t/b}$ is the tissue/ blood partition coefficient of drug then the first-order distribution rate constant, K_t, is given by following equation:

$$K_t = \text{Perfusion Rate}/K_{t/b} \qquad ... (3.8)$$

The tissue distribution half-life is given by equation

Distribution half-life $= 0.693/K_t = 0.693\, k_{t/b}/\text{Perfusion rate}$ ... (3.9)

The extent to which a drug is distributed in a particular tissue or organ depends upon the size of the tissue (i.e. tissue volume) and the tissue/blood partition coefficient of the drug. Consider the classic example of thiopental. This lipophilic drug has a high tissue/blood partition coefficient towards the brain and still higher for adipose tissue. Since the brain (site of action) is a highly perfused organ, following i.v. injection, thiopental readily diffuses into the brain showing a rapid onset of action.

Adipose tissue being poorly perfused, takes longer to get distributed with the same drug. But as the concentration of thiopental in the adipose proceeds towards equilibrium, the drug rapidly diffuses out of the brain and localizes in the adipose tissue whose volume is more than 5 times that of brain and has greater affinity for the drug. The result is rapid termination of action of thiopental due to such tissue redistribution.

Binding of drugs to tissue components

This topic is dealt comprehensively in chapter 4 on protein binding of drugs.

Miscellaneous factors affecting drug distribution

Age

Differences in distribution pattern of a drug in different age groups are mainly due to differences in

a. Total body water (both intracellular and extracellular) – is much greater in infants

b. Fat content – is also higher in infants and elderly

c. Skeletal muscles – are lesser in infants and in elderly

d. Organ composition - the BBB is poorly developed in infants, the myelin content is low and cerebral blood flow is high, hence greater penetration of drugs in the brain.

e. Plasma protein content – low albumin content in both infants and in elderly

Pregnancy

During pregnancy, the growth of uterus, placenta and fetus increases the volume available for distribution of drugs. The fetus represents a separate compartment in which a drug can distribute. The plasma and the ECF volume also increase but there is a fall in albumin content.

Obesity

In obese persons, the high adipose tissue content can take up a large fraction of lipophilic drug despite the fact that perfusion through it is low. The high fatty acid levels in obese persons alter the binding characteristics of acidic drugs.

Diet

A diet high in fats will increase the free fatty acid levels in circulation thereby affecting binding of acidic drugs such as NSAIDs to albumin.

Disease States

A number of mechanisms may be involved in the alteration of drug distribution characteristics in disease states:

a. Altered albumin and other drug-binding protein concentration

b. Altered or reduced perfusion to organs or tissues

c. Altered tissue pH

An interesting example of altered permeability of the physiologic barriers is that of BBB. In meningitis and encephalitis, the BBB becomes more permeable and thus polar antibiotics such as penicillin G and ampicillin which do not normally cross it, gain access to the brain. In a patient suffering from CCF, the perfusion rate to the entire body decreases affecting distribution of all drugs.

Drug Interactions

Drug interactions that affect distribution are mainly due to differences in plasma protein or tissue binding of drugs.

Questions

Essay questions

1. Define distribution of drugs. Discuss briefly physiological factors of distribution.

2. Explain factor influencing drug distribution.

3. What is apparent and real volume of distribution? Explain it briefly.

Short questions

1. The tracers used to determine the volume of body fluids have V_d same as their true volume. Why?

2. Explain physiologic barriers that restrict diffusion of drug into tissues.

3. Polar drugs such as penicillin normally do not cross BBB but do so in meningitis. Explain.

4. Why is the placental barrier not as effective as BBB?

5. What are the various mechanisms involved in the alteration of drug distribution characteristics in disease states?

Chapter—4

PROTEIN BINDING OF DRUGS

Many drugs interact with plasma or tissue proteins or with other macromolecules, such as melanin and DNA, to form a **drug–macromolecule complex.** The formation of a drug protein complex is often named **drug–protein binding.** Drug–protein binding may be a reversible or an irreversible process. **Irreversible** drug–protein binding is usually a result of chemical activation of the drug, which then attaches strongly to the protein or macromolecule by covalent chemical bonding. Irreversible drug binding accounts for certain types of drug toxicity that may occur over a long time period, as in the case of chemical carcinogenesis, or within a relatively short time period, as in the case of drugs that form reactive chemical intermediates. For example, the hepatotoxicity of high doses of acetaminophen is due to the formation of reactive metabolite intermediates that interact with liver proteins.

Most drugs bind or complex with proteins by a reversible process. **Reversible drug–protein binding** implies that the drug binds the protein with weaker chemical bonds, such as hydrogen bonds or vander Waals forces. The amino acids that compose the protein chain have hydroxyl, carboxyl, or other sites available for reversible drug interactions. Reversible drug–protein binding is of major interest in pharmacokinetics. The protein-bound drug is a large complex that cannot easily transverse cell or possibly even capillary membranes and therefore has a restricted distribution. Moreover, the protein-bound drug is usually pharmacologically inactive. In contrast, the free or unbound drug crosses cell membranes and is therapeutically active. Studies that critically evaluate drug–protein binding are usually performed *in vitro* using a purified protein such as albumin. Methods for studying protein binding, including equilibrium dialysis and ultra filtration, make use of a semipermeable membrane that separates the protein and protein-bound drug from the free or unbound drug. By these *in-vitro* methods, the concentrations of bound drug, free drug, and total protein may be determined. Each method for the investigation of drug–protein binding *in vitro* has advantages and disadvantages in terms of cost, ease of measurement, time, instrumentation, and other considerations. Various experimental factors for the measurement of protein binding are listed in.

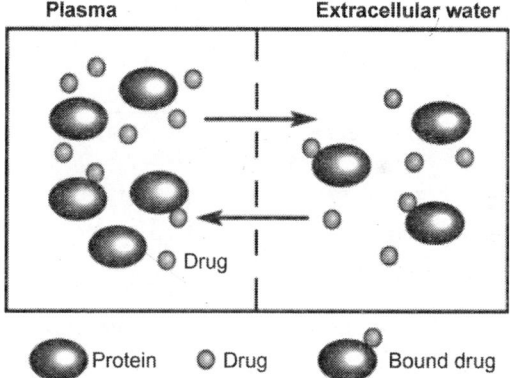

Fig. 4.1: Diagram showing that bound drugs will not diffuse across membrane but free drug will diffuse freely between the plasma and extracellular water.

Table 4.1: Methods for studying drug–protein binding

Equilibrium dialysis	Gel chromatography
Dynamic dialysis	Spectrophotometry
Diafiltration	Electrophoresis
Ultra filtration	Optical rotatory dispersion and circulatory dichroism

Table 4.2: Considerations in the study of drug–protein binding

Equilibrium between bound and free drug must be maintained.
The method must be valid over a wide range of drug and protein concentrations.
Extraneous drug binding or drug adsorption onto the apparatus walls, membranes, or other components must be avoided or considered in the method.
Denaturation of the protein or contamination of the protein must be prevented.
The method must consider pH and ionic concentrations of the media and Donnan effects due to the protein.
The method should be capable of detecting both reversible and irreversible drug binding, including fast- and slow-phase associations and dissociations of drug and protein.
The method should not introduce interfering substances, such as organic solvents.
The results of the *in vitro* method should allow extrapolation to the *in vivo* situation.

Relationship of Plasma Drug–Protein Binding to Distribution and Elimination

In general, drugs that are highly bound to plasma protein have reduced overall drug clearance. For a drug that is metabolized mainly by the liver, binding to plasma proteins prevents the drug from entering the hepatocytes, resulting in reduced drug metabolism by the liver. In addition, molecularly bound drugs may not be available as substrates for liver enzymes, thereby further reducing the rate of metabolism.

Protein-bound drugs act as larger molecules that cannot diffuse easily through the capillary membranes in the glomeruli. The elimination half-lives of some drugs, such as the cephalosporins, which are excreted mainly by renal excretion, are generally increased when the percent of drug bound to plasma proteins increases. The effect of serum protein binding on the renal clearance and elimination half-life on several tetracycline analogs is shown in. For example, doxycycline, which is 93% bound to serum proteins, has an elimination half-life of 15.1 hours, whereas Oxytetracycline, which is 35.4% bound to serum proteins, has an elimination half-life of 9.2 hours. On the other hand, drug that is both extensively bound and actively secreted by the kidneys, such as penicillin, has a short elimination half-life, because active secretion takes preference in removing or stripping the drug from the proteins as the blood flows through the kidney.

Table 4.3: Influence of protein binding on the pharmacokinetics of primarily glomerular filtrated cephalosporins

	Protein Bond (%)	$t_{1/2}$ (hr)	Renal Clearance (mL/min/1.73m^2)
Ceftriaxone	96	8.0	10
Cefoperazone	90	1.8	19
Cefotetan	85	3.3	28
Ceforanide	81	3.0	44
Cefazolin	70	1.7	56
Moxalactam	52	2.3	64
Cefsulodin	26	1.5	90
Ceftazidime	22	1.9	85
Cephaloridine	21	1.5	125

Table 4.4: Comparison of serum protein binding of several tetracycline analogs with their half-life in serum renal clearance and urinary recovery after intravenous injection

Tetracycline Analogs	Tetracycline Analogs	Half-Life (hr)	Renal Clear-ance (mL/min)	Urinary Re-covery (%)
Oxytetracycline	35.4	9.2	98.6	70
Tetracycline	64.6	8.5	73.5	60
Demeclocycline	90.8	12.7	36.5	45
Doxycycline	93.0	15.1	16.0	45

Some cephalosporins are excreted by both renal and biliary secretion. The half-lives of drugs that are significantly excreted in the bile and do not correlate well with the extent of plasma protein binding.**Relationship between v_d and drug elimination half-life**Drug elimination is governed mainly by renal and other metabolic processes in the body. However, extensive drug distribution has the effect of diluting the drug in a large volume, making it harder for the kidney to filter the drug by glomerular filtration. Thus, the $t_{1/2}$ of the drug is prolonged if clearance (Cl) is constant and V_D is increased according to Equation 4.2. Cl is related to apparent volume of distribution, V_D, and the elimination constant k, as shown in Equation 4.1 (see also).

$$Cl = kV_D \qquad \text{... (4.1)}$$

$$t_{1/2} = 0.693 \; V_D/Cl \qquad \text{... (4.2)}$$

For a first-order process, Cl is the product of V_D and the elimination rate constant, k, according to Equation 4.1. The equation is derived for a given drug dose distributed in a single volume of body fluid without protein binding. The equation basically describes the empirical observation that a large clearance or large volume of distribution both leads to low plasma drug concentrations after a given dose. Mechanistically, a low plasma drug concentration may be due to (1) extensive distribution into tissues due to favorable lipophilicity, (2) extensive distribution into tissues due to protein binding in peripheral tissues, or (3) lack of drug plasma protein binding.

Two drug examples are selected to illustrate further the relationship between elimination half-life, clearance, and the volume of distribution. Although the kinetic relationship is straightforward, there is more than one way of explaining the observations.

Clinical examples

Drug with a large volume of distribution and a long elimination $t_{1/2}$
The macrolide antibiotic dirithromycin is extensively distributed in tissues, resulting in a large steady-state volume of distribution of about 800 L (range 504–1041 L). The elimination $t_{1/2}$ in humans is about 44

hours (range 16–65 hours). The drug has a relatively large total body clearance of 226–1040 mL/min (13.6–62.4 L/hr) and is given once daily. In this case, clearance is large due to a large V_D, whereas k is relatively small. In this case, Cl is large but the elimination half-life is longer because of the large V_D. Intuitively, the drug will take a long time to be removed when the drug is distributed extensively over a large volume; despite a relatively large clearance, $t_{1/2}$ accurately describes drug elimination alone.

Drug with a small volume of distribution and a long elimination $t_{1/2}$

Tenoxicam is a nonsteroidal anti-inflammatory drug that is about 99% bound in human plasma protein. The drug has low lipophilicity, is highly ionized (approximately 99%), and is distributed in blood. Because tenoxicam is very polar, the drug penetrates cell membranes slowly. The synovial fluid peak drug level is only one-third that of the plasma drug concentration and occurs 20 hours (range 10–34 hours) later than the peak plasma drug level. In addition, the drug is poorly distributed to body tissues and has an apparent volume of distribution, V_D, of 9.6 L (range 7.5–11.5 L). Tenoxicam has a low total plasma clearance of 0.106 L/hr (0.079 – 0.142 L/hr) and an elimination half-life of 67 hours (range 49–81 hours), undoubtedly related to the extensive drug binding to plasma proteins.

According to Equation 4.1, drug clearance from the body is small if V_D is small and k is not too large. This relationship is consistent with a small Cl and a small V_D observed for tenoxicam. However, predicts that a small V_D would result in a small elimination $t_{1/2}$. In this case, the actual elimination half-life is long (67 hours) because the plasma tenoxicam clearance is so small. The long elimination half-life of tenoxicam is better explained by restrictive drug clearance due to its binding to plasma protein, making it difficult for the drug to clear rapidly.

Clearance

Cl and V_D are regarded as independent model variables by some physiologic pharmacokineticists, based on Equation 4.2. Actually, Equation 4.1 and its equivalent, Equation 4.2, are rooted in classical pharmacokinetics. Initially, it may be difficult to understand why a drug such as dirithromycin, with a rapid clearance of 226–1040 mL/min, has a long half-life. In pharmacokinetics, the elimination constant $k = 0.0156$ hr^{-1} implies that 1/64 (i.e., 0.0156 hr^{-1} = 1/64) of the drug is cleared per hour (a low efficiency elimination factor). From the elimination rate constant k, one can estimate that it takes 44 hours ($t_{1/2}$ = 44 hours) to eliminate half the drug in the body, regardless of V_D. While $t_{1/2}$ is dependent on clearance and V_D, clearance is clearly affected by the volume of distribution and by many variables of the drug in the biological system. In patients with ascites, clearance is increased but with no increase in half-life, reflecting the increase in volume of distribution in ascitic patients.

Elimination of protein-bound drug: restrictive versus nonrestrictive elimination

When a drug is tightly bound to a protein, only the unbound drug is assumed to be metabolized; drugs belonging to this category are described as restrictively eliminated. On the other hand, some drugs may be eliminated even when they are protein bound; drugs in this category are described as nonrestrictively eliminated. When some drugs with different fractions of plasma protein binding are examined, the expected reduction in clearance is sometimes absent or very minor because some drugs are nonrestrictively cleared. The effect of protein binding on the kinetics of drug clearance in an organ system is discussed in detail in.

In practice, the molecular effect of protein binding on elimination is not always predictable. Drugs with restrictive elimination are recognized by very small plasma clearances and extensive plasma protein binding. The hepatic extraction ratios (ERs) for drugs that are restrictively eliminated are generally small, because of strong protein binding. Their hepatic extraction ratios are generally smaller than their unbound fractions in plasma (i.e. ER < f_u). For example, phenylbutazone and the oxicams, including piroxicam, isoxicam, and tenoxicam, all have hepatic extraction ratios smaller than their unbound fraction in plasma. The hepatic elimination for these drugs is therefore restrictive. A series of nonsteroid anti-inflammatory drugs (NSAIDs) were reported by the same authors to be nonrestrictive with the following characteristics: (1) drug elimination is exclusively hepatic, (2) bioavailability of the drug from an oral dosage form is complete, and (3) these drugs do not undergo extensive reversible biotransformation or enterohepatic circulation.

Propranolol is a drug that has low bioavailability with a hepatic extraction ratio, ER, of 0.7–0.9. Propranolol is 89% bound, i.e. 11% free (or $f_u = 0.11$) so that the ER > f_u. Thus, propranolol is considered to be nonrestrictively eliminated. The bioavailability of propranolol is very low because of the large first-pass effect, and its elimination half-life is relatively short. In contrast, diazepam is 98% bound ($f_u < 0.02$). Diazepam has a small ER of 0.1, because of extensive drug protein binding. Therefore, diazepam is considered restrictively eliminated. Diazepam has a long elimination half-life of 37 hours.

Determinants of Protein Binding

Drug–protein binding is influenced by a number of important factors, including the following:

1. The drug
    ❖ Physicochemical properties of the drug.
    ❖ Total concentration of the drug in the body.
2. The protein
    ❖ Quantity of protein available for drug–protein binding.
    ❖ Quality or physicochemical nature of the protein synthesized.
3. The affinity between drug and protein
    ❖ Includes the magnitude of the association constant.
4. Drug interactions
    ❖ Competition for the drug by other substances at a protein-binding site
    ❖ Alteration of the protein by a substance that modifies the affinity of the drug for the protein; for example, aspirin acetylates lysine residues of albumin

5. The pathophysiologic condition of the patient

   ❖ For example, drug–protein binding may be reduced in uremic patients and in patients with hepatic disease

Plasma drug concentrations are generally reported as the total drug concentration in the plasma, including both protein-bound drug and unbound (free) drug concentrations. Most literature values for the therapeutic effective drug concentrations refer to the total plasma or serum drug concentration. For therapeutic drug monitoring, the total plasma drug concentrations are generally used in the development of the appropriate drug dosage regimen for the patient. In the past, measurement of free drug concentration was not routinely performed in the laboratory. More recently, free drug concentrations may be measured quickly using ultra filtration. Because of the high plasma protein binding of phenytoin and the narrow therapeutic index of the drug, more hospital laboratories are measuring both free and total phenytoin plasma levels.

Kinetics of Protein Binding

If P represents proteins and D the drug, then applying law of mass action to reversible protein-drug binding, we can write:

$$P + D \underset{K_d}{\overset{K_a}{\rightleftharpoons}} PD \qquad \text{... (4.3)}$$

At equilibrium,

$$K_a = \frac{[PD]}{[P][D]} \qquad \text{... (4.4)}$$

$$[PD] = K_a [P][D] \qquad (4.5)$$

Where,

[P] = concentration of free protein

[D] = concentration of free drug

[PD] = concentration of protein-drug complex

K_a = association rat constant

K_d = dissociation rate constant

$K_a > K_d$ indicates forward reaction i.e. protein-drug binding is favored. If P_T is the total concentration of protein present, bound and unbound, then:

$$P_T = [PD] + [P] \qquad ... (4.6)$$

If r is the number of moles of drug bound to total moles of protein then,

$$r = \frac{[PD]}{[P_r]} = \frac{[PD]}{[PD]+[P]} \qquad ... (4.7)$$

Substituting the value of [PD] from equation in equation we get:

$$r = \frac{K_a[P][D]}{K_a[P][D]+[P]} = \frac{K_a[D]}{K_a[D]+1} \qquad ... (4.8)$$

Equation holds when there is only one binding site on the protein and the protein-drug complex is a 1:1 complex. If more than one or N number of binding sites are available per mole of the protein them:

$$r = \frac{NK_a[D]}{K_a[D]+1} \qquad ... (4.9)$$

The value of association constant, K_a and the number of binding sites N can be obtained by plotting equation in three different ways as shown below.

1. **Direct Plot** is made by plotting r versus [D] as shown in Fig 4.2.
2. **Scatchard plot** is made by transforming equation 4.9 into a linear form. Thus,

$$r = \frac{r}{[D]} \qquad ... (4.10)$$

$$r + r\,K_a[D] = N\,K_a[D] \qquad ... (4.11)$$

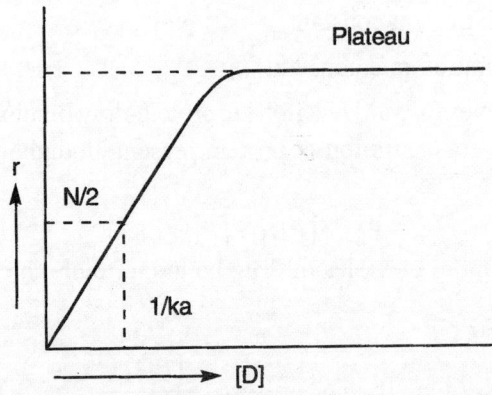

Fig. 4.2: Direct plot of r versus [D]. Note that when all the binding sites are occupied by the drug, the protein is saturated and plateau is reached. At the plateau, $r = N$. When $r = N/2$, $[D] = 1/ka$

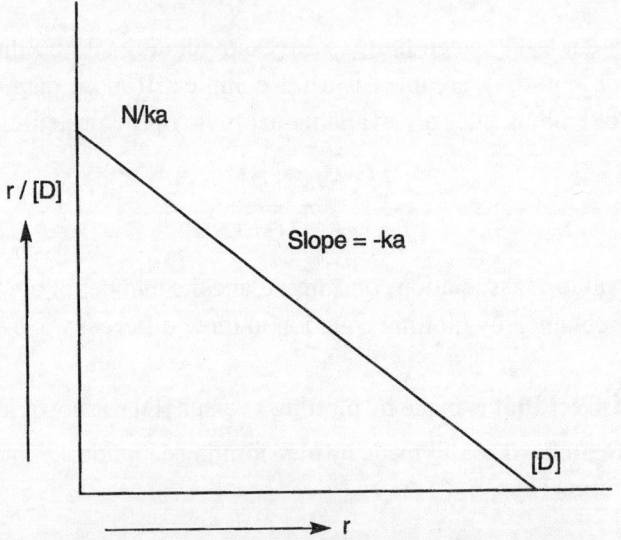

Fig. 4.3: Scatchard plot for protein - drug binding

$$r = N K_a [D] - r K_a [D] \qquad \qquad ... (4.12)$$

Therefore, $\dfrac{r}{[D]} = N K_a - r K_a$ ... (4.13)

A plot of $r/[D]$ versus r yields a straight line (Fig. 4.13) slope of the line $= -K_a$, y-intercept $= NK_a$ and x-intercept $= N$.

3. **Double Reciprocal Plot (Line weaver-Burk Plot):** The reciprocal of equation yields.

$$\frac{1}{r} = \frac{1}{NK_a[D]} + \frac{1}{N} \qquad ... (4.14)$$

A plot of $1/r$ versus $1/[D]$ yields a straight line with slope $1/NK_a$ and y-intercept $1/N$ (Fig. 4.4).

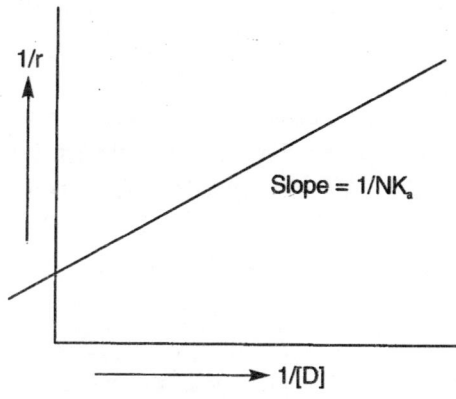

Fig. 4.4: Double Reciprocal Plot for Protein-Drug Binding

Significance of Protein/Tissue Binding of Drugs

Most drugs bind reversibly to plasma proteins to some extent. When the clinical significance of the fraction of drug bound is considered, it is important to know whether the study was performed using pharmacologic or therapeutic plasma drug concentrations. As mentioned previously, the fraction of drug bound can change with plasma drug concentration and dose of drug administered. In addition, the patient's plasma protein concentration should be considered. If a patient has a low plasma protein concentration, then, for any given dose of drug, the concentration of free (unbound) bioactive drug may be higher than anticipated. The plasma protein concentration is controlled by a number of variables, including (1) protein synthesis, (2) protein catabolism, (3) distribution of albumin between intravascular and extravascular space, and (4) excessive elimination of plasma protein, particularly albumin. A number of diseases, age, trauma, and related circumstances affect the plasma protein concentration (Tables).

For example, liver disease results in a decrease in plasma albumin concentration due to decreased protein synthesis. In nephrotic syndrome, an accumulation of waste metabolites, such as urea and uric acid, as well as an accumulation of drug metabolites, may alter protein binding of drugs. Severe burns may cause an increased distribution of albumin into the extracellular fluid, resulting in a smaller plasma albumin concentration. In certain genetic diseases, the quality of the protein that is synthesized in the plasma may be altered due to a change in the amino acid sequence. Both chronic liver disease and renal disease, such as uremia, may cause an alteration in the quality of plasma protein synthesized. An alteration in the protein quality may be demonstrated by an alteration in the association constant or affinity of the drug for the protein.

When a highly protein-bound drug is displaced from binding by a second drug or agent, a sharp increase in the free drug concentration in the plasma may occur, leading to toxicity. For example, an increase in free warfarin level was responsible for an increase in bleeding when warfarin was co-administered with phenylbutazone, which competes for the same protein-binding site. Recently, studies and reviews have shown that the clinical significance of warfarin protein binding and its impact on bleeding are less prominent, adding other factors and explanations.

Albumin has two known binding sites that share the binding of many drugs. Binding site I is shared by phenylbutazone, sulfonamides, phenytoin, and valproic acid. Binding site II is shared by the semi synthetic penicillins, probenecid, medium-chain fatty acids, and the benzo-diazepines. Some drugs bind to both sites. Displacement occurs when a second drug is taken that competes for the same binding site in the protein as the initial drug.

Although it is generally assumed that binding sites are preformed, there is some evidence pointing to the allosteric nature of protein binding. This means that the binding of a drug modifies the conformation of protein in such a way that the drug binding influences the nature of binding of further molecules of the drug. The binding of oxygen to hemoglobin is a well studied biochemical example in which the initial binding of other oxygen to the iron in the heme portion influences the binding of other oxygen molecules.

Absorption

The absorption equilibrium is attained by transfer of free drug from the site of administration into the systemic circulation and when the concentration in these two compartments becomes equal. Following equilibrium, the process may stop. However, binding of the absorbed drug to plasma proteins decreases free drug concentration and disturbs such equilibrium. Thus, sink conditions and the concentration gradient are reestablished which now act as the driving force for further absorption. This is particularly useful in cases of ionized drugs which are transported with difficulty.

Systemic Solubility of Drugs

Water insoluble drugs, neutral endogenous macromolecules such as heparin and several steroids and oil soluble vitamins are circulated and distributed to tissues by binding especially to lipoproteins which act as a vehicle for such hydrophobic compounds.

Distribution

Plasma protein binding restricts the entry of drugs that have specific affinity for certain tissues. This prevents accumulation of a large fraction of drug in such tissues and thus, subsequent toxic reactions. Plasma protein-drug binding thus favors uniform distribution of drugs throughout the body by its buffer function (maintains equilibrium between the free and the bound drug). A protein bound drug in particular does not cross the BBB, the placental barrier and the glomerulus.

Tissue Binding, Apparent Volume of Distribution and Drug Storage

A drug that is extensively bound to blood components remains confined to blood. Such a drug has a small volume of distribution. A drug that shows extravascular tissue binding has a large volume of distribution. A tissue or blood component that has great affinity for a particular drug acts as a depot or storage site for that drug; for example, RBC is a storage site for the lipophilic compound tetrahydrocannabinol.

The relationship between tissue-drug binding and apparent volume of distribution can be established as follows:

$$V_d = \frac{\text{Amount of drug in the boxy}}{\text{Plasma drug concentration}} = \frac{X}{C} \qquad \text{... (4.15)}$$

or, the amount of drug in the body,

$$X = V_d C \qquad \text{... (4.16)}$$

Similarly, we can write,

Amount of drug in plasma $= V_p C$ ... (4.17)

and,

Amount of drug in extravascular tissues $= V_t C$ ... (4.18)

The total amount of drug in the body is the sum of amount of drug in plasma and the amount of drug in extravascular tissues. Thus,

$$V_d C = V_p C + V_t C_t \qquad \text{... (4.19)}$$

Where,

V_d = apparent volume of distribution of drug

V_p = volume of plasma

V_t = volume of extravascular tissues

C_t = tissue drug concentration

Dividing equation with C we get:

$$V_d = V_p + V_t C_t / C \qquad \qquad ...(4.20)$$

The fraction of drug unbound (f_u) in plasma is given as:

f_u = Concentration of Unbound Drug in Plasma = C_u ... (4.21)

Total Plasma Drug Concentration $\qquad\qquad$ C

Similarly, fraction of drug unbound to tissues is:

$$f_{ut} = C_{ut} / C_t \qquad\qquad ...(4.22)$$

Assuming that at distribution equilibrium, the unbound or free drug concentration in plasma equals that in extravascular tissues i.e. $C_u = C_{ut}$, equations can be combined to give:

$$\frac{C_t}{C} = \frac{f_u}{f_{ut}} \qquad\qquad ...(4.23)$$

Substitution of equation yields:

$$V_d = V_p + \frac{V_t \cdot f_u}{f_{ut}} \qquad\qquad ...(4.24)$$

From equation it is clear that greater the unbound or free concentration of drug in plasma, larger its V_d.

Elimination

Only the unbound or free drug is capable of being eliminated. This is because the drug-protein complex cannot penetrate into the metabolizing organ (liver). The large molecular size of the complex also prevents it from getting filtered through the glomerulus. Thus, drugs which are more than 95% bound are eliminated slowly i.e. they have long elimination half-lives; for example, tetracycline, which is only 65% bound, has an elimination half-life of 8.5 hours in comparison to 15.1 hours of doxyeycline which is 93% bound to plasma proteins. However, penicillins have short elimination half-lives despite being extensively bound to plasma proteins. This is because rapid equilibration occurs between the free and the bound drug and the free drug is equally rapidly excreted by active secretion in renal tubules.

Displacement Interactions and Toxicity

As stated earlier, displacement interactions are significant in case of drugs which are more than 95% bound. This is explained from the example given in Table 4.3. A displacement of just 1% of a 99% bound drug results in doubling of the free drug concentration i.e. a 100% rise. For a drug that is bound to a lesser extent e.g. 90%, displacement of 1% results in only a 10% rise in free drug concentration which may be insignificant clinically.

Table 4.5: Influence of percent binding and displacement on change in free concentration of drugs

	Drug A	Drug B
% drug before displacement		
bound	99	90
Free	1	10
% drug after displacement		
bound	98	89
Free	2	11
% increase in free drug concentration	100	10

Kernicterus in infants is an example of a disorder caused by displacement of bilirubin from albumin binding sites by the NSAIDs. Another example discussed earlier was that of interaction between warfarin and phenylbutazone. Yet another example of displacement is that of digoxin with quinidine. Yet another example of displacement is that of digoxin bution (i.e. shows extensive extravascular tissue binding). Since displacement interactions may precipitate toxicity of displaced drug, a reduction in its dose may be called for. This may become necessary for a drug having a small V_d such as warfarin since displacement can result in a large increase in free drug concentration in plasma. With a drug of large V_d such as digoxin, even a substantial increase in the degree of displacement of drug in plasma may not effect a large increase in free drug concentration and dose adjustment may not be required. This is for two reasons-one, only a small fraction of such a drug is present in plasma whereas most of it is localized in extravascular tissues, and secondly, following displacement, the free drug, because of its large V_d, redistributes in a large pool of extravascular tissues. The extent to which the free plasma drug concentration of drugs with different V_d values will change when displaced, can be computed from Equation.

Diagnosis

The chlorine atom of chloroquine when replaced with radiolabeled I-131 can be used to visualize melanomas of the eye since chloroquine has a tendency to interact with the melanin of eyes. The thyroid gland has great affinity for iodine containing compounds; hence any disorder of the same can be detected by tagging such a compound with a radioisotope of iodine.

Therapy and drug targeting

The binding of drugs to lipoproteins can be used for site-specific delivery of hydrophilic moieties. This is particularly useful in cancer therapies since certain tumor cells have greater affinity for LDL than normal tissues. Thus, binding of a suitable antineoplastic to it can be used as a therapeutic tool. HDL is similarly transported more to adrenal and testes. An example of site-specific drug delivery in cancer treatment is that of estramustine. Estradiol binds selectively and strongly to prostrate and thus prostate cancer can be treated by attaching nitrogen mustard to estradiol for targeting of prostate glands. Drug targeting prevents normal cells from getting destroyed.

Clinical examples

Protein concentration may change during some acute disease states. For example, plasma á$_1$-acid glycoprotein (AAG) levels in patients may increase due to the host's acute-phase response to infection, trauma, inflammatory processes, and some malignant diseases. The acute-phase response is a change in various plasma proteins that is observed within hours or days following the onset of infection or injury. The acute-phase changes may be also indicative of chronic disease.

AAG binds to many basic drugs, and a change in AAG protein concentration can contribute to more fluctuation in free drug concentrations among patients during various stages of infection or disease. Amprenavir (Agenerase), a protease inhibitor of human immunodeficiency virus type 1 (HIV-1), is highly bound to human plasma proteins, mostly to AAG (approximately 90%). AAG levels are known to vary with infection, including HIV disease. Sadler et al (2001) showed a significant inverse linear relationship between AAG levels and amprenavir clearance as estimated by CL/F. Unbound, or free, amprenavir concentrations were not affected by AAG concentrations even though the apparent total drug clearance was increased. The intrinsic clearance of the drug was not changed. The authors cautioned that incorrect conclusions could be drawn about the pharmacokinetics of highly protein-bound drugs if AAG concentration is not included in the analysis.

In addition, race, age, and weight were also found to affect AAG levels. African-American subjects had significantly lower AAG concentrations than Caucasian subjects. AAG in African-Americans was 77.2 ± 13.8 mg/dL versus 90 ± 20.2 mg/dL in Caucasians, $p < 0.0001$). Pharmacokinetic analysis showed that AAG correlated significantly with age and race and was a significant predictor of amprenavir CL/F.

Interestingly, in spite of a statistically significant difference in total plasma amprenavir level, a dose adjustment for racial differences was not indicated, because the investigators found the unbound amprenavir concentrations to be similar.

Protein binding can lead to nonlinear or dose-dependent kinetics. It was interesting to note that amprenavir CL/F was dose dependent in the analysis without AAG data, but that no dose dependence was observed when AAG concentration was considered in the analysis. The higher doses of amprenavir, which produce the greatest antiviral activity, resulted in the largest decrease in AAG concentration, which led to the greatest changes in total drug concentration.

In evaluating change in protein binding and its impact on free plasma drug, it is important to realize that protein changes or displacement often result in changes in free plasma drug concentration. Nonetheless, the free drug is not necessarily increasingly eliminated unless the change in free drug concentration facilitates metabolism, accompanied by a change in Cl_{int} (Cl_{int} measures the inherent capacity to metabolize the drug). For some drugs, the change in protein binding may be sufficiently compensated by a redistribution of the drug from one tissue to another within the body. In contrast, a change in drug protein binding accompanied by metabolism (Cl_{int}) will invariably result in an increased amount of drug needed to maintain a steady-state level because the total drug concentration is continuously being eliminated. The maintenance of an adequate therapeutic free drug level through re-equilibration is difficult in such a case.

Table 4.6: Factors that decrease plasma protein concentration

Mechanism	Disease State
Decreased protein synthesis	Liver disease
Increased protein catabolism	Trauma, surgery
Distribution of albumin into extra vascular space	Burns
Excessive elimination of protein	Renal disease

Table 4.7: Physiologic and pathologic conditions altering protein concentrations in plasma

	Albumin	α_1-Glycoprotein	Lipoprotein
Decreasing	Age (geriatric, neonate)	Fetal concentrations	Hyperthyroidism
	Bacterial Pneumonia	Nephrotic syndrome	Injury
	Bums	Oral contraceptives	Liver disease?
	Cirrhosis of liver		Trauma
	Cystic fibrosis		
	GI disease		
	Histoplasmosis		
	Leprosy		
	Liver abscess		
	Malignant neoplasms		
	Malnutrition (severe)		
	Multiple myeloma		
	Nephrotic syndrome		
	Pancreatitis (acute)		
	Pregnancy		
	Renal failure		
	Surgery		
	Trauma		
Increasing	Benign tumor	Age (geriatric)	Diabetes
	Exercise	Celiac disease	Hypothyroidism
	Hypothyroidism	Crohn's disease	Liver disease?
	Neurological disease?	Injury	Nephrotic syndrome
	Neurosis	Myocardial infarction	
	Paranoia	Renal failure	

Table 4.8: Protein binding in normal renal function, end-stage renal disease, during hemodialysis, and in nephrotic syndrome

	Norm (% Bound)	ESRD (% Bound)	HD (% Bound)	NS (% Bound)
Azlocillin	28	25		
Bilirubin		Decreased		
Captopril	24	18		
Cefazolin	84	73	22	
Cefoxitin	73	20		
Chloramphenicol	53	45	30	
Chlorpromazine	98	98		
Clofibrate	96			89
Clonidine	30	30		
Congo red		Decreased		
Dapsone		Normal		
Desipramine	80	Normal		
N-Desmethyldazepam	98	94		
Desmethyldiazepam	89	88		
Diazepam	99	94		
Diazoxide (30µg/mL)	92	86	83	
(300µg/mL)	77	72		
Dicloxacillin	96	91		
Diflunisal	88	56		39
Digitoxin	97	96	90	96
Digoxin	25		22	
Doxycycline	88	71		
Erythromycin	75	77		
Etomidate	75	57		
Fluorescein	86	Decreased		
Furosemid	96	94		93
Indomethacin		Normal		
Maprotiline	90	Normal		
β-Methyldigoxin	30		19	
Methylorange		Decreased		
Methyl red		Decreased		
Morphine	35	31		
Nafcillin	88	81		
Naproxen	75	21		
Oxazepam	95	88		

	Norm (% Bound)	ESRD (% Bound)	HD (% Bound)	NS (% Bound)
Papaverine	97	94		
Penicillin G	72	36		
Pentobarbital	66	59		
Phenobarbital	55	Decreased		
Phenol red		Decreased		
Phenylbutazone	97	88		
Phenytoin	90	80	93	81
Pindolol	41	Normal		
Prazosin	95	92		
Prednisolone (50 mg)	74		65	64
(15 mg)	87	88		85
D-Propoxyphene	76	80		
Propranolol	88	89	90	
Quinidine	88	86	88	
Salicylate	94	85		
Sulfadiazine		Decreased		
Sulfamethoxazole	74	50		

Binding Sites

(1) Binding of drugs to blood components

(a) **Plasma protein-drug binding:** Following entry of a drug into the systemic circulation, the first things with which it can interact are blood components like plasma proteins, Blood cells and hemoglobin. The main interaction of drug in the blood compartment is with the plasma proteins which are present in abundant amounts and in large variety. The binding of drugs to plasma Proteins is reversible. The extent or order of binding of drugs to various plasma proteins is:

albumin > α1-acid glycoprotein > lipoproteins > globulins.

(b) **Binding of drugs to human serum albumin:** The human serum albumin (HAS), having a molecular weight of 65,000, is the most abundant plasma protein (59%) of total plasma

Table 4.9: Blood proteins to which drugs bind

Protein	Molecular Weight	Concentration (g%)	Drugs that bind
Human Serum Albumin	65,000	3.5-5.0	large verity of all types of drugs
α_1-Acid Glycoprotein	44,000	0.04-0.1	basic drugs such as imipramine, lidocaine, quinidine, etc.
Lipoproteins	200,000 to 3,400,000	variable	basic, lipophilic drugs like chlorpromazine
α_1- Globulin	59,000	0.003-0.007	steroids like corticosterone, and thyroxine and cyanocobalamin
α_1- Globulin	1,34,000	0.015-015-0.06	vitamins A, D, E and K and cupric ions
Hemoglobin	64,500	11-16	phenytoin, pentobarbital, and phenothiazines

and 3.5 To 5.0 g%) with a large drug binding capacity. The therapeutic doses of most drugs are relatively much smaller and their plasma concentrations do not normally reach equimolar concentration with GSA. The HAS can Bind several compounds having varied structures. Both endogenous com-Pounds such as fatty acids, bilirubin and tryptophan as well as drugs bind to GSA. A large variety of drugs ranging from weak acids, neutral compounds to weak

bases bind to HSA. Four different sites on GSA have been identified for drug-binding. They are:

Site I: Also called as warfarin and azapropazone binding site, it Represents the region to which large number of drugs are bound, e.g. Several NSAIDs (phenylbutazone, naproxen, indomethacin), sulfonamides (sulfadimethoxine, sulfamethizole), phenytoin, sodium valproate and bilirubin.

Site II: It is also called as the diazepam binding site. Drugs which bind to this region include benzodiazepines, medium chain fatty acids, ibuprofen, ketoprofen, tryptophan, cloxacillin, probenicid, etc.

Site I and **site II** are responsible for the binding of most drugs.

Site III: is also called as digitoxin binding site.

Site IV: is also called as tamoxifen binding site.

Very few drugs bind to **sites III** and **IV**.

A drug can bind to more than one site in which case the main binding site is called as the primary site and the other as the secondary site; for Example, site I is the primary site for dicoumarol and site II the secondary site. Groups of drugs that bind to the same site, compete with each other for binding, but drugs that bind to one site do not competitively inhibit Binding of drugs to other sites, However, they may either promote or retard binding of a drug to another site by energetic coupling mechanisms.

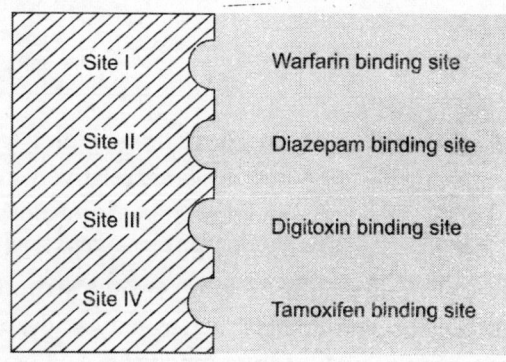

Fig. 4.5: Four major drug binding sites on human serum albumin

(c) Binding of drugs to - acid glycoprotein

Also called as the orosomucoid, it has a molecular weight of 44,000 and a plasma concentration range of 0.04 to 0.1g%. It binds to a number of basic drugs like imipramine, amitriptyline, nortriptyline, lidocaine propranolol, quinidine and disopyramide.

(d) Binding of drugs to lipoproteins

Binding of drugs to HAS and AAG involve hydrophobic bonds. Since only lipophilic drugs can undergo hydrophobic bonding, lipoproteins can also bind to such drugs because of their high lipid content. However, the Plasma concentration of lipoproteins is much less in comparison to HAS And AAG.

A drug that binds to lipoproteins does so by dissolving in the lipid core of the protein and thus its capacity to bind depends upon its lipid content. The molecular weights of lipoproteins vary from 2 lakhs to 34 lakhs depending on their chemical composition. They are classified on the basis of their density. The 4 classes of lipoproteins are:

1. Chylomicrons
2. Very low density lipoproteins (VLDL)
3. Low density lipoproteins (LDL) (Predominant in humans)
4. High density lipoproteins (HDL)

The lipid core of these macromolecules consists of triglycerides and cholesteryl esters and the outside is made of apoproteins (free cholesterol and proteins). Predictably, VLDL is rich in triglycerides and HDL is rich in apoproteins.

The binding of drugs to lipoproteins is noncompetitive. A number of acidic (diclofenac), neutral (cyclosporin A) and basic drugs (chlorpromazine) bind to lipoproteins. Basic, lipophilic drugs have relatively more affinity lipoprotein binding becomes significant in cases of drugs that predominantly bind to them, and secondly, when levels of HAS and AAG in plasma are decreased.

(e) Binding of drugs to globulins

Several plasma globulins have been identified and are labeled as $\alpha 1^-$, α_2^-, β_1^-, $\beta 2^-$ and γ-globulins.

1. **α_1- globulin:** Also called as transcortin or CBG (corticosteroid binding globulin), it binds a number of steroidal drugs such as cortisone and prednisone. It also binds to thyroxine and cyanocobalamin.

2. **α_1- globulin:** also called as ceruloplasmin, it binds vitamins A, D, E and K and cupric ions.

3. **β_1- globulin:** also called as transferrin, it binds to ferrous ions.

4. **β_1- globulin:** binds to carotinoids.

5. **γ-globulin:** binds specifically to antigens.

(f) Binding of drugs to blood cells

More than 40% of the blood comprises of blood cells of which the major cell component is the RBC. The RBCs constitute 95% of the total blood cells. Thus, significant RBC drug binding is possible. The red cell is 500 times in diameter as the major plasma protein binding component, Albumin. The RBC comprises of 3 components each of which can bind to drugs:

1. **Hemoglobin:** It has a molecular weight of 64,500 (almost equal to that of HSA) but is 7 to 8 times the concentration of albumin in blood. Drugs like phenytoin, pentobarbital and phenothiazines bind to hemoglobin.

2. **Carbonic anhydrase:** Drugs known to bind to it are acetzolamide and chlorthalidone (i.e. carbonic anhydrase inhibitors).

3. **Cell membranes:** Imipramine and chlorpromazine are reported to bind with the RBC membrane.

It has been shown that the rate and extent of entry into RBC is more for lipophilic drugs, e.g. phenytoin. Hydrophilic drugs like ampicillin do not enter RBC.

2. Tissue binding of drugs (tissue localization of drugs)

The body tissues, apart from HAS, comprise 40% of the body weight which is 100 times that of HAS. Hence, tissue-drug binding is much more significant that thought to be.

A drug can bind to one or more of the several tissue components. Tissue-drug binding is important is distribution from two viewpoints: Firstly, it increases the apparent volume of distribution of drugs in contrast to plasma protein binding which decreases it; this is because the parameter is related to the ratio of amount of drug in the body to the plasma concentration of free drug and the latter is decreased under conditions of extensive tissue binding of drugs, and secondly, tissue-drug binding results in localization of a drug at a specific site in the body (with a Subsequent increase in biological half-life). This is more so because a Number of drugs bind irreversibly with the tissues (contrast to plasma Protein-drug binding); for example, oxidation products of paracetamol, Phenacetin, chloroform, carbon tetrachloride and bromobenzene bind co-valently to hepatic tissues.

Factors influencing localization of drugs in tissues include lipophilicity and structural features of the drug, perfusion rate, P^H differences, etc. Extensive tissue-drug binding suggests that a tissue can act as the storage site for drugs. Drugs that bind to both tissue and plasma components result in competition between drug binding sites.

For majority of drugs that bind to extravascular tissues, the order of binding is: liver > kidney > lung > muscle. Several examples of extravascular tissue-drug binding are:

1. **Liver:** As stated earlier, epoxides of a number of halogenated hydrocarbons and paracetamol bind irreversibly to liver tissues resulting in Hepatotoxicity.

2. **Lungs:** Basic drugs like imipramine, chlorpromazine and anti-histamines accumulate in lungs.

3. **Kidneys:** Metallothionin, a protein present in kidneys, binds to heavy metals such as lead, mercury, and cadmium and results in their renal accumulation and toxicity.

4. **Skin:** Chloroquine and phenothiazines accumulate in skin by interacting with melanin.

5. **Eyes:** The retinal pigments of the eye also contain melanin. binding of chloroquine and phenothiazines to it is responsible for retinopathy.

6. **Hairs:** Arsenicals, chloroquine and phenothiazines are reported to deposit in hair shafts

7. **Bones:** Tetracycline is a well known example of a drug that binds to bones, and teeth. Administration of this antibiotic to infants or children during odontogeneses results in permanent brown-yellow discoloration of teeth. Lead is known to replace calcium from bones and cause their brittleness.

8. **Fats:** Lipophilic drugs such as thiopental and the pesticide DDT accumulate in adipose tissues by partitioning into it. However, high o/w partition coefficient is not the only criteria for adipose distribution of drugs since several highly lipophilic (more than thiopental) basic drugs like imipramine and chlorpromazine are not localized in fats. The poor perfusion of adipose could be the reason for such an ambiguity. Reports have stated that adipose localization of drugs is a result of binding competition between adipose and non-adipose tissues (lean tissues like muscles, skin and viscera) and not partitioning.

9. **Nucleic Acids:** Molecular components of cells such as DNA interact strongly with drugs like chloroquine and quinacrine resulting in distortion of its double helical structure.

Factors Affecting Protein-Drug Binding

Factors affecting protein-drug binding can be broadly category as:

1. Factors relating to the drug
   a. Physicochemical characteristics of the drug
   b. Concentration of drug in the body
   c. Affinity of a drug for a particular binding component

2. Factors relating to the protein and other binding components
   a. Physicochemical characteristics of the protein or binding agent
   b. Concentration of protein or binding component
   c. Number of binding sites on the binding agent
3. Drug interactions
   a. Competition between drugs for the binding site (displacement interactions)
   b. Competition between drugs and normal, body constituents
   c. Allosteric changes in protein molecule
4. Patient related factors
   a. Age
   b. Intersubject variations
   c. Disease states

1. Factors relating to the drug

(a) **Physicochemical characteristics of the drug:** As mentioned earlier, protein binding is directly related to the lipophilicity of drug. An increase in lipophilicity increases the extent of binding; for example, the slow absorption of cloxacillin in comparison to ampicillin after i.m. injection is attributed to its higher lipophilicity and larger (95%) Binding to proteins while the latter is les lipophilic and just 20% bound to proteins. Highly lipophilic drugs such as thiopental tend to localize in adipose tissues. Anionic or acidic drugs such as penicillins and sulfonamides bind more to HAS whereas cationic or basic drugs such as imipramine and alprenolol bind to AAG. Neutral, unionized drugs bind more to lipoproteins.

(b) **Concentration of drug in the body:** The extent of protein-drug binding can change with both changes in drug as well as protein concentration. The concentration of drugs that bind to HAS does not have much of an influence as the therapeutic concentration of any drug is insufficient to saturate it. However, therapeutic concentration of lidocaine can saturate AAG which it binds as the concentration of AAG is much less in comparison to that of GSA in Blood.

(c) **Drug-protein/tissue affinity:** Lidocaine has greater affinity for AAG than for HAS. Digoxin has more affinity for proteins of cardiac muscles than those of skeletal muscles or plasma. Iophenoxic acid, a radio opaque medium, has so great an affinity for plasma proteins that it has a half-life of $2\ ^{1/2}$ years.

2. **Protein/tissue related factors**

(a) **Physicochemical properties of protein/Binding component:** Lipoproteins and adipose tissue tend to bind lipophilic drugs by dissolving them in their lipid core. The physiologic pH determines the presence of active anionic and cationic groups on the albumin molecules to bind a variety of drugs.

(b) **Concentration of protein/Binding component:** Among the plasma proteins, binding predominantly occurs with albumin as it is present in a higher concentration in comparison to other plasma proteins. The amount of several proteins and tissue components available for binding, changes during disease states. This effect will be discussed in the subsequent sections.

(c) **Number of Binding Sites on the Protein:** Albumin has a large number of binding sites as compared to other proteins and is a high capacity binding component. Several drugs are capable of binding at more than one site on albumin, e.g. fluocloxacillin, flurbiprofen, ketoprofen, tamoxifen and dicoumarol bind to both primary and secondary sites on albumin. Indomethacin is known to bind to 3 different sites. AAG is a protein with limited binding capacity because of its low concentration and low molecular size. Though pure AAG has only one binding site for lidocaine, in presence of HAS, two binding sites have been reported which was suggested to be due to direct interaction between HAS and AAG.

3. Drug interactions

(a) **Competition between drugs for the binding sites (displacement interactions):** When two or more drugs can bind to the same site, competition between them for interaction with the binding site results. If one of the drugs (drug A) is bound to such a site, then administration of another drug (drug B) having affinity for the same site results in displacement of drug A from its binding site. Such a drug-drug interaction for the common binding site is called as displacement interaction. The drug A here is called as the **displaced drug** and drug B as the **displacer**. Warfarin and phenylbutazone have same degree of affinity for HSA. Administration of phenylbutazone to a patient on warfarin therapy results in displacement of latter from its binding site. The free warfarin may cause adverse hemorrhagic reactions which may be lethal. Phenylbutazone is also known to displace sulfonamides from their HAS binding sites. Displacement interactions can result in unexpected rise in free concentration of the displaced drug which may enhance clinical response or toxicity even a drug metabolite can affect displacement interaction.

Clinically significant interactions will result when:

1. The displaced drug (e.g. warfarin) —
   a. is more than 95% bound
   b. has a small volume of distribution (less than 0.15 L/Kg
   c. shows a rapid onset of therapeutic or adverse effects
   d. has a narrow therapeutic index
2. The displacer drug (e.g. phenylbutazone)
   a. has a high degree of affinity as the drug to be displaced

b. competes for the same binding sites.

c. the drug/protein concentration ratio is high (above 0.10) and

d. shows a rapid and large increase in plasma drug concentration.

It will be worthwhile to mention here that, both the concentration of the displacer drug and its affinity for the binding site with respect to that of the drug to be displaced, will determine the extent to which displacement will occur.

For a drug that is 95% bound a displacement of just 5% of the bound drug results in a 100% rise in free drug concentration. If the displaced drug has a small volume of distribution, it remains confined to the blood compartment and shows serious toxic responses. On the contrary, if such a drug has a large V_d, redistributes into a large volume of body fluids and clinical effects may be negligible or insignificant. The increase in free drug concentration following displacement also makes it more available for elimination by the liver and the kidneys. If the drug is easily metabolizable or excretable, its displacement results in significant reduction in elimination half-life.

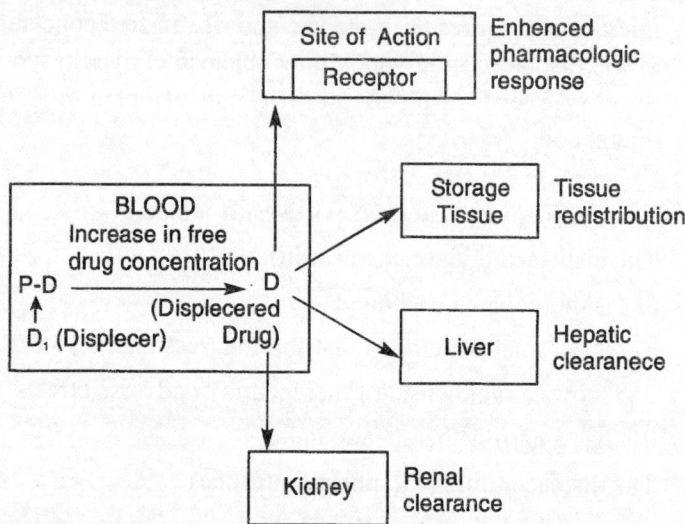

Fig. 4.6: Fate of a drug after displacement interaction

Displacement also becomes insignificant with the use of more selective, potent, low dose drugs.

(b) **Competition between drugs and normal body constituents:** Among the various normal, body constituents, the free fatty acids are known to interact with a number of drugs that bind primarily to HAS. The free fatty acid level is increased in several physiologic (fasting), pathologic (diabetes, myocardial infarction, alcohol abstinence) and pharmacologically induced conditions (after heparin and caffeine Administration). The fatty acids, which also bind to albumin, influence Binding of several benzodiazepines and propranolol (decreased binding) and warfarin (increased binding). Bilirubin binding to HAS can be impaired by certain drugs and is of great concern in neonates whose BBB and bilirubin metabolizing capacity are not very efficient. Acidic drugs such as sodium salicylate, sodium benzoate and sulfonamides displace bilirubin from its albumin binding site. The free bilirubin is not conjugated by the liver of the neonates and thus crosses the BBB and precipitates the condition called as **Kernicterus** (characterized by degeneration of brain and mental retardation).

(c) **Allosteric changes in protein molecule:** This is yet another mechanism by which drugs can affect protein binding interactions. The process involves alteration of the protein structure by the drug or its metabolite thereby modifying its binding capacity. The agent that produces such an effect is called as **allosteric effector**, e. g. Aspirin acetylates the lysine fraction of albumin thereby modifying its capacity to bind NSAIDs like phenylbutazone (increased affinity) and flufenamic acid (decreased affinity).

4. Patient related factors

(a) **Age:** Modification in protein-drug binding as influenced by age of the patient is mainly due to differences in the protein content in various age groups.

i. **Neonates**: Albumin content is low in newborn; as a result, the unbound concentration of drug that primarily binds to albumin, for example phenytoin and diazepam, is increased.

ii. **Young infants**: An interesting example of differences in protein drug binding in infants is that of digoxin. Infants suffering from congestive cardiac failure are given a digitalizing dose 4 to 6 times the adult dose on body weight basis. This is contrary to one's belief that infants should be given low doses considering their poorly developed drug eliminating system. The reason attributed for use of a large digoxin dose is greater binding of the drug in infants (the other reason is abnormally large renal clearance of digoxin in infants).

iii. **Elderly:** In old age, the albumin content is lowered and free concentration of drugs that bind primarily to it is increased. Old age is also characterized by an increase in the levels of AAG and thus decreased free concentration is observed for drugs that bind to it. The situation is complex and difficult to generalize for drugs that bind to both HAS and AAG, e.g. lidocaine and propranolol.

(b) **Intersubject variations:** Intersubject variability in drug binding as studied with few drugs showed that the difference is small and no more than two fold. These differences have been attributed to genetic and environmental factors.

(c) **Disease states:** Several pathologic conditions are associated with alteration in protein content. Since albumin is the major drug binding protein, hypoalbuminemia can severely impair protein-drug binding. Hypoalbuminemia is caused by several conditions like aging, CCF, trauma, burns, inflammatory states, serious renal and hepatic disorders, pregnancy, surgery, cancer, etc. Almost every serious chronic illness is characterized by decreased albumin content. Some of the diseases that modify protein-drug binding are depicted in Table. Hyperlipoproteinemia, caused by hypothyroidism, obstructive liver disease, alcoholism, etc., affects binding of lipophilic drugs.

Table 4.10: Influence of disease states on protein-drug binding

Disease	Influence on Plasma Protein	Influence on Protein-Drug Binding
1. Renal failure	Decreased albumin content	Decreased binding of acidic drugs; neutral and basic drugs unaffected.
2. Hepatic failure	Decreased albumin synthesis	Decreased binding of acidic drugs; binding of basic drugs is normal or reduced depending on AAG levels.
3. Inflammatory states (trauma, surgery,	Increased AAG levels	Increased binding of basic drugs; neutral and burns, infections, etc.) acidic drugs; unaffected.

Putting in a nutshell, all factors, especially drug interactions and patient related factors that affect protein or tissue binding if drugs, influence:

1. **Pharmacokinetics of drugs:** A decrease in plasma protein-drug binding i.e. an increase in unbound drug concentration, favors tissue redistribution and/or clearance of drugs from the body (enhanced biotransformation and excretion).

2. **Pharmacodynamics of drugs:** An increase in concentration of free or unbound drug results in increased intensity of action (therapeutic/toxic).

Questions

Essay questions

1. Define protein binding of drugs. Explain kinetics of protein-drug binding.
2. Explain factor influencing protein binding of drug.
3. What is reversible and irreversible protein drug binding? Explain relationship of plasma drug-protein binding to distribution and elimination.

Short questions

1. What is the significance of protein drug binding? Explain briefly.
2. Explain determinants of protein binding.
3. Why HSA is considered a versatile protein for drug binding?
4. With examples, name the various drug binding sites on HSA.
5. Define displacement interaction. What characteristics of the displacer and the displaced drug are important for displacement interactions to be clinically significant?
6. What is the influence of protein binding and displacement interaction on the elimination half-life of a drug?

Chapter—5

PHARMACOKINETICS

Pharmacokinetics: Basic Consideration

Pharmacokinetics is defined as the study of drug absorption, distribution, metabolism and excretion (ADME) and their relationship with the pharmacology, therapeutic or toxicological response in human beings and animals. Absorption depends on the route of administration. Drug distribution depends on how soluble the drug molecule is in fat (to pass through membranes) and on the extent to which the drug binds to blood proteins (albumin). Drug elimination is accomplished by excretion into urine and/or by inactivation by enzymes in the liver.

Because of pharmacokinetics:

- Individualize patient drug therapy monitor medications with a narrow therapeutic index.
- Decrease the risk of adverse effects while maximizing pharmacologic response of medications.
- Evaluate PK/PD as a diagnostic tool for underlying disease states.

Dosage regimen is defined as the frequency of drug administration in a particular dose. Depending on the therapeutic objective, the duration of drug therapy; dosage regimen is decided. Rational and optimal therapy with drug depends upon:

1. Choice of suitable drug.

2. A balance between therapeutic and toxic effects.

The plasma drug concentration between these two limits is called as **therapeutic concentration range or therapeutic window** (the ratio of maximum safe concentration to minimum effective concentration of the drug is called as the **therapeutic index**). Thus, in order to achieve therapeutic success, plasma concentration of drug should be maintained within the therapeutic window. For this, knowledge is needed not only of the mechanisms of drug absorption, distribution, metabolism and excretion, but also of the kinetics of these processes i.e. pharmacokinetics.

Plasma drug concentrations-time profile

A direct relationship exists between the concentration of a drug at the biophase (site of action) and the concentration of drug in plasma. A typical plasma drug concentration-time curve obtained after a single oral dose

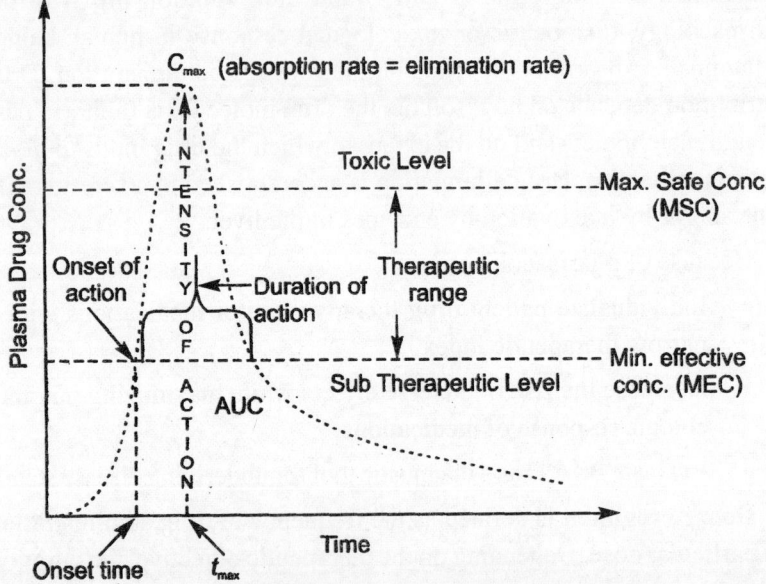

Fig. 5.1: A typical plasma concentration-time profile showing pharmacokinetic and pharmacodynamic parameters obtained after oral administration of single dose of drug.

of a drug and showing various pharmacokinetic and Pharmacodynamic parameters is depicted in fig. 5.1.

The three important **pharmacokinetic parameters** that describe the plasma level-time curve and useful in assessing the bioavailability of a drug from its formulation is:

(1) **Peak plasma concentration (C_{max}):**

> The point of maximum concentration of drug in plasma is called as the **peak** and the concentration of drug at peak is known as **peak plasma concentration** and **maximum drug concentration.**

> It is expressed in mcg/ml.

> The peak represents point of time when absorption rate equals elimination rate of drug.

(2) **Time of peak concentration (t_{max})**

> The time for drug to reach peak concentration in plasma (after extravascular administration) is called as the **time of peak concentration.**

> It is expressed in hours.

> Onset time and duration of action depends on t_{max}

(3) **Area under curve (AUC)**

> It represents the total integrated area under the plasma level–time profile and expresses the total amount of drug that comes into the systemic circulation after its administration.

> It is expressed in mcg/ml × hours.

> It is most important parameter in evaluating bioavailability of drug from its dosage form as it represents extent of absorption.

The various pharmacodynamic parameters are:

(1) **Minimum effective concentration (MEC):**

> Minimum concentration of drug in plasma required to produce the therapeutic effect.

➢ It reflects the minimum concentration of drug at the receptor site to elicit the desired pharmacologic response.

➢ The concentration of drug below MEC is said to be **sub-therapeutic level**.

➢ In case of antibiotics, the term **Minimum inhibitory concentration (MIC)** is used.

(2) Maximum safe concentration (MSC):

➢ The concentration of drug in plasma above which adverse or unwanted effects are precipitated.

➢ Concentration of drug above MSC is said to be in the toxic level.

(3) Onset of action:

➢ The beginning of pharmacological response.

➢ It occurs when plasma drug level concentration just exceeds required MEC.

(4) Onset time:

➢ The time required for the drug to start producing pharmacological response.

(5) Duration of action:

➢ The time period for which the plasma concentration of drug remains above the MEC level

(6) Intensity of action:

➢ The maximum pharmacological response produced by the peak plasma concentration of drug.

➢ It is also called as **peak response**.

(7) Therapeutic range:

➢ The drug concentration between MEC and MSC represents the **therapeutic range**.

Rate, Rate constant and order of reaction

Pharmacokinetics is the mathematical analysis of processes of ADME. The movement of drug molecules from the site of application to the systemic circulation, through various barriers, their conversion into another chemical form and finally their exit out of the body can be expressed mathematically by rate at which they proceed. The velocity with which a reaction or a process occurs is called as its rate. Consider the following chemical reaction:

$$\text{Drug } A \rightarrow \text{Drug } B \qquad \text{... (5.1)}$$

The rate of forward reaction is expressed as:

$$- dA/dt \qquad \text{... (5.2)}$$

Negative sign indicates the concentration of drug A decreases with time t. As the reaction proceeds, the concentration of drug B increases and rate can be expressed as:

$$dB/dt \qquad \text{... (5.3)}$$

The manner in which the concentration of drug (or reactants) influences the rate of reaction or process is called as **order of reaction** or **order of process**. If C is the concentration of drug A, the rate of decrease in C of drug A as it is changed to B can be described by:

$$dC/dt = -KC^n \qquad \text{... (5.4)}$$

Where,

K = Rate constant

n = order of reaction

If n = 0, its a Zero order process. If n = 1, its a first order process.

Zero – order kinetics (constant rate process)

If n = 0, the equation 5.4 becomes,

$$dC/dt = -K_0 C^0 = -K_0 \qquad \text{... (5.5)}$$

Where K_0 = zero order rate constant (in mg/min)

From the equation 5.5, zero order process can be defined as the one whose rate is independent of drug undergoing reaction i.e. rate of reaction cannot be increased by increasing the concentration of reaction.

Rearranging the equation 5.5, we get,

$$dC = -K_0 \, dt \qquad \text{... (5.6)}$$

Integrating the equation 5.6 we get,

$$C - C_0 = - K_0 t$$

or

$$C = C_0 - K_0 t \qquad \text{... (5.7)}$$

Where C_0 = concentration of drug at time $t = 0$

C = concentration of drug to undergo reaction at time t.

When graph plot against time with concentration, straight line obtained and shows concentration decreases linearly.

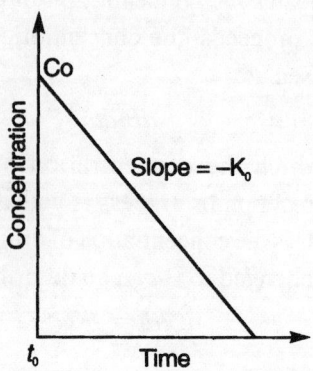

Fig. 5.2: Graph of zero-order kinetics

Zero-order half life

Half life is defined as the time period required for the concentration of drug to decreases by one-half. When $t = t_{1/2}$, $C = C_{0/2}$ then equation 5.7 becomes:

$$\frac{C_0}{2} = C_0 - K_0 t_{1/2} \qquad \text{... (5.8)}$$

Solving 5.8, we get:

$$t1/2 = \frac{C_0}{2K_0} = \frac{0.5C_0}{K_0} \qquad \text{... (5.9)}$$

The equation 5.9 shows that $t_{1/2}$ of zero order process is not constant but proportional to the initial concentration of drug C_0 and inversely proportional to the zero order rate constant. Examples of zero order processes are:

- ✓ Metabolism/protein drug binding/enzyme or carrier –mediated transport under saturated condition.
- ✓ Administration of drug as a constant rate i.v. infusion.
- ✓ Controlled drug delivery such as that from i.m. implants or osmotic pumps.

First order kinetics (linear kinetics)

If $n = 1$, then equation 5.4 can be written as,

$$dC/dt = -KC \qquad \text{... (5.10)}$$

Where K = first order rate constant.

From equation 5.10, it is clear that first order process is the one whose rate is directly proportional to the concentration of drug undergoing reaction i.e., greater the concentration, faster the reaction. It is because of such proportionality between rate of reaction and the concentration of drug that a first-order process is said to follow linear kinetics.

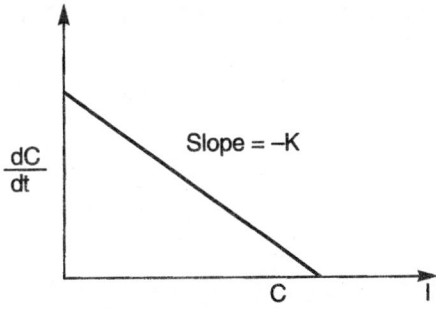

Fig. 5.3: Graph of first-order kinetics showing linear relationship between rate of reaction and concentration of drug

Rearranging the equation 5.10, we get,

$$dc/c = -Kdt \qquad \qquad ...(5.11)$$

Integrating the equation 5.11, we get,

$$\ln C = \ln C_0 - Kt \qquad \qquad ...(5.12)$$

In the exponential form the above equation 5.12 can be written as:

$$C = C_0 e^{-Kt} \qquad \qquad ...(5.13)$$

Where e = natural (Naperian) log base.

The equation 5.13 has only one exponent, therefore the first order process is also called as **monoexponential rate process.**

Since $\ln = 2.303 \log$, equation 5.12 can be written as:

$$\log C = \log C_0 - \frac{Kt}{2.303} \qquad \qquad ...(5.14)$$

or

$$\log C = \log C_0 - 0.434 \, Kt \qquad \qquad ...(5.15)$$

A semi log plot of equation 5.14 yields a straight line with slope $= -K$ and intercept, $y = \log C_0$

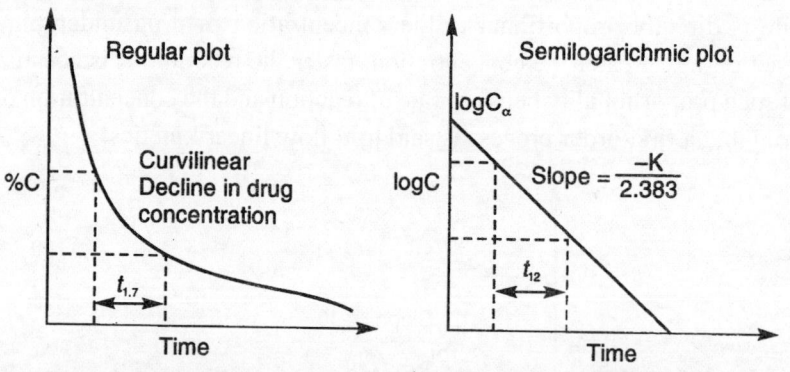

Fig. 5.4: Regular and semilog graphs of first-order kinetics

First order half life

Substituting the value of $C = C_0/2$ at $t_{1/2}$ in equation 5.14 and solving it, we get,

$$t_{1/2} = 0.693/k \qquad \dots (5.16)$$

The equation 5.16 shows that, in contrast to zero –order process, the half life of first-order is a constant and independent of initial drug concentration. Most pharmacokinetic process viz. absorption, distribution and elimination follow first-order kinetics.

Mixed order kinetics (nonlinear kinetics)

In some instances, the kinetics of pharmacokinetics process change from predominantly first-order to predominantly zero-order with increasing dose or chronic medication. A mixture of both first and zero-order kinetics is observed in such cases and therefore the process is said to be mixed-order kinetics. Since deviation from an originally linear pharmacokinetic profile is observed, rate process of such drug is called as **non-linear kinetics**. Mixed order is also termed as **dose dependent kinetics** as it is absorbed at increased or multiple doses of some drug. The phenomena is seen when particular pharmacokinetic process involves presence of carriers or enzymes which are substitute specific and have definite capacities and can get saturated at high drug conc.(i.e., capacity limited). Kinetics of such capacity limited process can be described by **Michaelis-Menten kinetics**.

Significance of Plasma Drug Concentrations Measurement

- The intensity of the pharmacologic or toxic effect of a drug is often related to the concentration of the drug at the receptor site, usually located in the tissue cells. Because most of the tissue cells are richly perfused with tissue fluids or plasma, measuring the plasma drug level is a responsive method of monitoring the course of therapy.

- Clinically, individual variations in the pharmacokinetics of drugs are quite common. Monitoring the concentration of drugs in the blood or plasma ascertains that the calculated dose actually delivers the plasma level required for therapeutic effect. With some drugs, receptor expression and/or sensitivity in individuals varies, so monitoring of plasma levels is needed to distinguish the patient who is receiving too much of a drug from the patient who is supersensitive to the drug. Moreover, the patient's physiologic functions may be affected by disease, nutrition, environment, concurrent drug therapy, and other factors. Pharmacokinetic models allow more accurate interpretation of the relationship between plasma drug levels and pharmacologic response.

• In the absence of pharmacokinetic information, plasma drug levels are relatively useless for dosage adjustment. For example, suppose a single blood sample from a patient was assayed and found to contain 10 mg/mL. According to the literature, the maximum safe concentration of this drug is 15 mg/mL. In order to apply this information properly, it is important to know when the blood sample was drawn, what dose of the drug was given, and the route of administration. If the proper information is available, the use of pharmacokinetic equations and models may describe the blood level–time curve accurately.

• Monitoring of plasma drug concentrations allows for the adjustment of the drug dosage in order to individualize and optimize therapeutic drug regimens. In the presence of alteration in physiologic functions due to disease, monitoring plasma drug concentrations may provide a guide to the progress of the disease state and enable the investigator to modify the drug dosage accordingly. Clinically, sound medical judgment and observation are most important. Therapeutic decisions should not be based solely on plasma drug concentrations.

• In many cases, the pharmacodynamic response to the drug may be more important to measure than just the plasma drug concentration. For example, the electrophysiology of the heart, including an electrocardiogram (ECG), is important to assess in patients medicated with cardiotonic drugs such as digoxin. For an anticoagulant drug, such as dicumarol, prothrombin clotting time may indicate whether proper dosage was achieved. Most diabetic patients taking insulin will monitor their own blood or urine glucose levels.

• For drugs that act irreversibly at the receptor site, plasma drug concentrations may not accurately predict pharmacodynamic response. Drugs used in cancer chemotherapy often interfere with nucleic acid or protein biosynthesis to destroy tumor cells. For these drugs, the plasma drug concentration does not relate directly to the pharmacodynamic response. In this case, other pathophysiologic parameters and side effects are monitored in the patient to prevent adverse toxicity.

Compartment Model: Definition and Scope

If the tissue drug concentrations and binding are known, physiologic pharmacokinetic models, which are based on actual tissues and their respective blood flow, describe the data realistically. Physiologic pharmacokinetic models are frequently used in describing drug distribution in animals, because tissue samples are easily available for assay. On the other hand, tissue samples are often not available for human subjects, so most physiological models assume an average set of blood flow for individual subjects.

In contrast, because of the vast complexity of the body, drug kinetics in the body are frequently simplified to be represented by one or more tanks, or compartments, that communicate reversibly with each other. A compartment is not a real physiologic or anatomic region but is considered as a tissue or group of tissues that have similar blood flow and drug affinity. Within each compartment, the drug is considered to be uniformly distributed. Mixing of the drug within a compartment is rapid and homogeneous and is considered to be "well stirred," so that the drug concentration represents an average concentration, and each drug molecule has an equal probability of leaving the compartment. Rate constants are used to represent the overall rate processes of drug entry into and exit from the compartment. The model is an open system because drug can be eliminated from the system. Compartment models are based on linear assumptions using linear differential equations.

Mammillary Model

A compartmental model provides a simple way of grouping all the tissues into one or more compartments where drugs move to and from the central or plasma compartment. The **mammillary model** is the most common compartment model used in pharmacokinetics. The mammillary model is a strongly connected system, because one can estimate the amount of drug in any compartment of the system after drug is introduced into a given compartment. In the one-compartment model, drug is both added to and eliminated from a central compartment. The central compartment is assigned to represent plasma and highly perfused tissues that rapidly equilibrate with drug. When an intravenous dose of drug is given, the drug enters directly into the central compartment. Elimination of drug occurs from the central compartment because the organs involved in drug elimination, primarily kidney and liver, are well-perfused tissues.

In a two-compartment model, drug can move between the central or plasma compartment to and from the tissue compartment. Although the tissue compartment does not represent a specific tissue, the mass balance accounts for the drug present in all the tissues. In this model, the total amount of drug in the body is simply the sum of drug present in the central compartment plus the drug present in the tissue compartment. Knowing the parameters of either the one- or two-compartment model, one can estimate the amount of drug left in the body and the amount of drug eliminated from the body at any time. The compartmental models are particularly useful when little information is known about the tissues.

Several types of compartment models are described in. The pharmacokinetic rate constants are represented by the letter k. Compartment 1 represents the plasma or central compartment, and compartment 2 represents the tissue compartment. The drawing of models has three functions. The model (1) enables the pharmacokineticist to write differential equations to describe drug concentration changes in each compartment, (2) gives a visual representation of the rate processes, and (3) shows how many pharmacokinetic constants are necessary to describe the process adequately.

Model 1. One-compartment open model, IV injection.

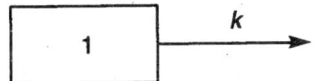

Model 2. One-compartment open model with first-order absorption.

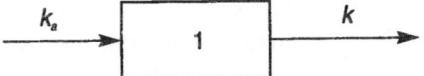

Model 3. Two-compartment open model, IV injection.

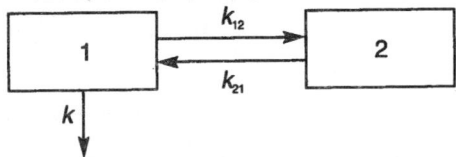

Model 4. Two-compartment open model with first-order absorption.

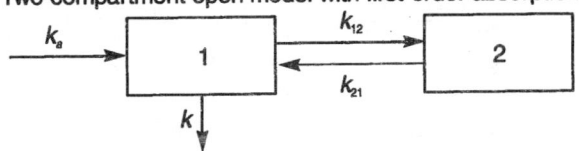

Fig. 5.5: Various mammillary compartment models.

Example

Two parameters are needed to describe model 1: the volume of the compartment and the elimination rate constant, k. In the case of model 4, the pharmacokinetic parameters consist of the volumes of compartments 1 and 2 and the rate constants—k_a, k, k_{12}, and k_{21}—for a total of six parameters.

In studying these models, it is important to know whether drug concentration data may be sampled directly from each compartment. For models 3 and 4, data concerning compartment 2 cannot be obtained easily because tissues are not easily sampled and may not contain homogeneous concentrations of drug. If the amount of drug absorbed and eliminated per unit time is obtained by sampling compartment 1, then the amount of drug contained in the tissue compartment 2 can be estimated mathematically.

Caternary model

In pharmacokinetics, the mammillary model must be distinguished from another type of compartmental model called **the caternary model**. The caternary model consists of compartments joined to one another like the compartments of a train. In contrast, the mammillary model consists of one or more compartments around a central compartment like satellites. Because the caternary model does not apply to the way most functional organs in the body are directly connected to the plasma, it is not used as often as the mammillary model.

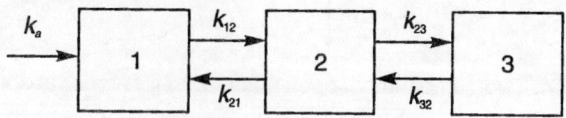

Fig. 5.6: A caternary model

Pharmacokinetics of Drug Absorption

The pharmacokinetics of drugs following intravenous drug administration are more simple to model compared to extravascular delivery. Extravascular delivery routes, particularly oral dosing, are important and popular means of drug administration. Unlike intravenous administration, in which the drug is injected directly into the plasma, pharmacokinetic models after extravascular drug administration must consider systemic drug absorption from the site of administration, eg, the lung, the gut, etc., into the plasma. Extravascular drug delivery is further complicated by variables at the absorption site, including possible drug degradation and significant inter- and intrapatient differences in the rate and extent of absorption. Absorption and metabolic variables are characterized using pharmacokinetic methods. The variability in systemic drug absorption can be minimized to some extent by proper biopharmaceutical design of the dosage form to provide predictable and reliable drug therapy. The major advantage of intravenous administration is that the rate and extent of systemic drug input is carefully controlled.

The systemic drug absorption from the gastrointestinal (GI) tract or from any other extravascular site is dependent on (1) the physicochemical properties of the drug, (2) the dosage form used, and (3) the anatomy and physiology of the absorption site. Although this chapter will focus primarily on oral dosing, the concepts discussed here may be easily extrapolated to other extravascular routes. For oral dosing, such factors as surface area of the GI tract, stomach-emptying rate, GI mobility, and blood flow to the absorption site all affect the rate and the extent of drug absorption. In pharmacokinetics, the overall rate of drug absorption may be described as either a first-order or zero-order input process. Most pharmacokinetic models assume first-order absorption unless an assumption of zero-order absorption improves the model significantly or has been verified experimentally.

The rate of change in the amount of drug in the body, dD_B/dt, is dependent on the relative rates of drug absorption and elimination. The net rate of drug accumulation in the body at any time is equal to the rate of drug absorption less the rate of drug elimination, regardless of whether absorption is zero-order or first-order.

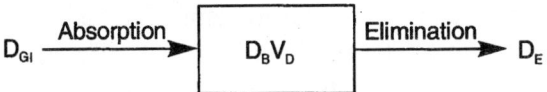

Fig. 5.7: Model of drug absorption and elimination.

$$\frac{dD_{GI}}{dt} > \frac{dD_E}{dt} \qquad \qquad ... (5.17)$$

At the peak drug concentration in the plasma the rate of drug absorption just equals the rate of drug elimination, and there is no net change in the amount of drug in the body.

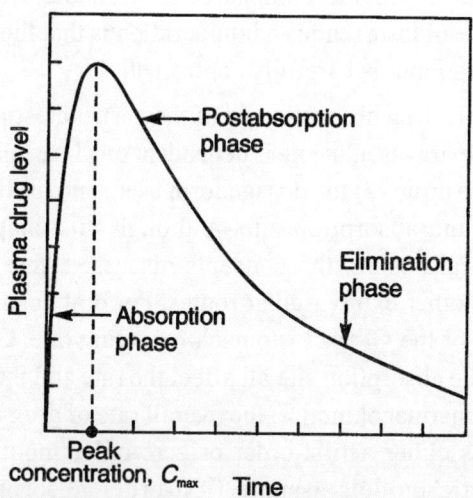

Fig. 5.8: Plasma level–time curve for a drug given in a single oral dose. The drug absorption and elimination phases of the curve are shown.

$$\frac{dD_{GI}}{dt} = \frac{dD_E}{dt} \qquad \text{... (5.18)}$$

Immediately after the time of peak drug absorption, some drug may still be at the absorption site (i.e., in the GI tract or other site of administration). However, the rate of drug elimination at this time is faster than the rate of absorption, as represented by the post absorption phase in.

$$\frac{dD_{GI}}{dt} > \frac{dD_E}{dt} \qquad \text{... (5.19)}$$

When the drug at the absorption site becomes depleted, the rate of drug absorption approaches zero, or $dD_{GI}/dt = 0$. The plasma level–time curve (now the elimination phase) then represents only the elimination of drug from the body, usually a first-order process. Therefore, during the elimination phase the rate of change in the amount of drug in the body is described as a first-order process,

$$\frac{dD_B}{dt} = -KD_B \qquad \qquad ... (5.20)$$

Where, k is the first-order elimination rate constant.

Zero order and first order absorption rate constant using Wagner Nelson method

The method involves determination of ka from % unabsorbed – time plots and does not require the assumption of zero or first order absorption.

After oral administration of a single dose of drug, at any given time, the amount of drug absorbed into systemic circulation X_A, is sum of amount of drug in the body X and the amount of drug eliminated from the body X_E. Thus:

$$X_A = X + X_E \qquad \qquad ... (5.21)$$

The amount of drug in the body is $X = V_d C$. The amount of drug eliminated at any time t can be calculated as follows:

$$X_E = K_E V_D \left[AUC \right]_0^t \qquad \qquad ... (5.22)$$

Substitution of values X and X_E in equation 5.21 yields:

$$X_A = V_D C + K_E V_d \left[AUC \right]_0^t \qquad \qquad ... (5.23)$$

The total amount of drug absorbed into the systemic circulation from time zero to infinity X_A^∞ can be given as:

$$X_A^\infty = V_D C^\infty + K_E V_d \left[AUC \right]_0^\infty \qquad \qquad ... (5.24)$$

Since at $t = \infty$, $c^\infty = 0$, the above equation reduces to:

$$X_A^\infty = K_E V_d \left[AUC \right]_0^\infty \qquad \qquad ... (5.25)$$

The fraction of drug absorbed at any time t is given as:

$$\frac{X_A}{X_A^\infty} = \frac{V_d C + K_E V_d \left[AUC \right]_0^t}{K_E V_d \left[AUC \right]_0^\infty}$$

$$= \frac{C + K_E [AUC]_0^t}{K_E [AUC]_0^\infty} \qquad \dots (5.26)$$

Percent drug unabsorbed at any time is therefore:

$$\% \, ARA = \left[1 - \frac{X_A}{X_A^\infty} \right] 100 = \left[1 - \frac{C + K_E [AUC]_0^t}{K_E [AUC]_0^\infty} \right] 100$$

$$\dots (5.27)$$

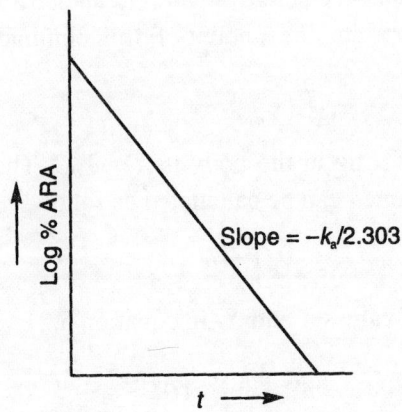

Fig. 5.9: Semi-log plot of %ARA versus *t* according to Wagner-Nelson method

The method requires collection of blood sample after administration of single oral dose at regular interval of time till entire amount of drug is eliminated from the body. K_e is obtained from log c versus t. $[AUC]_0^t$ and $[AUC]_0^\infty$ are obtained from plot of c versus t.

Disadvantage of Wagner–Nelson method is that it applies only to drug with one-compartment characteristics. Problem arise when a drug that obeys one-compartment model after e.v. administration shows multi – compartment characteristics on i.v. injection.

Zero order and first order absorption rate constant using loo -riegelman method

Plotting the percent of drug unabsorbed versus time to determine the k_a may be calculated for a drug exhibiting a two-compartment kinetic model. This method does require that the drug be given intravenously as well as orally to obtain all the necessary kinetic constants.

After oral administration of a dose of a drug that exhibits two-compartment model kinetics, the amount of drug absorbed is calculated as the sum of the amounts of drug in the central compartment (D_p) and in the tissue compartment (D_t) and the amount of drug eliminated by all routes (D_u).

$$A_b = D_P + \text{Dt} + \text{Du} \qquad \qquad ...(5.28)$$

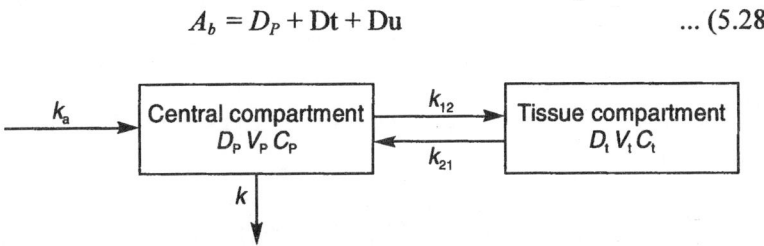

Fig. 5.10: Two-compartment pharmacokinetic mode. Drug absorption and elimination occur from the central compartment.

Each of these terms may be expressed in terms of kinetics constants and plasma drug concentrations, as follows:

$$D_P = V_P C_P \qquad \qquad ...(5.29)$$

$$D_t = V_t C_t \qquad \qquad ...(5.30)$$

$$\frac{dD_u}{dt} = K V_P C_P \qquad \qquad ...(5.31)$$

$$D_u = K V_P [AUC]_0^t$$

The fraction of drug absorbed at any time t is equal to the amount of drug absorbed at this time, Ab_t, divided by the total amount of drug absorbed, Ab^∞.

$$\frac{Ab_t}{Ab^\infty} = \frac{(dD_u/dt)_t + K(D_u)t}{KD_u^\infty} \qquad \ldots (5.32)$$

Substituting the expression for D_p and D_u into equation 5.32,

$$Ab = V_P C_P + D_t + KV_P \left[AUC \right]_0^t \qquad \ldots (5.33)$$

By dividing this equation by V_p to express the equation on drug concentrations, we obtain

$$\frac{Ab}{V_P} = C_P + \frac{D_t}{V_P} + K \left[AUC \right]_0^t \qquad \ldots (5.34)$$

At $t = \infty$ this equation becomes

$$\frac{Ab}{V_P} = K \left[AUC \right]_0^\infty \qquad \ldots (5.35)$$

Equation 5.35 divided by Equation 5.36 gives the fraction of drug absorbed at any time.

$$\frac{Ab}{Ab^\infty} = \frac{C_P + \left(\dfrac{D_t}{V_P} \right) + K \left[AUC \right]_0^t}{K \left[AUC \right]_0^\infty} \qquad \ldots (5.36)$$

A plot of the fraction of drug unabsorbed, $1 - Ab/Ab^\infty$, versus time gives $-k_a/2.3$ as the slope from which the value for the absorption rate constant is obtained.

C_p and $k \left[AUC \right]_0^t$ are calculated from a plot of C_p versus time. Values for (D_t/V_p) can be approximated by the Loo–Riegelman method, as follows:

$$(C_t)t_n = \frac{K_{12}\Delta C_P \Delta t}{2} + \frac{K_{12}}{K_{21}}(C_P)t_{n-1}\left(1 - e^{-K_{21}\Delta t}\right) + (C_t)t_{n-1}e^{-K_{21}\Delta t} \qquad \ldots (5.37)$$

Where C_t is D_t/V_p, or apparent tissue concentration; t = time of sampling for sample n; t_{n-1} = time of sampling for the sampling point preceding sample n; and $(C_p)_{m-1}$ = concentration of drug at central compartment for sample $n - 1$.

Calculation of C_t values is shown in, using a typical set of oral absorption data. After calculation of C_t values, the percent of drug unabsorbed is calculated with Equation 5.36, as shown in. A plot of percent of drug unabsorbed versus time on semilog graph paper gives a k_a of approximately 0.5 hr^{-1}.

Table 5.1: Calculation of C_t Values

$(C_p)_{tn}$	$(t)_{tn}$	ΔC_P	Δt	$\dfrac{K_{12}\Delta C_P\Delta t}{2}$	$(C_p)_{m-1}$	(k_{12}/k_{21}) x $(1-e^{-k_{21}\Delta t})$	$(C_p)_{t\,n-1}$ k_{12}/k_{21} x $(1-e^{-k_{21}\Delta t})$	$(C_t)_{t\,n-1}$ $xe^{-k_{21}\Delta t}$	$(C_t)_{t_n}$
3.00	0.5	3.0	0.5	0.218	0	0.134	0	0	0.218
5.20	1.0	2.2	0.5	0.160	3.00	0.134	0.402	0.187	0.749
6.50	1.5	1.3	0.5	0.094	5.20	0.134	0.697	0.642	1.433
7.30	2.0	0.8	0.5	0.058	6.50	0.134	0.871	1.228	2.157
7.60	2.5	0.3	0.5	0.022	7.30	0.134	0.978	1.849	2.849
7.75	3.0	0.15	0.5	0.011	7.60	0.134	1.018	2.442	3.471
7.70	3.5	−0.05	0.5	−0.004	7.75	0.134	1.039	2.976	4.019
7.60	4.0	−0.10	0.5	−0.007	7.70	0.134	1.032	3.444	4.469
7.10	5.0	−0.50	1.0	−0.073	7.60	0.250	1.900	3.276	5.103
6.60	6.0	−0.50	1.0	−0.073	7.10	0.250	1.775	3.740	5.442
6.00	7.0	−0.60	1.0	−0.087	6.60	0.250	1.650	3.989	5.552
5.10	9.0	−0.90	2.0	−2.261	6.00	0.432	2.592	2.987	5.318
4.40	11.0	−0.70	2.0	−0.203	5.10	0.432	2.203	2.861	4.861
3.30	15.0	−1.10	4.0	−0.638	4.40	0.720	3.168	1.361	3.891

Table 5.2: Calculation of percentage unabsorbed

Time (hr)	$(C_p)_{tn}$	$[AUC]^t_{ntn-1}$	$[AUC]^t_{nt0}$	$k[AUC]^t_{nt0}$	$(C_t)_{tn}$	Ab/V_p	$\%Ab/V_p$	$100\% -Ab/V_p\%$
0.5	3.00	0.750	0.750	0.120	0.218	3.338	16.6	83.4
1.0	5.20	2.050	2.800	0.448	0.749	6.397	31.8	68.2
1.5	6.50	2.925	5.725	0.916	1.433	8.849	44.0	56.0
2.0	7.30	3.450	9.175	1.468	2.157	10.925	54.3	45.7
2.5	7.60	3.725	12.900	2.064	2.849	12.513	62.2	37.8
3.0	7.75	3.838	16.738	2.678	3.471	13.889	69.1	30.9
3.5	7.70	3.863	20.601	3.296	4.019	15.015	74.6	25.4
4.0	7.60	3.825	24.426	3.908	4.469	15.977	79.4	20.6
5.0	7.10	7.350	31.726	5.084	5.103	17.287	85.9	14.1
6.0	6.60	6.850	38.626	6.180	5.442	18.222	90.6	9.4
7.0	6.00	6.300	44.926	7.188	5.552	18.740	93.1	6.9
9.0	5.10	11.100	56.026	8.964	5.318	19.382	96.3	3.7
11.0	4.40	9.500	65.526	10.484	4.861	19.745	98.1	1.9
15.0	3.30	15.400	80.926	12.948	3.891	20.139	100.0	0

For calculation of the k_a by this method, the drug must be given intravenously to allow evaluation of the distribution and elimination rate constants. For drugs that cannot be given by the IV route, the k_a cannot be calculated by the Loo–Riegelman method. For these drugs, given by the oral route only, the Wagner–Nelson method, which assumes a one-compartment model, may be used to provide an initial estimate of k_a. If the drug is given intravenously, there is no way of knowing whether there is any variation in the values for the elimination rate constant k and the distributive rate constants k_{12} and k_{21}. Such variations alter the rate constants. Therefore, a one-compartment model is frequently used to fit the plasma curves after an oral or intramuscular dose. The plasma level predicted from the k_a obtained by this method does deviate from the actual plasma level. However, in many instances, this deviation is not significant.

Volume of Distribution: (see apparent volume distribution in chapter 3)

Distribution Coefficient

In chemistry and the pharmaceutical sciences, **distribution co-efficient** (D) is the ratio of concentrations of a compound in the two phases of a mixture of two immiscible solvents at equilibrium. Hence these coefficients are a measure of differential solubility of the compound between these two solvents. The phrase "Partition Coefficient" is now considered obsolete by IUPAC, and the appropriate alternative ("partition constant", "partition ratio" or "distribution ratio") should be used as appropriate.

Normally one of the solvents chosen is water while the second is hydrophobic such as octanol. Hence both the partition and distribution coefficient are measures of how hydrophilic ("water loving") or hydrophobic ("water fearing") a chemical substance is. A partition coefficient can also be used when one or both solvents is a solid though. In medical practice, partition coefficients are useful for example in estimating distribution of drugs within the body. Hydrophobic drugs with high partition coefficients are preferentially distributed to hydrophobic compartments such as lipid bilayers of cells while hydrophilic drugs (low partition coefficients) preferentially are found in hydrophilic compartments such as blood serum.

Distribution coefficient and log d

The distribution coefficient is the ratio of the sum of the concentrations of all forms of the compound (ionized plus un-ionized) in each of the two phases. For measurements of distribution coefficient, the pH of the aqueous phase is buffered to a specific value such that the pH is not significantly perturbed by the introduction of the compound. The logarithm of the ratio of the sum of concentrations of the solute's various forms in one solvent, to the sum of the concentrations of its forms in the other solvent is called **Log D**:

$$LogD_{oct/wat} = Log\left(\frac{[solute]_{octanol}}{[solute]_{ionized\ water} + [solute]_{neutral\ water}}\right)$$

$$... (5.38)$$

In addition, log D is pH dependent; hence the one must specify the pH at which the log D was measured. Of particular interest is the log D at pH = 7.4 (the physiological pH of blood serum). For un-ionizable compounds, log P = log D at any pH.

Applications

(1) Pharmacology

A drug's distribution coefficient strongly affects how easily the drug can reach its intended target in the body, how strong an effect it will have once it reaches its target, and how long it will remain in the body in an active form.

(2) Pharmacokinetics

In the context of pharmacokinetics (what the body does to a drug), the distribution coefficient has a strong influence on ADME properties (Absorption, Distribution, Metabolism, and Excretion) of the drug. Hence the hydrophobicity of a compound (as measured by its distribution coefficient) is a major determinant of how drug-like it is. More specifically, in order for a drug to be orally absorbed, it normally must first pass through lipid bilayers in the intestinal epithelium (a process known as transcellular transport). For efficient transport, the drug must be hydrophobic enough to partition into the lipid bilayer, but not so hydrophobic, that once it is in the bilayer, it will not partition out again. Likewise, hydrophobicity plays a major role in determining where drugs are distributed within the body after adsorption and as a consequence in how rapidly they are metabolized and excreted.

(3) Pharmacodynamics

In the context of pharmacodynamics (what a drug does to the body), the hydrophobic effect is the major driving force for the binding of drugs to their receptor targets. On the other hand, hydrophobic drugs tend to be more toxic because they in general are retained longer, have a wider distribution within the body (*e.g.*, intracellular, are somewhat less selective in their binding to proteins, and finally are often extensively metabolized. In some cases the metabolites may be chemically reactive. Hence it is advisable to make the drug as hydrophilic as possible while it still retains adequate binding affinity to the therapeutic protein target. Therefore the ideal distribution coefficient for a drug is usually intermediate (not too hydrophobic nor too hydrophilic).

(4) Consumer Products

Many other industries take into account distribution coefficients for example in the formulation of make-up, topical ointments, dyes, hair colors and many other consumer products.

(5) Agrochemicals

Hydrophobic insecticides and herbicides tend to be more active. Hydrophobic agrochemicals in general have longer half lives and therefore display increased risk of adverse environmental impact.

(6) Metallurgy

In metallurgy, the partition coefficient is an important factor in determining how different impurities are distributed between molten and solidified metal. It is a critical parameter for purification using zone melting, and determines how effective an impurity can be removed using directional solidification, described by the Scheil equation.

(7) Environmental

The hydrophobicity of a compound can give scientists an indication of how easily a compound might be taken up in groundwater to pollute waterways, and its toxicity to animals and aquatic life. Distribution coefficients may be measured or predicted for compounds currently causing problems or with foresight to gauge the structural modifications necessary to make a compound environmentally friendlier in the research phase.

In the field of hydrogeology, the octanol water partition coefficient, or K_{ow}, is used to predict and model the migration of dissolved hydrophobic organic compounds in soil and groundwater.

Comparative Kinetics

The time course of drug concentration determined after its administration can be satisfactorily explained by assuming the body as a single, well mixed compartment with first-order disposition processes. In case of other drugs two body compartments may be postulated to describe mathematically the data collected.

One-compartment Open Model: Intravenous Bolus Administration

The most common and most desirable route of drug administration is orally—by mouth—using tablets, capsules, or oral solutions. In developing pharmacokinetic models to describe and predict drug disposition kinetically, the model must account for both the route of administration and the kinetic behavior of the drug in the body.

The one-compartment open model offers the simplest way to describe the process of drug distribution and elimination in the body. This model assumes that the drug can enter or leave the body (ie, the model is "open"), and the body acts like a single, uniform compartment. The simplest route of drug administration from a modeling perspective is a rapid intravenous injection (IV bolus). The simplest kinetic model that describes drug disposition in the body is to consider that the drug is injected all at once into a box, or compartment, and that the drug distributes instantaneously and homogenously throughout the compartment. Drug elimination also occurs from the compartment immediately after injection.

Of course, this model is a simplistic view of drug disposition in the body, which in reality is infinitely more complex than a single compartment. In the body, when a drug is given in the form of an IV bolus, the entire dose of drug enters the bloodstream immediately, and the drug absorption process is considered to be instantaneous. In most cases, the drug distributes via the circulatory system to potentially all the tissues in the body. Uptake of drugs by various tissue organs will occur at varying rates, depending on the blood flow to the tissue, the lipophilicity of the drug, the molecular weight of the drug, and the binding affinity of the drug for the tissue mass. Most drugs are eliminated from the body either through the kidney and/or by being metabolized in the liver. Because of rapid drug equilibration between the blood and tissue, drug elimination occurs as if the dose is all dissolved in a tank of uniform fluid (a single compartment) from which the drug is eliminated. The volume in which the drug is distributed is termed the **apparent volume of distribution, V_D.** The apparent volume of distribution assumes that the drug is uniformly distributed in the body. The V_D is determined from the preinjected amount of the dose in the syringe and the plasma drug concentration resulting immediately after the dose is injected.

The apparent volume of distribution is a parameter of the one-compartment model and governs the plasma concentration of the drug after a given dose. A second pharmacokinetic parameter is the elimination rate constant, k, which governs the rate at which the drug concentration in the body declines over time. The one-compartment model that describes the distribution and elimination after an IV bolus dose is given in.

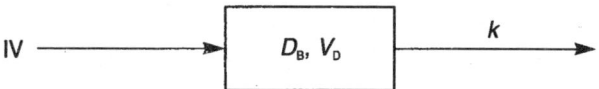

Fig. 5.11: Pharmacokinetic model for a drug administered by rapid intravenous injection. D_B =drug in body; V_D = apparent volume of distribution; k = elimination rate constant.

The one-compartment open model does not predict actual drug levels in the tissues. However, the model assumes that changes in the plasma levels of a drug will result in proportional changes in tissue drug levels, since their kinetic profile is consistent with inclusion within the vascular compartment and the various drug concentrations within the compartment are in equilibrium. The drug in the body, D_B, cannot be measured directly; however, accessible body fluids (such as blood) can be sampled to determine drug concentrations.

• Elimination rate constant

The rate of elimination for most drugs from a tissue or from the body is a first-order process, in which the rate of elimination is dependent on the amount or concentration of drug present. The elimination rate constant, k, is a first-order elimination rate constant with units of time^{-1} (e.g., hr^{-1} or 1/hr). Generally, the parent or active drug is measured in the vascular compartment. Total removal or elimination of the parent drug from this compartment is effected by metabolism (biotransformation) and excretion. The elimination rate constant represents the sum of each of these processes:

$$K = K_m + K_e \qquad \qquad \dots (5.39)$$

Where k_m = first-order rate process of metabolism and k_e = first-order rate process of excretion. There may be several routes of elimination of drug by metabolism or excretion. In such a case, each of these processes has its own first-order rate constant.

A rate expression for is

$$\frac{dD_B}{dt} = -KD_B \qquad \qquad \dots (5.40)$$

This expression shows that the rate of elimination of drug in the body is a first-order process, depending on the overall elimination rate constant, k, and the amount of drug in the body, D_B, remaining at any given time, t. Integration of equation 5.40 gives the following expression:

$$\log DB = \frac{-Kt}{2.3} + \log D_B^0 \qquad \qquad \dots (5.41)$$

Where D_B = drug in the body at time t and $D_B{}^0$ = drug in the body at $t = 0$. When log D_B is plotted against t for this equation, a straight line is obtained. In practice, instead of transforming values of D_B to their corresponding logarithms, each value of D_B is placed at logarithmic intervals on semilog paper.

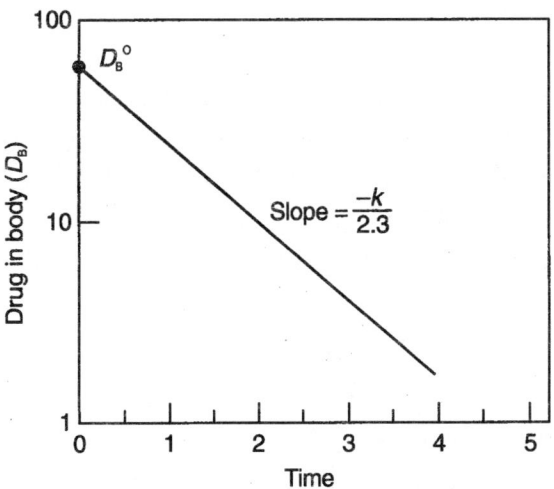

Fig. 5.12: Semilog graph of the rate of drug elimination in a one compartment model.

Equation 5.41 can also be expressed as:

$$D_B = D_B^0 e^{-Kt} \qquad \dots (5.42)$$

• Apparent volume of distribution

In general, drug equilibrates rapidly in the body. When plasma or any other biologic compartment is sampled and analyzed for drug content, the results are usually reported in units of concentration instead of amount. Each individual tissue in the body may contain a different concentration of drug due to differences in drug affinity for that tissue. Therefore, the amount of drug in a given location can be related to its concentration by a proportionality constant that reflects the volume of fluid the drug is dissolved in. The volume of distribution represents a volume that must be considered in estimating the amount of drug in the body from the concentration of drug found in the sampling compartment. The volume of distribution is also the apparent volume (V_D) in which the drug is dissolved (Eq. 5.43). Because the value of the volume of distribution does not have a true physiologic meaning in terms of an anatomic space, the term apparent volume of distribution is used.

The amount of drug in the body is not determined directly. Instead, a blood sample is removed at periodic intervals and analyzed for its concentration of drug. The V_D relates the concentration of drug in plasma (C_p) and the amount of drug in the body (D_B), as in the following equation:

$$D_B = V_D + C_P \qquad \text{... (5.43)}$$

By substituting equation 5.43 into equation 5.41, a similar expression based on drug concentration in plasma is obtained for the first-order decline of drug plasma levels:

$$\log C_P = \frac{-Kt}{2.3} + \log C_P^0 \qquad \text{... (5.44)}$$

Where C_p = concentration of drug in plasma at time t and C_p^0 = concentration of drug in plasma at $t = 0$. Equation 5.44 can also be expressed as:

$$CP = \frac{-Kt}{2.3} + \log C_p^0 e^{-kt} \qquad \text{... (5.45)}$$

The relationship between apparent volume, drug concentration, and total amount of drug may be better understood by the following example.

➤ **Example**

Exactly 1g of a drug is dissolved in an unknown volume of water. Upon assay, the concentration of this solution is 1 mg/mL. What is the original volume of this solution?

The original volume of the solution may be obtained by the following proportion, remembering that 1 g = 1000 mg:

1000 mg / *x* mL = 1 mg / mL

$$X = 1000 \text{ mL}$$

Therefore, the original volume was 1000 mL or 1 L.

If, in the above example, the volume of the solution is known to be 1 L and the concentration of the solution is 1 mg/mL, then, to calculate the total amount of drug present,

$$X \text{ mg}/1000 \text{ mL} = 1 \text{ mg} / \text{mL}$$

$$X = 1000 \text{ mg}$$

Therefore, the total amount of drug in the solution is 1000 mg, or 1 g.

From the preceding example, if the volume of solution in which the drug is dissolved and the drug concentration of the solution are known, then the total amount of drug present in the solution may be calculated. This relationship between drug concentration, volume in which the drug is dissolved, and total amount of drug present is given in the following equation:

$$V_D = \frac{\text{Dose}}{C_P^0} = \frac{D_B^0}{C_P^0} \qquad \qquad \text{... (5.46)}$$

Where D = total amount of drug, V = total volume, and C = drug concentration. From Equation 5.46, which is similar to Equation 5.43, if any two parameters are known, then the third term may be calculated.

The body may be considered as a constant-volume system or compartment. Therefore, the apparent volume of distribution for any given drug is generally a constant. If both the concentration of drug in the plasma and the apparent volume of distribution for the drug are known, then the total amount of drug in the body (at the time in which the plasma sample was obtained) may be calculated from Equation 5.43.

➤ Calculation of volume of distribution

In a one-compartment model (IV administration), the V_D is calculated with the following equation:

$$V_D = \frac{\text{Dose}}{C_P^0} = \frac{D_B^0}{C_P^0} \qquad \text{... (5.47)}$$

When C_P^0 is determined by extrapolation, it represents the instantaneous drug concentration (concentration of drug at $t = 0$) after drug equilibration in the body. The dose of drug given by IV bolus (rapid IV injection) represents the amount of drug in the body, D_B^0, at $t = 0$.

Because both D_B^0 and C_P^0 are known at $t = 0$, then the apparent volume of distribution, V_D, may be calculated from Equation 5.47.

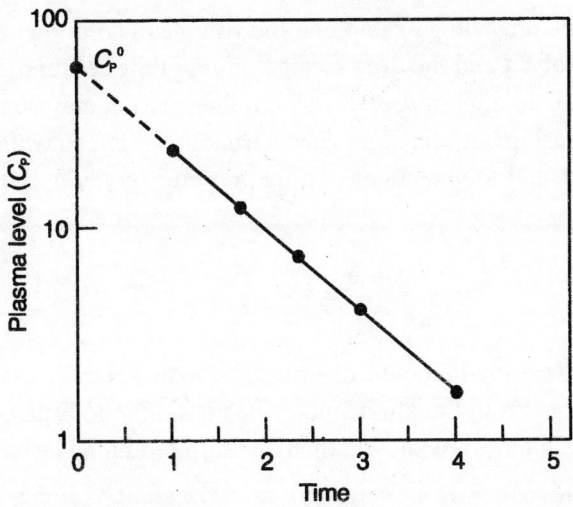

Fig. 5.13: Semilog graph giving the value of C_P^0 by extrapolation.

$$\frac{dD_B}{dt} = -KD_B$$

From equation 5.40 (repeated here), the rate of drug elimination is:

By substitution of equation 5.43, $D_B = V_D C_p$, into equation 5.40, the following expression is obtained:

$$\frac{dD_B}{dt} = -KV_DC_P \qquad \qquad ...(5.48)$$

Rearrangement of equation 5.48 gives

$$dD_B = -KV_DC_Pdt \qquad \qquad ...(5.49)$$

As both k and V_D are constants, Equation 5.48 may be integrated as follows:

$$\int_0^{D_0} dD_B = -KV_D\int_0^\infty C_Pdt \qquad \qquad ...(5.50)$$

Equation 5.50 shows that a small change in time (dt) results in a small change in the amount of drug in the body, D_B.

The integral $+ \int_0^\infty C_Pdt$ represents the AUC^∞_0, which is the summation of the area under the curve from t = 0 to $t = \infty$. Thus, the apparent V_D may also be calculated from knowledge of the dose, elimination rate constant, and the area under the curve (AUC) from $t = 0$ to $t = \infty$. The AUC^∞_0 is usually estimated by the trapezoidal rule. After integration, equation 5.50 becomes:

$$D_0 = KV_D[AUC]_0^\infty \qquad \qquad ...(5.51)$$

Which upon rearrangement yields the following equation:

$$V_D = \frac{D_0}{K[AUC]_0^\infty} \qquad \qquad ...(5.52)$$

The calculation of the apparent V_D by means of equation 5.52 is a model-independent method, because no pharmacokinetic model is considered and the AUC is determined directly by the trapezoidal rule.

> ### ➤ Significance of the apparent volume of distribution

The apparent volume of distribution is not a true physiologic volume. Most drugs have an apparent volume of distribution smaller than, or equal to, the body mass. For some drugs, the volume of distribution may be several times the body mass. Equation 5.47 shows that the apparent V_D is dependent on C_P^0. For a given dose, a very small C_P^0 may occur in the body due to concentration of the drug in peripheral tissues and organs. For this dose, the small C_P^0 will result in a large V_D.

Drugs with a large apparent V_D are more concentrated in extravascular tissues and less concentrated intravascularly. If a drug is highly bound to plasma proteins or remains in the vascular region, then C_P^0 will be higher, resulting in a smaller apparent V_D. Consequently, binding of a drug to peripheral tissues or to plasma proteins will significantly affect V_D.

The apparent V_D is a volume term that can be expressed as a simple volume or in terms of percent of body weight. In expressing the apparent V_D in terms of percent of body weight, a 1-L volume is assumed to be equal to the weight of 1 kg. For example, if the V_D is 3500 mL for a subject weighing 70 kg, the V_D expressed as percent of body weight is

$$\frac{3.5 \text{ kg}}{70 \text{ kg}} \times 100 = 5\% \text{ of body weight}$$

If V_D is a very large number—ie, >100% of body weight—then it may be assumed that the drug is concentrated in certain tissue compartments. Thus, the apparent V_D is a useful parameter in considering the relative amounts of drug in the vascular and in the extravascular tissues.

Pharmacologists often attempt to conceptualize the apparent V_D as a true physiologic or anatomic fluid compartment. By expressing the V_D in terms of percent of body weight, values for the V_D may be found that appear to correspond to true anatomic volumes. However, it may be only fortuitous that the value for the apparent V_D of a drug has the same value as a real anatomic volume. If a drug is to be considered to be distributed in a true physiologic volume, then an investigation is needed to test this hypothesis.

Table 5.3: Fluid in the Body

Water Compartment	Percent of Body Weight	Percent of Total Body Water
Plasma	4.5	7.5
Total extracellular water	27.0	45.0
Total intracellular water	33.0	55.0
Total body water	60.0	100.0

Given the apparent V_D for a particular drug, the total amount of drug in the body at any time after administration of the drug may be determined by the measurement of the drug concentration in the plasma (eq. 3.5). Because the magnitude of the apparent V_D is a useful indicator for the amount of drug outside the sampling compartment (usually the blood), the larger the apparent V_D, the greater the amount of drug in the extravascular tissues.

For each drug, the apparent V_D is a constant. In certain pathologic cases, the apparent V_D for the drug may be altered if the distribution of the drug is changed. For example, in edematous conditions, the total body water and total extracellular water increase; this is reflected in a larger apparent V_D value for a drug that is highly water soluble. Similarly, changes in total body weight and lean body mass (which normally occur with age) may also affect the apparent V_D.

- **Clearance**

Clearance is a measure of drug elimination from the body without identifying the mechanism or process. Clearance (drug clearance, systemic clearance, total body clearance, Cl_T) considers the entire body as a drug-eliminating system from which many elimination processes may occur.

➤ **Drug clearance in the one-compartment model**

The body is considered as a system of organs perfused by plasma and body fluids. Drug elimination from the body is an ongoing process due to both metabolism (biotransformation) and drug excretion through the kidney and other routes. The mechanisms of drug elimination are complex, but collectively drug elimination from the body may be quantitated using the concept of drug clearance. Drug clearance refers to the volume of plasma fluid that is cleared of drug per unit time. Clearance may also be considered as the fraction of drug removed per unit time multiplied by the V_D. The rate of drug elimination may be expressed in several ways, each of which essentially describes the same process, but with different levels of insight and application in pharmacokinetics.

➢ **Drug elimination expressed as amount per time unit**

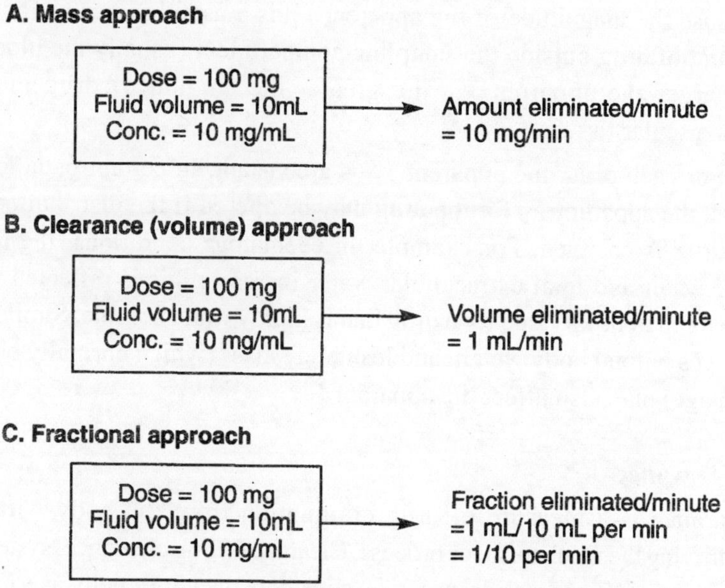

A. Mass approach

Dose = 100 mg
Fluid volume = 10mL
Conc. = 10 mg/mL ⟶ Amount eliminated/minute = 10 mg/min

B. Clearance (volume) approach

Dose = 100 mg
Fluid volume = 10mL
Conc. = 10 mg/mL ⟶ Volume eliminated/minute = 1 mL/min

C. Fractional approach

Dose = 100 mg
Fluid volume = 10mL
Conc. = 10 mg/mL ⟶ Fraction eliminated/minute = 1 mL/10 mL per min = 1/10 per min

Fig. 5.14: Diagram illustrating three different ways of describing drug elimination after a dose of 100 mg injected IV into a volume of 10 mL (a mouse, for example).

The expression of drug elimination from the body in terms of mass per unit time (eg, mg/min, or mg/hr) is simple, absolute, and unambiguous.

For a zero-order elimination process, expressing the rate of drug elimination as mass per unit time is convenient because the rate is constant. In contrast, the rate of drug elimination for a first-order elimination process is not constant and changes with respect to the drug concentration in the body. For a first-order elimination, drug clearance expressed as volume per unit time (eg, L/hr or mL/min) is convenient because it is a constant.

➢ Drug elimination expressed as volume per time unit

The concept of expressing a rate in terms of volume per unit time is common in pharmacy. For example, a patient may be dosed at the rate of 2 teaspoonsful (10 mL) of a liquid medicine (10 mg/mL) daily, or alternatively, a dose (weight) of 100 mg of the drug daily.

Clearance is a concept that expresses "the rate of drug removal" in terms of volume of drug solution removed per unit time (at whatever drug concentration in the body prevailing at that time). In contrast to a solution in a bottle, the drug concentration in the body will gradually decline by a first-order process such that the mass of drug removed over time is not constant. The plasma volume in the healthy state is relatively constant because water lost through the kidney is rapidly replaced with fluid absorbed from the gastrointestinal tract.

Since a constant volume of plasma (about 120 mL/min in humans) is filtered through the glomeruli of the kidneys, the rate of drug removal is dependent on the plasma drug concentration at all times. This observation is based on a first-order process governing drug elimination. For many drugs, the rate of drug elimination is dependent on the plasma drug concentration, multiplied by a constant factor ($dC/dt = kC$). When the plasma drug concentration is high, the rate of drug removal is high, and vice versa.

Clearance (volume of fluid removed of drug) for a first-order process is constant regardless of the drug concentration because clearance is expressed in volume per unit time rather than drug amount per unit time. Mathematically, the rate of drug elimination is similar to equation 5.48:

$$\frac{dD_B}{dt} = -KC_P V_D \qquad \qquad ...(5.53)$$

Dividing this expression on both sides by C_p yields Equation 5.54:

$$\frac{dD_B / dt}{C_P} = \frac{-KC_P V_D}{C_P} \qquad \qquad ...(5.54)$$

$$\frac{dD_B / dt}{C_P} = -KV_D = -Cl \qquad \qquad ...(5.55)$$

Where dD_B/dt is the rate of drug elimination from the body (mg/hr), C_p is the plasma drug concentration (mg/L), k is a first-order rate constant (hr^{-1} or 1/hr), and V_D is the apparent volume of distribution (L). Cl is clearance and has the units L/hr in this example. In the example in, Cl is in mL/min.

Clearance, Cl, is expressed as volume/time. Equation 5.55 shows that clearance is a constant because V_D and k are both constants. D_B is the amount of drug in the body, and dD_B/dt is the rate of change (of amount) of drug in the body with respect to time. The negative sign refers to the drug exiting from the body.

➢ Drug elimination expressed as fraction eliminated per time unit

Consider a compartment volume, containing V_D liters. If Cl is expressed in liters per minute (L/min), then the fraction of drug cleared per minute in the body is equal to Cl/V_D.

Expressing drug elimination as the fraction of total drug eliminated is applicable regardless of whether one is dealing with an amount or a volume. This approach is most flexible and convenient because of its dimensionless nature. Thus, it is valid to express drug elimination as a fraction (e.g., one-tenth of the amount of drug in the body is eliminated or one-tenth of the drug volume is eliminated). Pharmacokineticists have incorporated this concept into the first-order equation (i.e., k) that describes drug elimination from the one-compartment model. Indeed, the universal nature of many processes forms the basis of the first-order equation of drug elimination (eg, a fraction of the total drug molecules in the body will perfuse the glomeruli, a fraction of the filtered drug molecules will be reabsorbed at the renal tubules, and a fraction of the filtered drug molecules will be excreted from the body giving an overall first-order drug elimination rate constant, k). The rate of drug elimination is the product of k and the drug concentration (eq. 5.53). The first-order equation of drug elimination can be also based on probability and a consideration of the statistical moment theory.

➢ **Clearance and volume of distribution ratio, Cl/v$_d$**

o **Example**

Consider that 100 mg of drug is dissolved in 10 mL of fluid and 10 mg of drug is removed in the first minute. The drug elimination process could be described as:

    a. Number of mg of drug eliminated per minute (mg/min)

    b. Number of mL of fluid cleared of drug per minute

    c. Fraction of drug eliminated per minute

The relationship of the three drug elimination processes is illustrated in. Note that in, the fraction Cl/V_D is dependent on both the volume of distribution and the rate of drug clearance from the body. This clearance concept forms the basis of classical pharmacokinetics and is later extended to flow models in pharmacokinetic modeling. If the drug concentration is C_p, the rate of drug elimination (in terms of rate of change in concentration, dC_p/dt) is:

$$\frac{dC_P}{dt} = -\left(\frac{Cl}{V_D}\right) \times C_P \qquad \ldots (5.56)$$

For a first-order process,

$$\frac{dC_P}{dt} = -KC_P = \text{rate of drug administration} \qquad \ldots (5.57)$$

Equating the two expressions yields:

$$KC_P = \frac{Cl}{V_D} \times C_P \qquad \ldots (5.58)$$

$$K = \frac{Cl}{V_D} \qquad \ldots (5.59)$$

Thus, a first-order rate constant is the fractional constant Cl/V_D. Some pharmacokineticists regard drug clearance and the volume of distribution as independent parameters that are necessary to describe the time course of drug elimination. Equation 5.59 is a rearrangement of equation 5.55 given earlier.

➤ One-compartment model equation in terms of cl and v_d

Equation 5.60 may be rewritten in terms of clearance and volume of distribution by substituting Cl/V_D for k. The clearance concept may also be applied a biologic system in physiologic modeling without the need of a theoretical compartment.

$$C_P = C_P^{0-Kt} \qquad \ldots (5.60)$$

$$C_P = D_0/V_D e^{-\left(\frac{Cl}{V_D}\right)t} \qquad \ldots (5.61)$$

Equation 5.61 is applied directly in clinical pharmacy to determine clearance and volume of distribution in patients. When only one sample is available, ie, C_p is known at one sample time point, t after a given dose, the equation cannot be determined unambiguously because two unknown parameters must be solved, ie, Cl and V_D. In practice, the mean values for Cl and V_D of a drug are obtained from the population values (derived from a large population of subjects or patients) in the literature. The values of Cl and V_D for the patient are adjusted using a computer program. Ultimately, a new pair of Cl and V_D values that better fit the observed plasma drug concentration is found. The process is repeated through iterations until the "best" parameters are obtained. Since many mathematical techniques (algorithms) are available for iteration, different results may be obtained using different iterative programs. An objective test to determine the accuracy of the estimated clearance and V_D values is to monitor how accurately those parameters will predict the plasma level of the drug after a new dose is given to the patient. In subsequent chapters, mean predictive error will be discussed and calculated in order to determine the performance of various drug monitoring methods in practice.

The ratio of Cl/V_D may be calculated regardless of compartment model type using minimal plasma samples. Clinical pharmacists have applied many variations of this approach to therapeutic drug monitoring and drug dosage adjustments in patients.

➢ Clearance from drug-eliminating tissues

Clearance may be applied to any organ that is involved in drug elimination from the body. As long as first-order elimination processes are involved, clearance represents the sum of the clearances for each drug-eliminating organ as shown in equation 5.62:

$$Cl_T = Cl_R + Cl_{NR} \qquad \qquad ... (5.62)$$

Where Cl_R is renal clearance or drug clearance through the kidney, and Cl_{NR} is nonrenal clearance through other organs. Generally, clearance is considered as the sum of renal, Cl_R, and nonrenal drug clearance, Cl_{NR}. Cl_{NR} is assumed to be due primarily to hepatic clearance (Cl_H) in the absence of other significant drug clearances, such as elimination through the lung or the bile, as shown in equation 5.63:

$$Cl_T = Cl_R + Cl_H \qquad \qquad ... (5.63)$$

Drug clearance considers that the drug in the body is uniformly dissolved in a volume of fluid (apparent volume of distribution, V_D) from which drug concentrations can be measured easily. Typically, plasma fluid concentration is measured and drug clearance is then calculated as the fixed volume of plasma fluid (containing the drug) cleared of drug per unit of time. The units for clearance are volume/time (eg, mL/min, L/hr).

Alternatively, Cl_T may be defined as the rate of drug elimination divided by the plasma drug concentration. Thus, clearance is expressed in terms of the volume of plasma containing drug that is eliminated per unit time. This clearance definition is equivalent to the previous definition and provides a practical way to calculate clearance based on plasma drug concentration data.

$$Cl_T = \frac{\text{elimination rate}}{\text{plasma concentration } (C_P)} \qquad \text{... (5.64)}$$

$$Cl_T = \frac{(dD_E / dt)}{C_P} = (\mu g / min) / (\mu g / mL) = mL / min$$

$$\text{... (5.65)}$$

Where D_E is the amount of drug eliminated and dD_E/dt is the rate of drug elimination.

Rearrangement of equation 5.65 gives equation 5.66:

$$\text{Drug elimination rate} = \frac{dD_E}{dt} \qquad \text{... (5.66)}$$

Therefore Cl_T is a constant for a specific drug and represents the slope of the line obtained by plotting dD_E/dt versus C_p, as shown in equation 5.66.

For drugs that follow first-order elimination, the rate of drug

$$\frac{dD_E}{dt} = KD_B = KC_P V_D \qquad \text{... (5.67)}$$

elimination is dependent on the amount of drug remaining in the body.

Substituting the elimination rate in equation 5.66 for kC_pV_D in equation 5.67 and solving for Cl_T gives equation 5.68:

$$Cl_T = \frac{KC_P V_D}{C_P} KV_D \qquad \text{... (5.68)}$$

Equation 5.68 shows that clearance, Cl_T, is the product of V_D and k, both of which are constant. This equation 5.68 is similar to equation 5.59 shown earlier. As the plasma drug concentration decreases during elimination, the rate of drug elimination, dD_E/dt, will decrease accordingly, but clearance will remain constant. Clearance will be constant as long as the rate of drug elimination is a first-order process.

For some drugs, the elimination rate process is more complex and a noncompartment method may be used to calculate certain pharmacokinetic parameters such as clearance. In this case, clearance can be determined directly from the plasma drug concentration-versus-time curve by

$$Cl_T = \frac{D_0}{[AUC]_0^\infty} \qquad \qquad ... (5.69)$$

Where D_0 is the dose and $[AUC]_0^\infty = \int_0^\infty C_p dt$

Because $[AUC]_0^\infty$ is calculated from the plasma drug concentration-versus-time curve from 0 to infinity (∞) using the trapezoidal rule, no compartmental model is assumed. However, to extrapolate the data to infinity to obtain the residual $[AUC]_0^\infty$ or ($C_p t/k$), first-order elimination is usually assumed. In this case, if the drug follows the kinetics of a one-compartment model, the Cl_T is numerically similar to the product of V_D and k obtained by fitting the data to a one-compartment model.

- **Calculation of k from urinary excretion data**

The elimination rate constant k may be calculated from urinary excretion data. In this calculation the excretion rate of the drug is assumed to be first order. The term k_e is the renal excretion rate constant, and D_u is the amount of drug excreted in the urine.

$$\frac{dD_u}{dt} = K_e D_B \qquad \qquad ... (5.70)$$

From Equation 5.70, D_B can be substituted for $D_B^0 e^{-kt}$:

$$\frac{dD_u}{dt} = K_e D_B^0 e^{-Kt} \qquad \qquad \ldots (5.71)$$

Taking the natural logarithm of both sides and then transforming to common logarithms, the following expression is obtained:

$$\log \frac{dD_u}{dt} = \frac{-Kt}{2.3} + \log K_e D_B^0 \qquad \qquad \ldots (5.72)$$

A straight line is obtained from this equation by plotting $\log dD_u/dt$ vs time on regular paper or on semilog paper dD_u/dt against time (and). The slope of this curve is equal to $-k/2.3$ and the y intercept is equal to $k_e D_B^0$. For rapid intravenous administration, D_B^0 is equal to the dose D_0. Therefore, if D_B^0 is known, the renal excretion rate constant (k_e) can be obtained. Because both k_e and k can be determined by this method, the nonrenal rate constant (k_{nr}) for any route of elimination other than renal excretion can be found as follows:

$$K - K_e = K_{nr} \qquad \qquad \ldots (5.73)$$

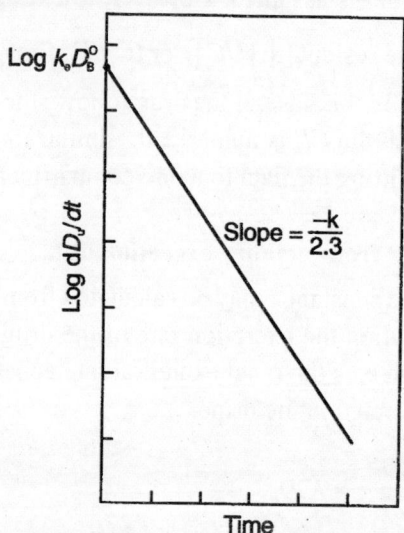

Fig. 5.15: Graph of equation 5.72: log rate of drug excretion versus *t* on regular paper.

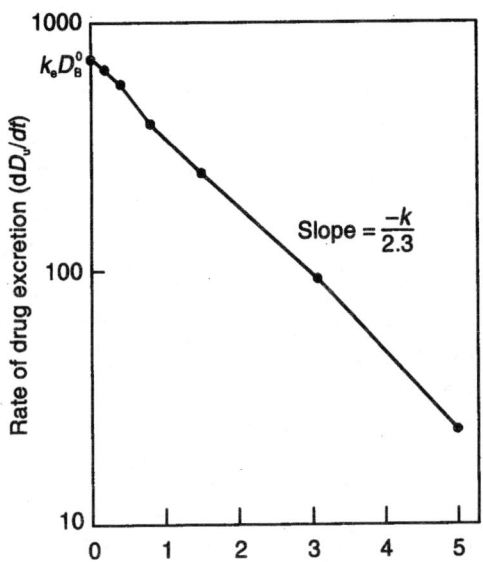

Fig. 5.16: Semilog graph of rate of drug excretion versus time according to equation 5.72 on semilog paper (intercept = $k_e D_B^0$).

Substitution of k_m for k_{nr} in equation 5.73 gives Equation 5.39. Because the major routes of elimination for most drugs are renal excretion and metabolism (biotransformation), k_{nr} is approximately equal to k_m.

$$K_{nr} = K_m \qquad \qquad \text{... (5.74)}$$

The drug urinary excretion rate (dD_u/dt) cannot be determined experimentally for any given instant. Therefore, the average rate of urinary drug excretion, D_u/t is plotted against the average time, t^*, for the collection of the urine sample. In practice, urine is collected over a specified time interval, and the urine specimen is analyzed for drug. An average urinary excretion rate is then calculated for that collection period. The average value of dD_u/dt is plotted on a semilogarithmic scale against the time that corresponds to the midpoint (average time) of the collection period.

One compartment open model: intravenous infusion

Drugs may be administered to patients by one of several routes, including oral, topical, or parenteral routes of administration. Examples of parenteral routes of administration include intravenous, subcutaneous, and intramuscular. Intravenous (IV) drug solutions may be given either as a bolus dose (injected all at once) or infused slowly through a vein into the plasma at a constant or zero-order rate. The main advantage for giving a drug by IV infusion is that IV infusion allows precise control of plasma drug concentrations to fit the individual needs of the patient. For drugs with a narrow therapeutic window (eg, heparin), IV infusion maintains an effective constant plasma drug concentration by eliminating wide fluctuations between the peak (maximum) and trough (minimum) plasma drug concentration. Moreover, the IV infusion of drugs, such as antibiotics, may be given with IV fluids that include electrolytes and nutrients. Furthermore, the duration of drug therapy may be maintained or terminated as needed using IV infusion.

The plasma drug concentration-versus-time curve of a drug given by constant IV infusion is shown in. Because no drug was present in the body at zero time, drug level rises from zero drug concentration and gradually becomes constant when a plateau or steady-state drug concentration is reached. At steady state, the rate of drug leaving the body is equal to the rate of drug (infusion rate) entering the body. Therefore, at steady state, the rate of change in the plasma drug concentration, $dC_p/dt = 0$, and

Rate of drug input = rate of drug output

(Infusion rate)   (Elimination rate)

Based on this simple mass balance relationship, a pharmacokinetic equation for infusion may be derived depending on whether the drug follows one- or two-compartment kinetics.

• One-compartment model drugs

The pharmacokinetics of a drug given by constant IV infusion follows a zero-order input process in which the drug is infused directly into the systemic blood circulation. Equation 5.76, below, gives the plasma drug

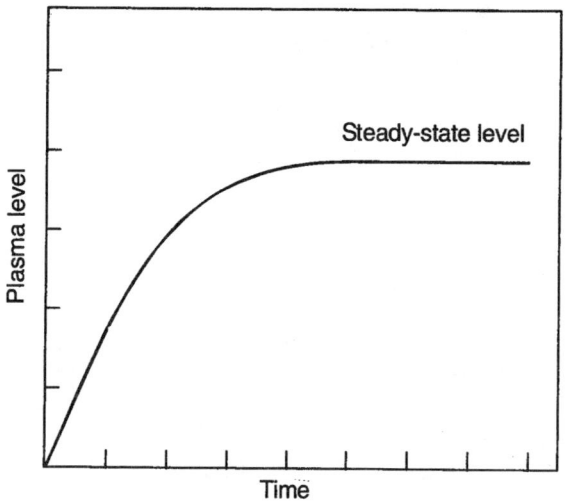

Fig. 5.17: Plasma level–time curve for constant IV infusion.

concentration at any time during the IV infusion, where t is the time for infusion. The graph of equation 5.76 appears in. For most drugs, elimination of drug from the plasma is a first-order process. Therefore, in this one-compartment model, the infused drug follows zero-order input and first-order output. The change in the amount of drug in the body at any time (dD_B/dt) during the infusion is the rate of input minus the rate of output.

$$\frac{dD_B}{dt} = R - KD_B \qquad \text{... (5.75)}$$

Where D_B is the amount of drug in the body, R is the infusion rate (zero order), and k is the elimination rate constant (first order).

Integration of equation 5.75 and substitution of $D_B = C_p V_D$ gives

$$C_P = \frac{R}{V_D^K}\left(1 - e^{-Kt}\right) \qquad \text{... (5.76)}$$

As the drug is infused, the value for time (t) increases in equation 5.76. At infinite time, $t = \infty$, e^{-kt} approaches zero, and equation 5.76 reduces

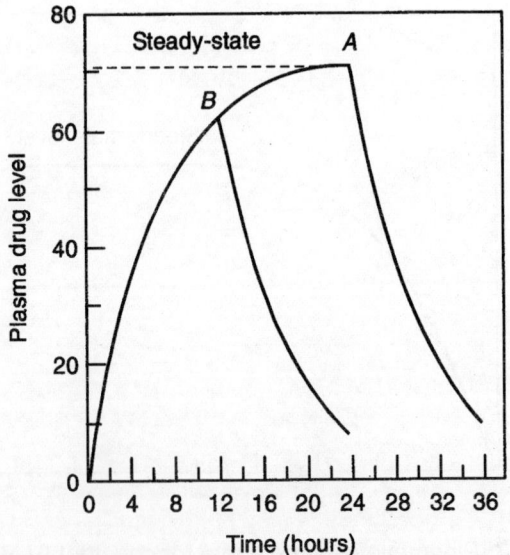

Fig. 5.18: Plasma drug concentrations versus time profiles after IV infusion. IV infusion is stopped at steady state (A) or prior to steady state (B). In both cases, plasma drug concentrations decline exponentially (first order) according to a similar slope.

to equation 5.78.

$$C_P = \frac{R}{V_D^K}\left(1 - e^{\infty}\right) \qquad \text{... (5.77)}$$

$$C_{SS} = \frac{R}{V_D^K} \qquad \text{... (5.78)}$$

$$C_{SS} = \frac{R}{V_D^K} = \frac{R}{Cl} \qquad \text{... (5.79)}$$

- **Steady-state drug concentration (c_{ss}) and time needed to reach c_{ss}**

As stated earlier, the rate of drug leaving the body is equal to the rate of drug entering the body (infusion rate) at steady state. In other words, there is no net change in the amount of drug in the body, D_B, as a function of time during steady state. Drug elimination occurs according to first-order elimination rate. Whenever the infusion stops either at steady state or before steady state is reached, the log drug concentration declines according to first-order kinetics with the slope of the elimination curve equal to $-k/2.3$. If the infusion is stopped before steady state is reached, the slope of the elimination curve remains the same.

Mathematically, the time to reach true steady-state drug concentration, C_{SS}, would take an infinite time. The time required to reach the steady-state drug concentration in the plasma is dependent on the elimination rate constant of the drug for a constant volume of distribution, as shown in Equation 5.78. Because drug elimination is exponential (first order), the plasma drug concentration becomes asymptotic to the theoretical steady-state plasma drug concentration. For a zero-order elimination process, if the rate of input is greater than the rate of elimination, plasma drug concentration will keep increasing and no steady state will be reached. This is a potentially dangerous situation that will occur when saturation of metabolic process occurs.

In clinical practice, a plasma drug concentration prior to, but asymptotically approaching, the theoretical steady state is considered the steady-state plasma drug concentration (C_{SS}). In a constant IV infusion, drug solution is infused at a constant or zero-order rate, R. During the IV infusion, the drug concentration increases in the plasma and the rate of drug elimination increases because rate of elimination is concentration dependent (i.e., rate of drug elimination = kC_p). C_p keeps increasing until steady state is reached, at which time the rate of drug input (IV infusion rate) equals the rate of drug output (elimination rate). The resulting plasma drug concentration at steady state (C_{SS}) is related to the rate of infusion and inversely related to the body clearance of the drug, as shown in Equation 5.79.

In clinical practice, the activity of the drug will be observed when the drug concentration is close to the desired plasma drug concentration, which is usually the target or desired steady-state drug concentration.

The time to reach 90%, 95%, and 99% of the steady-state drug concentration, C_{ss}, may be calculated. For therapeutic purposes, the time for the plasma drug concentration to reach more than 95% of the steady-state drug concentration in the plasma is often estimated. As detailed in, after IV infusion of the drug for 5 half-lives, the plasma drug concentration will be between 95% ($4.32t_{1/2}$) and 99% ($6.65t_{1/2}$) of the steady-state drug concentration. Thus, the time for a drug whose $t_{1/2}$ is 6 hours to reach at least 95% of the steady-state plasma drug concentration will be $5t_{1/2}$, or 5×6 hours = 30 hours. The calculation of the values in is given in the example that follows.

Table 5.4: Number of $t_{1/2}$ to reach a fraction of c_{ss}

Percent of C_{ss} Reached	Number of Half-Lives
90	3.32
95	4.32
99	6.65

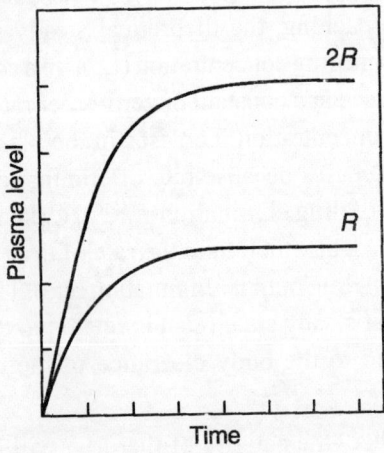

Fig. 5.19: Plasma level–time curve for IV infusions given at rates of R and $2R$, respectively.

An increase in the infusion rate will not shorten the time to reach the steady-state drug concentration. If the drug is given at a more rapid infusion rate, a higher steady-state drug level will be obtained, but the time to reach steady state is the same. This equation may also be obtained with the following approach. At steady state, the rate of infusion equals the rate of elimination. Therefore, the rate of change in the plasma drug concentration is equal to zero.

$$\frac{dC_P}{dt} = 0$$

$$\frac{dC_P}{dt} = \frac{R}{V_D} - KC_P = 0$$

$$(\text{Rate}_{in}) - (\text{rate}_{out}) = 0$$

$$\frac{R}{V_D} = KC_P$$

$$C_{SS} = \frac{R}{V_D^K} \qquad \qquad \text{... (5.80)}$$

Equation 5.80 shows that the steady-state concentration (C_{SS}) is dependent on the volume of distribution, the elimination rate constant, and the infusion rate. Altering any one of these factors can affect steady-state concentration.

• Infusion method for calculating patient elimination half-life

The C_P-versus-time relationship that occurs during an IV infusion (eq. 5.76) may be used to calculate k, or indirectly the elimination half-life of the drug in a patient. Some information about the elimination half-life of the drug in the population must be known, and one or two plasma samples must be taken at a known time after infusion. Knowing the half-life in the general population helps to determine if the sample is taken at steady state in the patient. To simplify calculation, Equation 5.76 is arranged to solve for k:

$$C_P = \frac{R}{V_D^K}\left(1 - e^{-Kt}\right) \qquad \ldots (5.76)$$

Since,

$$C_{SS} = \frac{R}{V_D^K}$$

Substituting into Equation 5.76;

$$C_P = C_{SS}\left(1 - e^{-Kt}\right)$$

Rearranging and taking the log on both sides,

$$\log\left(\frac{C_{SS} - C_P}{C_{SS}}\right) = -\frac{Kt}{2.3} \text{ and } K = \frac{-2.3}{t}\log\left(\frac{C_{SS} - C_P}{C_{SS}}\right) \quad \ldots (5.81)$$

Where C_p is the plasma drug concentration taken at time t; C_{SS} is the approximate steady-state plasma drug concentration in the patient.

• Loading dose plus iv infusion: one-compartment model

The loading dose, D_L, or initial bolus dose of a drug, is used to obtain desired concentrations as rapidly as possible. The concentration of drug in the body for a one-compartment model after an IV bolus dose is described by:

$$C_1 = C_0 e^{-Kt} = \frac{D_L}{V_D}e^{-Kt} \qquad \ldots (5.82)$$

and concentration by infusion at the rate R is

$$C_2 = \frac{D_L}{V_D}e^{-Kt} \qquad \ldots (5.83)$$

Assume that an IV bolus dose D_L of the drug is given and that an IV infusion is started at the same time. The total concentration C_p at t hours after the start of infusion is $C_1 + C_2$, due to the sum contributions of bolus and infusion, or

$$C_P = C_1 + C_2$$

$$C_P = \frac{D_L}{V_D}e^{-Kt} + \frac{R}{V_D K}\left(1 - e^{-Kt}\right)$$

$$C_P = \frac{D_L}{V_D}e^{-Kt} + \frac{R}{V_D K} - \frac{R}{V_D K}e^{-Kt}$$

$$C_P = \frac{R}{V_D K} + \left(\frac{D_L}{V_D}e^{-Kt} - \frac{R}{V_D K}e^{-Kt}\right) \qquad \text{... (5.84)}$$

Let the loading dose (D_L) equal the amount of drug in the body at steady state:

$$D_L = C_{SS}V_D$$

From equation 5.78, $C_{SS}V_D = R/k$. Therefore,

$$D_L = \frac{R}{K} \qquad \text{... (5.85)}$$

Substituting $D_L = R/k$ in Equation 5.11 makes the expression in parentheses in equation 5.84 cancel out. equation 5.84 reduces to equation 5.86, which is the same expression for C_{SS} or steady-state plasma concentration:

$$C_P = \frac{R}{V_D K} \qquad \text{... (5.86)}$$

$$C_{SS} = \frac{R}{V_D K} \qquad \text{... (5.87)}$$

Therefore, if an IV loading dose of R/k is given, followed by an IV infusion, steady-state plasma drug concentrations are obtained immediately and maintained. In this situation, steady state is also achieved in a one-compartment model, since rate in = rate out ($R = dD_B/dt$).

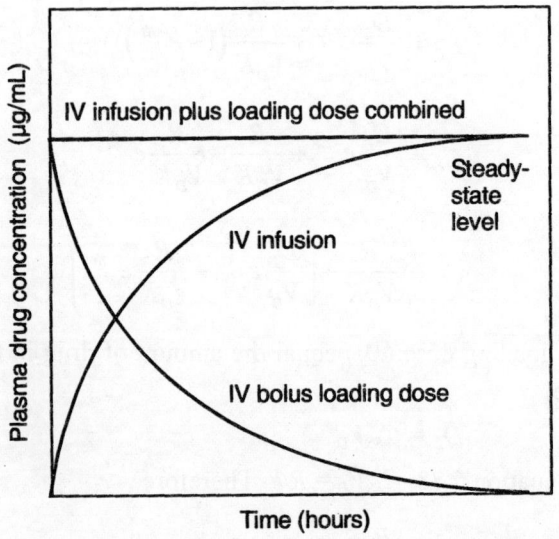

Fig. 5.20: IV Infusion with loading dose D_L. The loading dose is given by IV bolus injection at the start of the infusion. Plasma drug concentrations decline exponentially after D_L whereas they increase exponentially during the infusion. The resulting plasma drug concentration-versus-time curve is a straight line due to the summation of the two curves.

The loading dose needed to get immediate steady-state drug levels can also be found by the following approach.

Loading dose equation:

$$C_1 = \frac{D_L}{V_D} e^{-Kt}$$

Infusion equation:

$$C_2 = \frac{R}{V_D K}\left(1 - e^{-Kt}\right)$$

Adding up the two equations yields equation 5.88, an equation describing simultaneous infusion after a loading dose:

$$C_2 = \frac{R}{V_D K}\left(1 - e^{-Kt}\right)$$

$$C_2 = \frac{D_L}{V_D}e^{-Kt} + \frac{R}{V_D K}\left(1 - e^{-Kt}\right) \qquad \ldots (5.88)$$

By differentiating this equation at steady state, we obtain

$$\frac{dC_P}{dt} = 0 = \frac{-D_L K}{V_D}e^{-Kt} + \frac{RK}{V_D K}e^{-Kt} \qquad \ldots (5.89)$$

$$0 = e^{-Kt}\left(\frac{-D_L K}{V_D} + \frac{RK}{V_D K}\right)$$

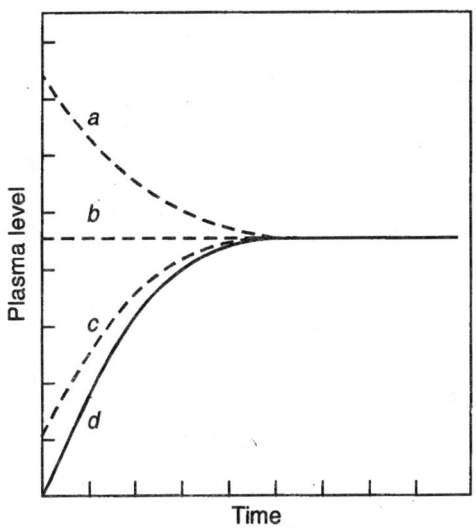

Fig. 5.21: Intravenous infusion with loading doses a, b, and c. Curve d represents an IV infusion without a loading dose.

$$\frac{D_L K}{V_D} + \frac{R}{V_D} \qquad \qquad \text{... (5.90)}$$

$$D_L = \frac{R}{K} = \text{ loading dose}$$

In order to maintain instant steady-state level $[(dC_p/dt) = 0]$, the loading dose should be equal to R/k.

For a one-compartment drug, if the D_L and infusion rate are calculated such that C_0 and C_{SS} are the same and both D_L and infusion are started concurrently, then steady state and C_{SS} will be achieved immediately after the loading dose is administered. Similarly, in, curve b shows the blood level after a single loading dose of R/k plus infusion from which the concentration desired at steady state is obtained. If the D_L is not equal to R/k, then steady state will not occur immediately. If the loading dose given is larger than R/k, the plasma drug concentration takes longer to decline to the concentration desired at steady state (curve a). If the loading dose is lower than R/k, the plasma drug concentrations will increase slowly to desired drug levels (curve c), but more quickly than without any loading dose.

Another method for the calculation of loading dose D_L is based on knowledge of the desired steady-state drug concentration C_{SS} and the apparent volume of distribution V_D for the drug, as shown in equation 5.91.

$$D_L = C_{SS} V_D \qquad \qquad \text{... (5.91)}$$

For many drugs, the desired C_{SS} is reported in the literature as the effective therapeutic drug concentration. The V_D and the elimination half-life are also available for these drugs.

• Estimation of drug clearance and v_d from infusion data

The plasma concentration of a drug during constant infusion was described in terms of volume of distribution and elimination constant k in equation 5.76. Alternatively, the equation may be described in terms of clearance by substituting for k into equation 5.76 with $k = Cl/V_D$.

$$C_P = \frac{R}{Cl} = \left(1 - e^{-\left(\frac{Cl}{V_D}\right)t}\right) \qquad \dots (5.92)$$

The drug concentration in this physiologic model is described in terms of volume of distribution of V_D and total body clearance (Cl). The independent parameters are clearance and volume of distribution; k is viewed as a dependent variable that depends on Cl and V_D. In this model, the time to reach steady state and the resulting steady-state concentration will be dependent on both clearance and volume of distribution. When a constant volume of distribution is evident, the time to reach steady state is then inversely related to clearance. Thus, drugs with small clearance will take a long time to reach steady state. Although this newer approach is preferred by some clinical pharmacists, the alternative approach to parameter estimation was known for some time in classical pharmacokinetics. Equation 5.92 has been applied in population pharmacokinetics to estimate both Cl and V_D in individual patients with one or more data points. However, clearance in patients may differ greatly from subjects in the population, especially subjects with different renal functions. Unfortunately, the plasma samples taken at time equivalent to less than one half-life after infusion was started may not be very discriminating, due to the small change in the drug concentration. Blood samples taken at 3–4 half-lives later are much more reflective of the difference in clearance.

One compartment open model: extravascular administration

The pharmacokinetics of drugs following intravenous drug administration are more simple to model compared to extravascular delivery. Extravascular delivery routes, particularly oral dosing, are important and popular means of drug administration. Unlike intravenous administration, in which the drug is injected directly into the plasma, pharmacokinetic models after extravascular drug administration must consider systemic drug absorption from the site of administration, eg, the lung, the gut, etc., into the plasma. Extravascular drug delivery is further complicated by variables at the absorption site, including possible drug degradation and significant inter- and intrapatient differences in the rate and extent of absorption. Absorption and metabolic variables are characterized using pharmacokinetic methods. The variability in systemic drug absorption can be minimized to some extent by proper biopharmaceutical design of the dosage form to provide predictable and reliable drug therapy. The major advantage of intravenous administration is that the rate and extent of systemic drug input is carefully controlled.

The systemic drug absorption from the gastrointestinal (GI) tract or from any other extravascular site is dependent on (1) the physicochemical properties of the drug, (2) the dosage form used, and (3) the anatomy and physiology of the absorption site. Although this chapter will focus primarily on oral dosing, the concepts discussed here may be easily extrapolated to other extravascular routes. For oral dosing, such factors as surface area of the GI tract, stomach-emptying rate, GI mobility, and blood flow to the absorption site all affect the rate and the extent of drug absorption. In pharmacokinetics, the overall rate of drug absorption may be described as either a first-order or zero-order input process. Most pharmacokinetic models assume first-order absorption unless an assumption of zero-order absorption improves the model significantly or has been verified experimentally.

The rate of change in the amount of drug in the body, dD_B/dt, is dependent on the relative rates of drug absorption and elimination. The net rate of drug accumulation in the body at any time is equal to the rate of drug absorption less the rate of drug elimination, regardless of whether absorption is zero-order or first-order.

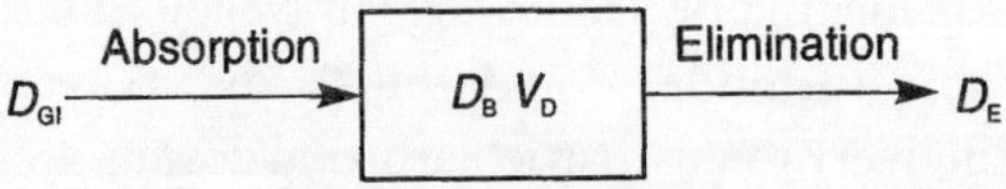

Fig. 5.22: Model of drug absorption and elimination.

$$\frac{dD_B}{dt} = \frac{dD_{GI}}{dt} - \frac{dD_E}{dt}$$

$$... (5.93)$$

Where D_{GI} is amount of drug in the gastrointestinal tract and D_E is amount of drug eliminated. A plasma level–time curve showing drug adsorption and elimination rate processes is given in. During the absorption phase of a plasma level–time curve, the rate of drug absorption is greater than the rate of drug elimination. Note that during the absorption phase, elimination occurs whenever drug is present in the plasma, even though absorption predominates.

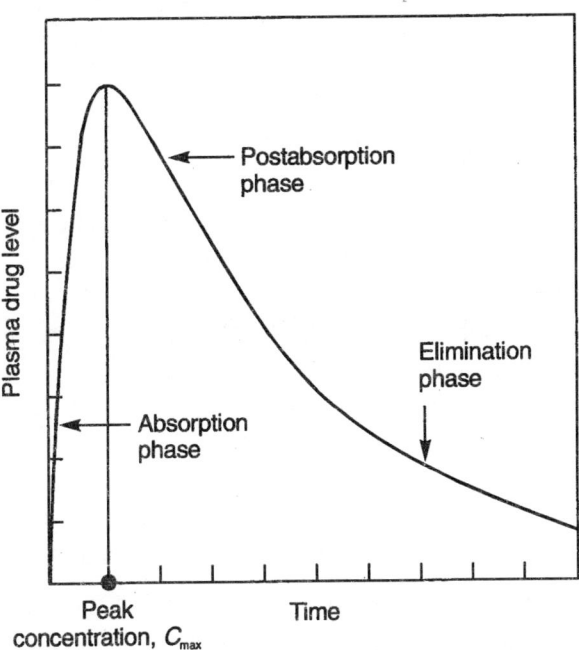

Fig. 5.23: Plasma level–time curve for a drug given in a single oral dose. The drug absorption and elimination phases of the curve are shown.

$$\frac{dD_{GI}}{dt} > \frac{dD_E}{dt}$$

... (5.94)

At the peak drug concentration in the plasma the rate of drug absorption just equals the rate of drug elimination, and there is no net change in the amount of drug in the body.

$$\frac{dD_{GI}}{dt} = \frac{dD_E}{dt} \qquad \qquad ... (5.95)$$

Immediately after the time of peak drug absorption, some drug may still be at the absorption site (ie, in the *GI* tract or other site of administration). However, the rate of drug elimination at this time is faster than the rate of absorption, as represented by the post absorption phase in.

$$\frac{dD_{GI}}{dt} < \frac{dD_E}{dt} \qquad \qquad ... (5.96)$$

When the drug at the absorption site becomes depleted, the rate of drug absorption approaches zero, or $dD_{GI}/dt = 0$. The plasma level–time curve (now the elimination phase) then represents only the elimination of drug from the body, usually a first-order process. Therefore, during the elimination phase the rate of change in the amount of drug in the body is described as a first-order process,

$$\frac{dD_B}{dt} = -KD_B \qquad \qquad ... (5.97)$$

Where, k is the first-order elimination rate constant.

• Zero-order absorption model

Zero-order drug absorption from the dosing site into the plasma usually occurs when either the drug is absorbed by a saturable process or a zero-order controlled-release delivery system is used. The pharmacokinetic model assuming zero-order absorption is described in. In this model, drug in the gastrointestinal tract, D_{GI}, is absorbed systemically at a constant rate, k_0. Drug is simultaneously and immediately eliminated from the body by a first-order rate process defined by a first-order rate constant, k. This model is analogous to that of the administration of a drug by intravenous infusion.

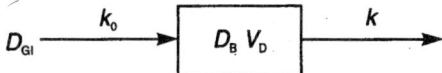

Fig. 5.24: One-compartment pharmacokinetic model for zero-order drug absorption and first-order drug elimination.

The rate of first-order elimination at any time is equal to $D_B k$. The rate of input is simply k_0. Therefore, the net change per unit time in the body can be expressed as:

$$\frac{dD_B}{dt} = K_0 - KD_B \qquad \qquad ... (5.98)$$

Integration of this equation with substitution of $V_D C_p$ for D_B produces:

$$C_P = \frac{K_0}{V_D K}\left(1 - e^{-Kt}\right) \qquad \qquad ... (5.99)$$

The rate of drug absorption is constant until the amount of drug in the gut, D_{GI}, is depleted. The time for complete drug absorption to occur is equal to D_{GI}/k_0. After this time, the drug is no longer available for absorption from the gut, and equation 5.99 no longer holds. The drug concentration in the plasma subsequently declines in accordance with a first-order elimination rate process.

● **First-order absorption model**

Although zero-order absorption can occur, absorption is usually assumed to be a first-order process. This model assumes a first-order input across the gut wall and first-order elimination from the body. This model applies mostly to the oral absorption of drugs in solution or rapidly dissolving dosage (immediate release) forms such as tablets, capsules, and suppositories. In addition, drugs given by intramuscular or subcutaneous aqueous injections may also be described using a first-order process.

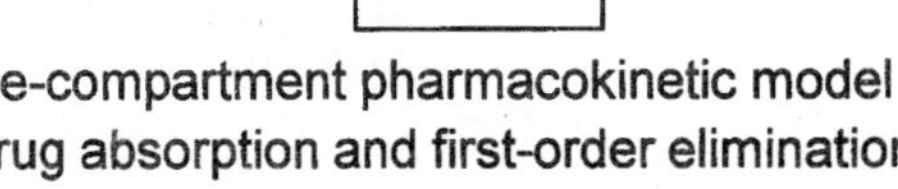

Fig. 5.25: One-compartment pharmacokinetic model for first-order drug absorption and first-order elimination.

In the case of a drug given orally, the dosage form first disintegrates if it is given as a solid, then the drug dissolves into the fluids of the GI tract. Only drug in solution is absorbed into the body. The rate of disappearance of drug from the gastrointestinal tract is described by:

$$\frac{dD_{GI}}{dt} = -K_a D_{GI} F \qquad \text{... (5.100)}$$

where k_a is the first-order absorption rate constant from the *GI* tract, F is the fraction absorbed, and D_{GI} is the amount of drug in solution in the *GI* tract at any time t. Integration of the differential equation (5.100) gives:

$$\frac{dD_{GI}}{dt} = D_0 e^{-K_2 t} \qquad \text{... (5.101)}$$

Where, D_0 is the dose of the drug.

The rate of drug elimination is described by a first-order rate process for most drugs and is equal to $-kD_B$. The rate of drug change in the body, dD $_B$/dt, is therefore the rate of drug in, minus the rate of drug out—as given by the differential equation, equation 5.102:

$$\frac{dD_B}{dt} = \text{rate in} - \text{rate out}$$

$$\frac{dD_B}{dt} = FK_a D_{GI} - KD_B \qquad \text{... (5.102)}$$

Where F is the fraction of drug absorbed systemically.

Since the drug in the gastrointestinal tract also follows a first-order decline (ie, the drug is absorbed across the gastrointestinal wall), the amount of drug in the gastrointestinal tract at any time t is equal to $D_0 e^{-k_a t}$.

$$\frac{dD_B}{dt} = FK_a D_0 e^{-K_2 t} - KD_B$$

The value of F may vary from 1 for a fully absorbed drug to 0 for a drug that is completely unabsorbed. This equation can be integrated to give the general oral absorption equation for calculation of the drug concentration (C_p) in the plasma at any time t, as shown below.

$$C_P = \frac{FK_1D_0}{V_D(K_a - K)}\left(e^{Kt} - e^{-K_a t}\right) \qquad ...(5.103)$$

A typical plot of the concentration of drug in the body after a single oral dose is presented in .

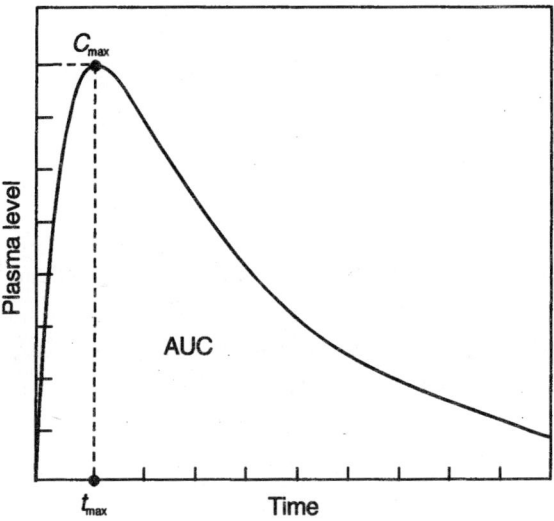

Fig. 5.26: Typical plasma level–time curve for a drug given in a single oral close.

The maximum plasma concentration after oral dosing is C_{max}, and the time needed to reach maximum concentration is t_{max}. The t_{max} is independent of dose and is dependent on the rate constants for absorption (k_a) and elimination (k) (eq. 5.106a). At C_{max}, sometimes called **peak concentration**, the rate of drug absorbed is equal to the rate of drug eliminated. Therefore, the net rate of concentration change is equal to zero. At C_{max}, the rate of concentration change can be obtained by differentiating equation 5.104, as follows:

$$dC_P/dt = \frac{FK_aD_0}{V_D(K_a - K)}\left(-Ke^{-Kt} + K_ae^{-K_at}\right) \qquad \text{... (5.104)}$$

This can be simplified as follows:

$$-Ke^{-Kt} + K_ae^{-K_at} = 0 \quad \text{or} \quad -Ke^{-Kt} + K_ae^{-K_at} \qquad \text{... (5.105)}$$

$$\ln K - Kt = \ln K_a - K_at$$

$$t_{max} = \frac{\ln K_a - \ln K}{K_a - K} = \frac{\ln\left(\dfrac{K_a}{K}\right)}{K_a - K}$$

$$t_{max} = \frac{2.3\log K_a / K}{K_a - K} \qquad \text{... (5.106)}$$

As shown in equation 5.106, the time for maximum drug concentration, t_{max}, is dependent only on the rate constants k_a and k. In order to calculate C_{max}, the value for t_{max} is determined via equation 5.106 and then substituted into equation 5.103, solving for C_{max}. Equation 5.103 shows that C_{max} is directly proportional to the dose of drug given (D_0) and the fraction of drug absorbed (F). Calculation of t_{max} and C_{max} is usually necessary, since direct measurement of the maximum drug concentration may not be possible due to improper timing of the serum samples.

The first-order elimination rate constant may be determined from the elimination phase of the plasma level–time curve. At later time intervals, when drug absorption has been completed, i.e., $e^{-k_at} \approx 0$, equation 5.103 reduces to:

$$C_P = \frac{FK_aD_0}{V_D(K_a - K)}e^{-Kt} \qquad \text{... (5.107)}$$

$$\ln C_P = \ln\frac{FK_aD_0}{V_D(K_a - K)}e^{-Kt} \qquad \text{... (5.108)}$$

Taking the natural logarithm of this expression,
Substitution of common logarithms gives

$$\log C_P = \log\frac{FK_aD_0}{V_D(K_a - K)} - \frac{Kt}{2.3} \qquad \text{... (5.109)}$$

With this equation, a graph constructed by plotting log C_p versus time will yield a straight line with a slope of $-k/2.3$.

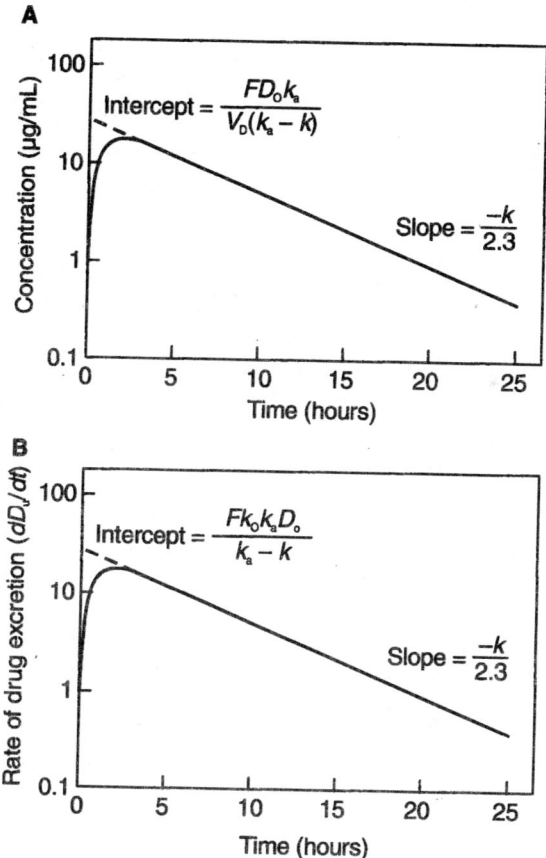

Fig. 5.27: **A.** Plasma drug concentration versus time, single oral dose. **B.** Rate of urinary drug excretion versus time, single oral dose.

With a similar approach, urinary drug excretion data may also be used for calculation of the first-order elimination rate constant. The rate of drug excretion after a single oral dose of drug is given by

$$\frac{dD_u}{dt} = \frac{FK_aK_eD_0}{K_a - K}-\left(e^{-Kt} - e^{-K_at}\right) \qquad \text{... (5.110)}$$

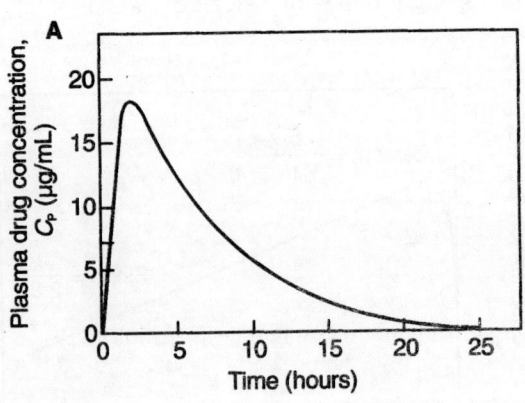

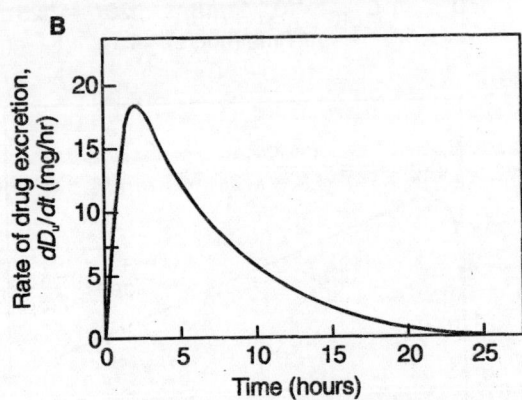

Fig. 5.28: **A.** Plasma drug concentration versus time, single oral dose.
B. Rate of urinary drug excretion versus time, single oral dose.

where dD_u/dt = rate of urinary drug excretion, k_e = first-order renal excretion constant, and F = fraction of dose absorbed.

A graph constructed by plotting dD_u/dt versus time will yield a curve identical in appearance to the plasma level–time curve for the drug. After drug absorption is virtually complete, $-e^{-k_a t}$ approaches zero, and equation 5.110 reduces to

$$\frac{dD_u}{dt} = \frac{FK_a K_e D_0}{K_a - K} e^{-Kt} \qquad \dots (5.111)$$

$$\log\frac{dD_u}{dt} = \log\frac{FK_a K_e D_0}{K_a - K} - \frac{Kt}{2.3} \qquad \dots (5.112)$$

When $\log (dD_u/dt)$ is plotted against time, a graph of a straight line is obtained with a slope of $-k/2.3$. Because the rate of urinary drug excretion, dD_u/dt, cannot be determined directly for any given time point, an average rate of urinary drug excretion is obtained, and this value is plotted against the midpoint of the collection period for each urine sample.

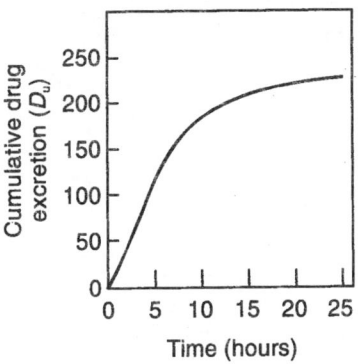

Fig. 5.29: Cumulative urinary drug excretion versus time, single oral dose. Urine samples are collected at various time periods after the dose. The amount of drug excreted in each sample is added to the amount of drug recovered in the previous urine sample (cumulative addition). The total amount of drug recovered after all the drug is excreted is D_u^∞.

To obtain the cumulative drug excretion in the urine, equation 5.110 must be integrated, as shown below.

$$D_u = \frac{FK_a K_e D_0}{K_a - K}\left(\frac{e^{-K_a t}}{K_a} - \frac{e^{-Kt}}{K}\right) + \frac{FK_e D_0}{K} \quad \dots (5.113)$$

A plot of D_u versus time will give the urinary drug excretion curve described in. When the entire drug has been excreted, at $t = \infty$. Equation 5.113 reduces to

$$D_u^\infty = \frac{FK_e D_0}{K} \quad \dots (5.114)$$

Where D_u^∞ is the maximum amount of active or parent drug excreted.

- **Determination of absorption rate constants from oral absorption data**

➢ **Method of residuals**

Assuming $k_a \gg k$ in equation 5.103, the value for the second exponential will become insignificantly small with time (i.e., $e^{-k_a t} \approx 0$) and can therefore be omitted. When this is the case, drug absorption is virtually complete. Equation 5.103 then reduces to equation 5.115.

$$C_P = \frac{FK_a D_0}{V_D(K_a - K)}e^{-Kt} \quad \dots (5.115)$$

From this, one may also obtain the intercept of the y axis.

$$\frac{FK_a D_0}{V_D(K_a - K)} = A$$

Where, A is a constant. Thus, equation 5.115 becomes:

$$C_P = Ae^{-Kt} \quad \dots (5.116)$$

This equation, which represents first-order drug elimination, will yield a linear plot on semilog paper. The slope is equal to $-k/2.3$. The value for k_a can be obtained by using the method of residuals or a feathering technique, as described in. The value of k_a is obtained by the following procedure:

1. Plot the drug concentration versus time on semilog paper with the concentration values on the logarithmic axis.

2. Obtain the slope of the terminal phase (line BC,) by extrapolation.

3. Take any points on the upper part of line BC (eg, $x'_1, x'_2, x'3,$) and drop vertically to obtain corresponding points on the curve (eg, $x_1, x_2, x_3, ...$).

4. Read the concentration values at x_1 and x'_1, x_2 and x'_2, x_3 and x'_3, and so on. Plot the values of the differences at the corresponding time points $\Delta_1, \Delta_2, \Delta_3$, A straight line will be obtained with a slope of $-k_a/2.3$.

When using the method of residuals, a minimum of three points should be used to define the straight line. Data points occurring shortly after t_{max} may not be accurate, because drug absorption is still continuing at that time. Because this portion of the curve represents the post absorption phase, only data points from the elimination phase should be used to define the rate of drug absorption as a first-order process.

If drug absorption begins immediately after oral administration, the residual lines obtained by feathering the plasma-time curve will intersect on the y-axis at point A. the value of this y intercept, A represents a hybrid constant composed of k_a, k, V_D, and FD_0. The value of A has no direct physiologic meaning (see eq. 5.116).

$$\frac{FK_a D_0}{V_D (K_a - K)} = A$$

The value for A, as well as the values for k and k_a, may be substituted back into equation 5.103 to obtain a general theoretical equation that will describe the plasma level–time curve.

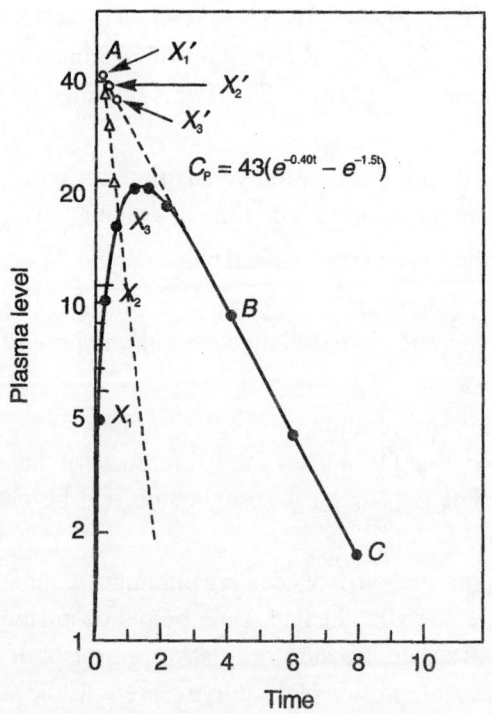

Fig. 5.30: Plasma level–time curve for a drug demonstrating first-order absorption and elimination kinetics. The equation of the curve is obtained by the method of residuals.

> **Lag time**

In some individuals, absorption of drug after a single oral dose does not start immediately, due to such physiologic factors as stomach-emptying time and intestinal motility. The time delay prior to the commencement of first-order drug absorption is known as lag time.

The lag time for a drug may be observed if the two residual lines obtained by feathering the oral absorption plasma level–time curve intersect at a point greater than $t = 0$ on the x axis. The time at the point of intersection on the x axis is the lag time.

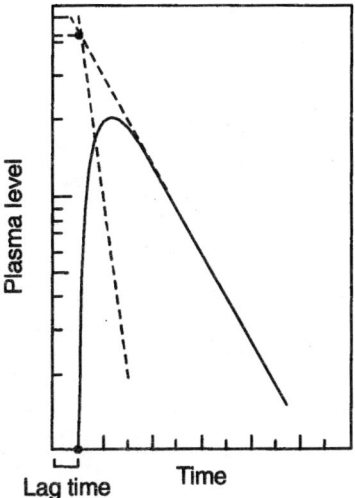

Fig. 5.31: The lag time can be determined graphically if the two residual lines obtained by feathering the plasma level–time curve intersect at a point where $t > 0$.

The lag time, t_0, represents the beginning of drug absorption and should not be confused with the pharmacologic term onset time, which represents latency, e.g., the time required for the drug to reach minimum effective concentration.

Two equations can adequately describe the curve in. In one, the lag time t_0 is subtracted from each time point, as shown in equation 5.117.

$$C_P = \frac{FK_a D_0}{V_D (K_a - K)} (e^{-K(t-t_0)} - (e^{-K_a(t-t_0)}) \qquad ...\,(5.117)$$

Where, $Fk_a D_0/V_D (k_a - k)$ is the y value at the point of intersection of the residual lines in.

The second expression that describes the curve in omits the lag time, as follows:

$$C_P = Be^{-Kt} - Ae^{-K_a t} \qquad ...\,(5.118)$$

Where A and B represents the intercepts on the y axis after extrapolation of the residual lines for absorption and elimination, respectively.

> **Flip-flop of k_a and k**

In using the method of residuals to obtain estimates of k_a and k, the terminal phase of an oral absorption curve is usually represented by k whereas the steeper slope is represented by k_a. In a few cases, the elimination rate constant k obtained from oral absorption data does not agree with that obtained after intravenous bolus injection. For example, the k obtained after an intravenous bolus injection of a bronchodilator was 1.72 hr^{-1}, whereas the k calculated after oral administration was 0.7 hr^{-1}. When k_a was obtained by the method of residuals, the rather surprising result was that the k_a was 1.72 hr^{-1}.

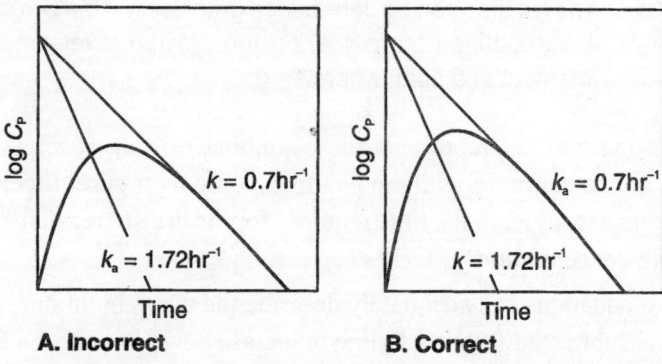

Fig. 5.32:   Flip-flop of k_a and k. Because $k > k_a$, the right-hand figure and slopes represent the correct values for k_a and k.

Apparently, the k_a and k obtained by the method of residuals has been interchanged. This phenomenon is called flip-flop of the absorption and elimination rate constants. Flip-flop, or the reversal of the rate constants, may occur whenever k_a and k are estimated from oral drug absorption data. Use of computer methods does not ensure against flip-flop of the two constants estimated.

In order to demonstrate unambiguously that the steeper curve represents the elimination rate for a drug given extravascularly, the drug must be given by intravenous injection into the same patient. After intravenous injection, the decline in plasma drug levels over time represents the true elimination rate. The relationship between k_a and k on the shape of the plasma drug concentration–time curve for a constant dose of drug given orally is shown in.

Most of the drugs observed to have flip-flop characteristics are drugs with fast elimination (i.e., $k > k_a$). Drug absorption of most drug solutions or fast-dissolving products are essentially complete or at least half-complete within an hour (ie, absorption half-life of 0.5 or 1hr, corresponding to a k_a of 1.38 hr^{-1} or 0.69 hr^{-1}). Because most of the drugs used orally have longer elimination half-lives compared to absorption half-lives, the assumption that the smaller slope or smaller rate constant (i.e., the terminal phase of the curve in) should be used as the elimination constant is generally correct.

For drugs that have a large elimination rate constant ($k > 0.69$ hr^{-1}), the chance for flip-flop of k_a and k is much greater. The drug isoproterenol, for example, has an oral elimination half-life of only a few minutes, and flip-flop of k_a and k has been noted. Similarly, salicyluric acid was flip-flopped when oral data were plotted. The k for salicyluric acid was much larger than its k_a. Many experimental drugs show flip-flop of k and k_a, whereas few marketed oral drugs do. Drugs with a large k are usually considered to be unsuitable for an oral drug product due to their large elimination rate constant, corresponding to a very short elimination half-life. An extended-release drug product may slow the absorption of a drug, such that the k_a is smaller than the k and producing a flip-flop situation.

- **Determination of k_a by plotting percent of drug unabsorbed versus time (wagner–nelson method):** (see zero order and first order absorption rate constant using Wagner-Nelson method)

- **Estimation of k_a from urinary data**

The absorption rate constant may also be estimated from urinary excretion data, using a plot of percent of drug unabsorbed versus time. For a one-compartment model:

Ab = total amount of drug absorbed – that is, the amount of drug in the body plus the amount of drug excreted

D_B = amount of drug in the body

D_u = amount of unchanged drug excreted in the urine

C_P = plasma drug concentration

D_E = total amount of drug eliminated (drug and metabolites)

$$Ab = D_B + D_E \qquad \qquad \text{... (5.119)}$$

The differential of Equation 5.119 with respect to time gives:

$$\frac{dAb}{dt} = \frac{dD_B}{dt} + \frac{dD_E}{dt} \qquad \qquad \text{... (5.120)}$$

Assuming first-order elimination kinetics with renal elimination constant k_e,

$$\frac{dD_u}{dt} = K_C D_B = K_C V_D C_P \qquad \qquad \text{... (5.121)}$$

Assuming a one-compartment model,

$$V_D C_P = D_B$$

Substituting $V_D C_P$ into equation 5.120,

$$\frac{dAb}{dt} = V_D \frac{dC_P}{dt} + \frac{dD_E}{dt} \qquad \qquad \text{... (5.122)}$$

And rearranging equation 5.121,

$$C_P = \frac{1}{K_C V_D} \left(\frac{dD_u}{dt} \right) \qquad \qquad \text{... (5.123)}$$

$$\frac{dC_P}{dt} = \frac{d\left(dD_u / dt \right)}{dt K_C V_D} \qquad \qquad \text{... (5.124)}$$

Substituting for dC_P/dt into equation 5.122 and kD_u/k_e for D_E,

$$\frac{dAb}{dt} = \frac{d\left(dD_u / dt\right)}{K_C dt} + \frac{K}{K_C}\left(\frac{dD_u}{dt}\right) \qquad \text{... (5.125)}$$

When the above expression is integrated from zero to time t,

$$Ab_t = \frac{1}{K_C}\left(\frac{dD_u}{dt}\right)t + \frac{K}{K_C}(D_U)t \qquad \text{... (5.126)}$$

At $t = \infty$ all the drug that is ultimately absorbed is expressed as Ab^∞ and $dD_u/dt = 0$. The total amount of drug absorbed is:

$$Ab^\infty = \frac{K}{K_C}D_u^\infty$$

Where D_u^∞ is the total amount of unchanged drug excreted in the urine.

The fraction of drug absorbed at any time t is equal to the amount of drug absorbed at this time, Ab_t, divided by the total amount of drug absorbed, Ab^∞.

$$\frac{Ab_t}{Ab^\infty} = \frac{\left(dD_u / dt\right)_t + K\left(D_u\right)t}{KD_u^\infty} \qquad \text{... (5.127)}$$

A plot of the fraction of drug unabsorbed, $1 - Ab/Ab^\infty$, versus time gives $-k_a/2.3$ as the slope from which the absorption rate constant is obtained.

When collecting urinary drug samples for the determination of pharmacokinetic parameters, one should obtain a valid urine collection as discussed in. If the drug is rapidly absorbed, it may be difficult to obtain multiple early urine samples to describe the absorption phase accurately. Moreover, drugs with very slow absorption will have low concentrations, which may present analytical problems.

• Effect of k_a and k on C_{max}, t_{max}, and AUC

Changes in k_a and k may affect t_{max}, C_{max}, and AUC as shown in. If the values for k_a and k are reversed, then the same t_{max} is obtained, but the

C_{max} and AUC are different. If the elimination rate constant is kept at 0.1 hr^{-1} and the k_a changes from 0.2 to 0.6 hr^{-1} (absorption rate increases), then the t_{max} becomes shorter (from 6.93 to 3.58 hr), the C_{max} increases (from 5.00 to 6.99 µg/mL), but the AUC remains constant (100 µg hr/mL). In contrast, when the absorption rate constant is kept at 0.3 hr^{-1} and k changes from 0.1 to 0.5 hr^{-1} (elimination rate increases), then the t_{max} decreases (from 5.49 to 2.55 hr), the C_{max} decreases (from 5.77 to 2.79 µg/mL), and the AUC decreases (from 100 to 20 µg hr/mL). Graphical representations for the relationships of k_a and k on the time for peak absorption and the peak drug concentrations are shown in Table 5.5.

Table. 5.5: Effects of the absorption rate constant and elimination rate

Absorption Rate Constant $k_a(\text{hr}^{-1})$	Elimination Rate Constant (hr^{-1})	t_{max} (hr)	C_{max} (µg/mL)	AUG (µg hr/mL)
0.1	0.2	6.93	2.50	50
0.2	0.1	6.93	5.00	100
0.3	0.1	5.49	5.77	100
0.4	0.1	4.62	6.29	100
0.5	0.1	4.02	6.69	100
0.6	0.1	3.58	6.99	100
0.3	0.1	5.49	5.77	100
0.3	0.2	4.05	4.44	50
0.3	0.3	3.33	3.68	33.3
0.3	0.4	2.88	3.16	25
0.3	0.5	2.55	2.79	20

Where, t_{max} = peak plasma concentration, C_{max} = peak drug concentration, AUC = area under the curve. Values are based on a single oral dose (100 mg) that is 100% bioavailable ($F = 1$) and has an apparent V_D of 10L. The drug follows a one-compartment open model. t_{max} is calculated by eq. 5.105 and C_{max} is calculated by eq. 5.103. The AUC is calculated by the trapezoidal rule from 0 to 24 hours.

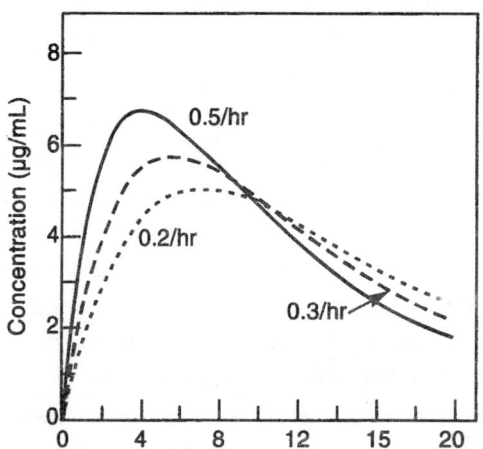

Fig. 5.33: Effect of a change in the absorption rate constant, k_a, on the plasma drug concentration-versus-time curve. Dose of drug is 100 mg, V_D is 10L, and k is 0.1 hr^{-1}.

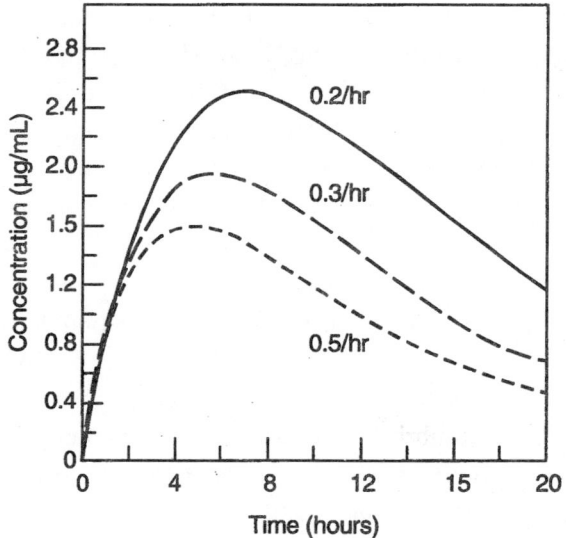

Fig. 5.34: Effect of a change in the elimination rate constant, k, on the plasma drug concentration-versus-time curve. Dose of drug is 100 mg, V_D is 10L, and k_a is 0.1 hr^{-1}.

Two compartment models: intravenous bolus administration

Pharmacokinetic models may be used to represent drug distribution and elimination in the body. Ideally, a model should mimic closely the physiologic processes in the body. In practice, models seldom consider all the rate processes ongoing in the body and are therefore simplified mathematical expressions. The inability to measure all the rate processes in the body, including the lack of access to biological samples from the interior of the body, limits the sophistication of a model. Compartmental models are classical pharmacokinetic models that simulate the kinetic processes of drug absorption, distribution, and elimination with little physiologic detail. In contrast, the more sophisticated physiologic model is discussed in. In compartmental models, drug tissue concentration is assumed to be uniform within a given hypothetical compartment. Hence, all muscle mass and connective tissues may be lumped into one hypothetical tissue compartment that equilibrates with drug from the central (or plasma) compartment. Since no data is collected on the tissue mass, the theoretical tissue concentration is unconstrained and cannot be used to forecast actual tissue drug levels. However, tissue drug uptake and tissue drug binding from the plasma fluid is kinetically simulated by considering the presence of a tissue compartment. Indeed, most drugs given by IV bolus dose decline rapidly soon after injection, and then decline moderately as some of the drug initially distributes into the tissue moves back into the plasma.

Multicompartment models were developed to explain this observation that, after a rapid IV injection, the plasma level–time curve does not decline linearly as a single, first-order rate process. The plasma level–time curve reflects first-order elimination of the drug from the body only after distribution equilibrium, or plasma drug equilibrium with peripheral tissues occurs. Drug kinetics after distribution is characterized by the first-order rate constant, b (or beta, β).

Nonlinear plasma level–time curves occur because some drugs distribute at various rates into different tissue groups. Multicompartment models were developed to explain and predict plasma and tissue concentrations for the behavior of these drugs. In contrast, a one-compartment model is used when the drug appears to distribute into tissues instantaneously and uniformly. For both one- and multicompartment models, the drug in the tissues that have the highest blood perfusion equilibrates rapidly with the drug in the plasma. These highly perfused tissues and blood make up the central compartment. While this initial drug distribution is taking place, multicompartment drugs are delivered concurrently to one or more peripheral compartments composed of groups of tissues with lower blood perfusion and different affinity for the drug. A drug will concentrate in a tissue in accordance with the affinity of the drug for that particular tissue. For example, lipid-soluble drugs tend to accumulate in fat tissues. Drugs that bind plasma proteins may be more concentrated in the plasma, because protein-bound drugs do not diffuse easily into the tissues. Drugs may also bind with tissue proteins and other macromolecules, such as DNA and melanin. Tissue sampling is invasive, and the drug concentration in the tissue sample may not represent the drug concentration in the entire organ. Occasionally, tissue samples may be collected after a drug-overdose episode. For example, the two-compartment model has been used to describe the distribution of colchicine, even though the drug's toxic tissue level after fatal overdoses has only been recently described. The drug isotretinoin has a long half-life because of substantial distribution into lipid tissues.

Kinetic analysis of a multicompartment model assumes that all transfer rate processes for the passage of drug into or out of individual compartments are first-order processes. On the basis of this assumption, the plasma level–time curve for a drug that follows a multicompartment model is best described by the summation of a series of exponential terms, each corresponding to first-order rate processes associated with a given compartment. Because of these distribution factors, drugs will generally concentrate unevenly in the tissues, and different groups of tissues will accumulate the drug at different rates. A summary of the approximate blood flow to major human tissues is presented in. Many different tissues and rate processes are involved in the distribution of any drug. However, limited physiologic significance has been assigned to a few groups of tissues.

Table 5.6: Blood flow to human tissues

Tissue	Percent Body Weight	Percent Cardiac Output	Blood Flow (mL/100 g tissue per min)
Adrenals	0.02	1	550
Kidneys	0.4	24	450
Thyroid	0.04	2	400
Liver			
Hepatic	2.0	5	20
Portal		20	75
Portal-drained viscera	2.0	20	75
Heart (basal)	0.4	4	70
Brain	2.0	15	55
Skin	7.0	5	5
Muscle (basal)	40.0	15	3
Connective tissue	7.0	1	1
Fat	15.0	2	1

Table 5.7: General grouping of tissues according to blood supply

Blood Supply	Tissue Group	Percent Body Weight
Highly perfused	Heart, brain, hepatic-portal system, kidney, and endocrine glands	9
	Skin and muscle	50
	Adipose (fat) tissue and marrow	19
Slowly perfused	Bone, ligaments, tendons, cartilage, teeth, and hair	22

The nonlinear profile of plasma drug concentration versus time is the result of many factors interacting together, including blood flow to the tissues, the permeability of the drug into the tissues, the capacity of the tissues to accumulate drug, and the effect of disease factors on these processes. Impaired cardiac function may produce a change in blood flow and in the drug distributive phase, whereas impairment of the kidney or the liver may decrease drug elimination as shown by a prolonged elimination half-life and corresponding reduction in the slope of the terminal elimination phase of the curve. Frequently, multiple factors can complicate the distribution profile in such a way that the profile can only be described clearly with the assistance of a simulation model.

Many drugs given in a single intravenous bolus dose demonstrate a plasma level–time curve that does not decline as a single exponential (first-order) process. The plasma level–time curve for a drug that follows a two-compartment model shows that the plasma drug concentration declines biexponentially as the sum of two first-order processes— distribution and elimination.

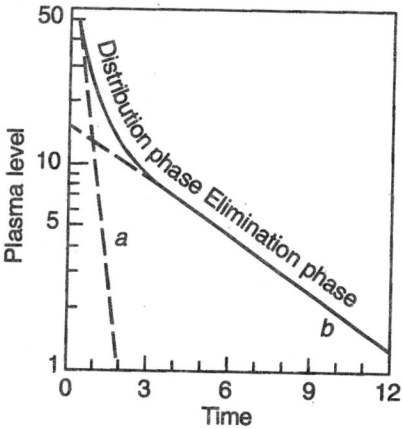

Fig. 5.35: Plasma level–time curve for the two-compartment open model (single IV dose) described in (model A).

A drug that follows the pharmacokinetics of a two-compartment model does not equilibrate rapidly throughout the body, as is assumed for a one-compartment model. In this model, the drug distributes into two compartments, the central compartment and the tissue, or peripheral compartment. The central compartment represents the blood, extracellular fluid, and highly perfused tissues. The drug distributes rapidly and uniformly in the central compartment. A second compartment, known as the tissue or peripheral compartment, contains tissues in which the drug equilibrates more slowly. Drug transfer between the two compartments is assumed to take place by first-order processes.

There are several possible two-compartment models. Model A is used most often and describes the plasma level–time curve observed in. By convention, compartment 1 is the central compartment and compartment 2 is the tissue compartment. The rate constants k_{12} and k_{21} represent the first-order rate transfer constants for the movement of drug from compartment 1 to compartment 2 (k_{12}) and from compartment 2 to compartment 1 (k_{21}). The transfer constants are sometimes termed microconstants, and their values cannot be estimated directly. Most two-compartment models assume that elimination occurs from the central compartment model, as shown in (model A), unless other information about the drug is known. Drug elimination is presumed to occur from the central compartment, because the major sites of drug elimination (renal excretion and hepatic drug metabolism) occur in organs, such as the kidney and liver, which are highly perfused with blood.

The plasma level–time curve for a drug that follows a two-compartment model may be divided into two parts, (a) a distribution phase and (b) an elimination phase. The two-compartment model assumes that, at $t = 0$, no drug is in the tissue compartment. After an IV bolus injection, drug equilibrates rapidly in the central compartment. The distribution phase of the curve represents the initial, more rapid decline of drug from the central compartment into the tissue compartment (, line a). Although drug elimination and distribution occur concurrently during the distribution phase, there is a net transfer of drug from the central compartment to the tissue compartment. The fraction of drug in the tissue

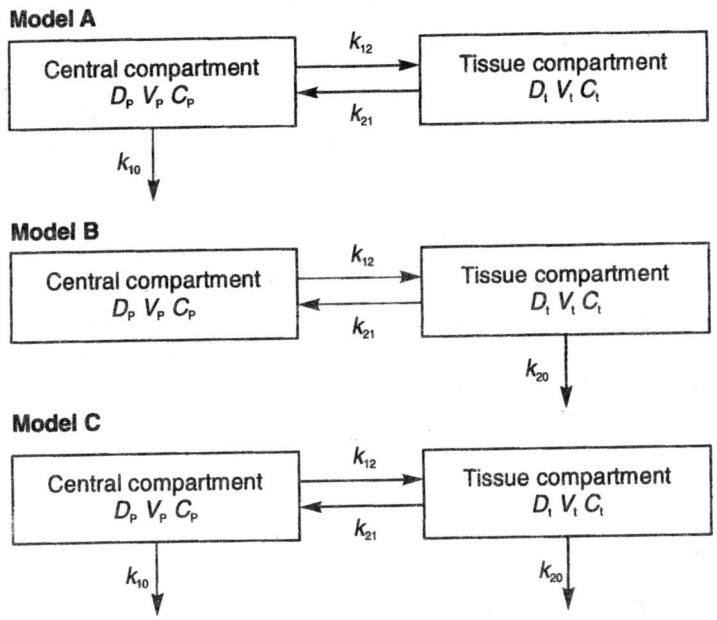

Fig. 5.36: Two-compartment open models, intravenous injection.

compartment during the distribution phase increases up to a maximum in a given tissue, whose value may be greater or less than the plasma drug concentration. At maximum tissue concentrations, the rate of drug entry into the tissue equals the rate of drug exit from the tissue. The fraction of drug in the tissue compartment is now in equilibrium (distribution equilibrium) with the fraction of drug in the central compartment, and the drug concentrations in both the central and tissue compartments decline in parallel and more slowly compared to the distribution phase. This decline is a first-order process and is called **the elimination phase** or **the beta (β) phase** (, line b). Since plasma and tissue concentrations decline in parallel, plasma drug concentrations provide some indication of the concentration of drug in the tissue. At this point, drug kinetics appears to follow a one-compartment model in which drug elimination is a first-order process described by b (also known as beta). A typical tissue drug level curve after a single intravenous dose is shown in.

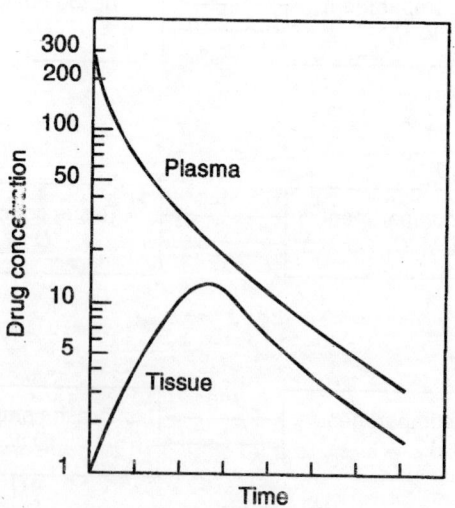

Fig. 5.37: Relationship between tissue and plasma drug concentrations for a two-compartment open model. The maximum tissue drug concentration may be greater or less than the plasma drug concentration.

Tissue drug concentrations are theoretical only. The drug level in the theoretical tissue compartment can be calculated once the parameters for the model are determined. However, the drug concentration in the tissue compartment represents the average drug concentration in a group of tissues rather than any real anatomic tissue drug concentration. In reality, drug concentrations may vary among different tissues and possibly within an individual tissue. These varying tissue drug concentrations are due to differences in the partitioning of drug into the tissues, as discussed in. In terms of the pharmacokinetic model, the differences in tissue drug concentration are reflected in the k_{12}/k_{21} ratio. Thus, tissue drug concentration may be higher or lower than the plasma drug concentrations, depending on the properties of the individual tissue. Moreover, the elimination of drug from the tissue compartment may not be the same as the elimination from the central compartment. For example, if $k_{12} \cdot C_p$ is greater than $k_{21} \cdot C_t$ (rate into tissue > rate out of tissue), the tissue drug concentrations will increase and plasma drug concentrations will decrease. Real tissue drug concentration can sometimes be calculated by the addition of compartments to the model until a compartment that mimics the experimental tissue concentrations is found.

In spite of the hypothetical nature of the tissue compartment, the theoretical tissue level is still valuable information for clinicians. The theoretical tissue concentration, together with the blood concentration, gives an accurate method of calculating the total amount of drug remaining in the body at any time.

In practice, a blood sample is removed periodically from the central compartment and the plasma is analyzed for the presence of drug. The drug plasma level–time curve represents a phase of initial rapid equilibration with the central compartment (the distribution phase) followed by an elimination phase after the tissue compartment has also been equilibrated with drug. The distribution phase may take minutes or hours and may be missed entirely if the blood is sampled too late or at wide intervals after drug administration.

In the model depicted above, k_{12} and k_{21} are first-order rate constants that govern the rate of drug change in and out of the tissues:

$$\frac{dC_t}{dt} = K_{12}C_P - K_{21}C_t \qquad \text{... (5.128)}$$

The relationship between the amount of drug in each compartment and the concentration of drug in that compartment is shown by equations 5.129 and 5.130:

$$C_P = \frac{D_P}{V_P} \qquad \text{... (5.129)}$$

$$C_t = \frac{D_t}{V_t} \qquad \text{... (5.130)}$$

Where D_p = amount of drug in the central compartment, D_t = amount of drug in the tissue compartment, V_p = volume of drug in the central compartment, and V_t = volume of drug in the tissue compartment.

$$\frac{dC_P}{dt} = K_{21}\frac{D_t}{V_t} - K_{12}\frac{D_P}{V_P} - K\frac{D_P}{V_P} \qquad \text{... (5.131)}$$

$$\frac{dC_t}{dt} = K_{12}\frac{D_P}{V_P} - K_{21}\frac{D_t}{V_t} \qquad \text{... (5.132)}$$

Solving equations 5.131 and 5.132 will give equations 5.133 and 5.134, which describe the change in drug concentration in the blood and in the tissue with respect to time:

$$C_P = \frac{D_P^0}{V_P}\left(\frac{K_{21}-a}{b-a}e^{-at} + \frac{K_{21}-b}{a-b}e^{-bt}\right) \qquad \text{... (5.133)}$$

$$C_t = \frac{D_P^0}{V_t}\left(\frac{K_{12}}{b-a}e^{-at} + \frac{K_{12}-b}{a-b}e^{-bt}\right) \qquad \text{... (5.134)}$$

$$D_P = D_P^0\left(\frac{K_{21}-a}{b-a}e^{-at} + \frac{K_{21}-b}{a-b}e^{-bt}\right) \qquad \text{... (5.135)}$$

$$D_t = D_P^0\left(\frac{K_{21}}{b-a}e^{-at} + \frac{K_{12}}{a-b}e^{-bt}\right) \qquad \text{... (5.136)}$$

Where D_P^0 = dose given intravenously, t = time after administration of dose, and a and b are constants that depend solely on k_{12}, k_{21}, and k. The amount of drug remaining in the plasma and tissue compartment at any time may be described realistically by equations 5.135 and 5.136.

The rate constants for the transfer of drug between compartments are referred to as microconstants or transfer constants, and relate the amount of drug being transferred per unit time from one compartment to the other. The values for these microconstants cannot be determined by direct measurement but can be estimated by a graphic method.

$$a + b = K_{12} + K_{21} + K \qquad \qquad ... (5.137)$$

$$ab = K_{12}K \qquad \qquad ... (5.138)$$

The constants a and b are hybrid first-order rate constants for the distribution phase and elimination phase, respectively. The mathematical relationship of a and b to the rate constants are given by equations 5.137 and 5.138, which are derived after integration of equations 5.131 and 5.132. Equation 5.133 can be transformed into the following expression:

$$C_P = Ae^{-at} + Be^{-bt} \qquad \qquad ... (5.139)$$

The constants a and b are rate constants for the distribution phase and elimination phase, respectively. The constants A and B are intercepts on the y axis for each exponential segment of the curve in equation 5.139. These values may be obtained graphically by the method of residuals or by computer. Intercepts A and B are actually hybrid constants, as shown in equations 5.140 and 5.141, and do not have actual physiologic significance.

$$A = \frac{D_0 (a - K_{21})}{V_P (1 - b)} \qquad \qquad ... (5.140)$$

$$B = \frac{D_0 (K_{21} - b)}{V_P (a - b)} \qquad \qquad ... (5.141)$$

- **Simulation of plasma and tissue level of a two-compartment model drug—digoxin in a normal patient and in a renal-failure patient**

The pharmacokinetic data for digoxin was calculated in a normal and in a renal-impaired, 70-kg subject using the parameters in as reported in the literature. The amount of digoxin remaining in the plasma and tissue compartment are tabulated in and plotted in. It can be seen that digoxin stored in the plasma declines rapidly during the initial distributive phase, while drug amount in the tissue compartment take 3–4 hours ($5t_{1/2} = 5$x 35 min) to accumulate. It is interesting that clinicians have recommended that digoxin plasma samples be taken at least several hours after IV bolus dosing, since the equilibrated level is more representative of myocardium digoxin level. In the simulation below, the amount of the drug in the plasma compartment at any time divided by V_p (54.6 L for the normal subject) will yield the plasma digoxin level. At 4 hours after an IV dose of 0.25 mg, $C_p = D_p/V_p = 24.43$ µg/54.6 L = 0.45 ng/mL, corresponding to 3 x 0.45 ng/mL = 1.35 ng/mL if a full loading dose of 0.75 mg is given in a single dose. Although the initial plasma drug levels were much higher than after equilibration, the digoxin plasma concentrations are generally regarded as not toxic, since drug distribution is occurring rapidly. The tissue drug levels were not calculated. The tissue drug concentration represents the hypothetical tissue pool, which may not represent actual drug concentrations in the myocardium. In contrast, the amount of drug remaining in the tissue pool is real, since the amount of drug is calculated using mass balance. The rate of drug entry into the tissue in micrograms per hour at any time is $k_{12}D_p$, while the rate of drug leaving the tissue is $k_{21}D_t$ in the same units. Both of these rates may be calculated from using k_{12} and k_{21} values listed in.

Table 5.8: Two-compartment model pharmacokinetic parameters of digoxin

Parameter	Unit	Normal	Renal Impaired
k_{12}	hr^{-1}	1.02	0.45
k_{21}	hr^{-1}	0.15	0.11
k	hr^{-1}	0.18	0.04
V_p	L/kg	0.78	0.73
D	µg/kg	3.6	3.6
a	1/hr	1.331	0.593
b	1/hr	0.019	0.007

Table 5.9: Amount of digoxin in plasma and tissue compartment after an IV dose of 0.252 mg in a normal and a renal-failure patient weighing 70 kg

| Time (hr) | Digoxin Amount | | | |
| | Normal Renal Function | | Renal Failure (RF) | |
	D_p (µg)	D_t (µg)	D_p (µg)	D_t (µg)
0.00	252.00	0.00	252.00	0.00
0.10	223.68	24.04	240.01	11.01
0.60	126.94	105.54	189.63	57.12
1.00	84.62	140.46	158.78	85.22
2.00	40.06	174.93	107.12	131.72
3.00	27.95	181.45	78.44	156.83
4.00	24.43	180.62	62.45	170.12
5.00	23.17	177.91	53.48	176.88
6.00	22.53	174.74	48.39	180.04
7.00	22.05	171.50	45.45	181.21
8.00	21.62	168.28	43.69	181.29
9.00	21.21	165.12	42.59	180.77
10.00	20.81	162.01	41.85	179.92
11.00	20.42	158.96	41.32	178.89
12.00	20.03	155.97	40.89	177.77
13.00	19.65	153.04	40.53	176.60
16.00	18.57	144.56	39.62	173.00
24.00	15.95	124.17	37.44	163.59

Although some clinicians assume that tissue and plasma concentrations are equal when at full equilibration, tissue and plasma drug ratios are determined by the partition coefficient (a drug-specific physical ratio that measures the lipid/water affinity of a drug) and the extent of protein binding of the drug. shows that the time for the RF (renal failure or renal impaired) patient to reach stable tissue drug levels is longer than the time for the normal subject due to changes in the elimination and transfer rate constants. As expected, a significantly higher

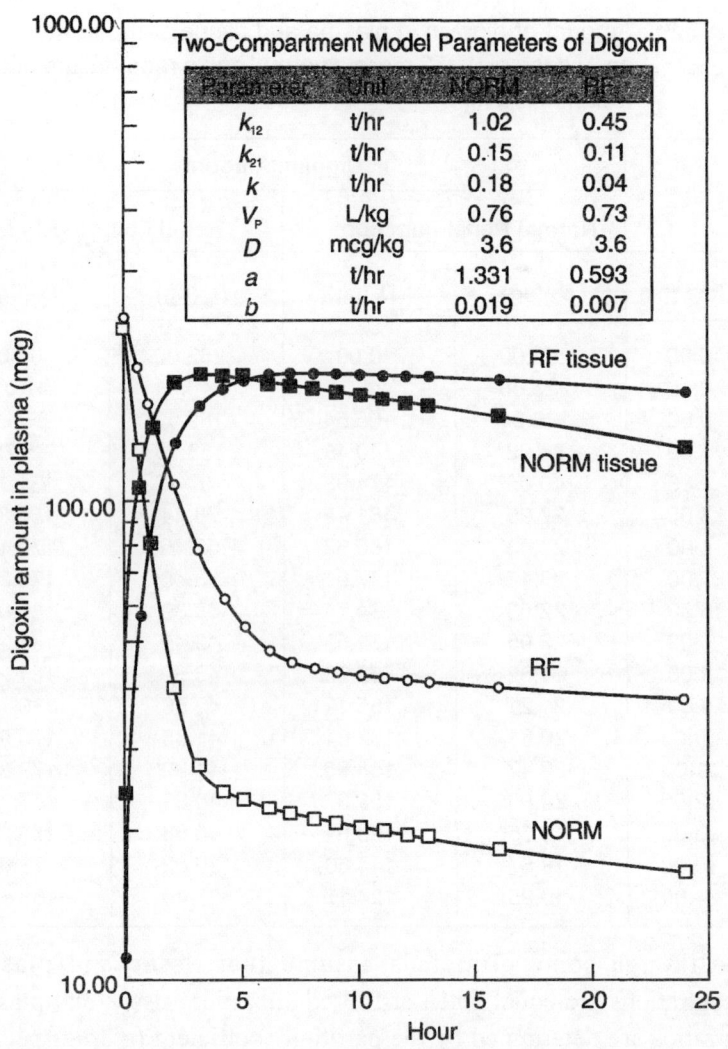

Fig. 5.38: Amount of digoxin (simulated) in plasma and tissue compartment after an IV dose to a normal and a renal-failure (RF) patient.

amount of digoxin remains in both the plasma and tissue compartment in the renally impaired subject compared to the normal subject.

• Apparent volumes of distribution

The apparent V_D is a useful parameter that relates plasma concentration to the amount of drug in the body. For drugs with large extravascular distribution, the apparent volume of distribution is generally large. Conversely, for polar drugs with low lipid solubility, the apparent V_D is generally small. Drugs with high peripheral tissue binding also contribute to a large apparent V_D. In multiple-compartment kinetics, such as the two-compartment model, several volumes of distribution can be calculated. Volumes of distribution generally reflect the extent of drug distribution in the body on a relative basis, and the calculations depend on the availability of data. In general, it is important to refer to the same volume parameter when comparing kinetic changes in disease states. Unfortunately, values of apparent volumes of distribution of drugs from tables in the clinical literature are often listed without specifying the underlying kinetic processes, model parameter, or method of calculation.

• Volume of the central compartment

The volume of the central compartment is useful for determining the drug concentration directly after an IV injection into the body. In clinical pharmacy, this volume is also referred to as V_i or the initial volume of distribution as the drug distributes within the plasma and other accessible body fluids. This volume is generally smaller than the terminal volume of distribution after drug distribution to tissue is completed. The volume of the central compartment is generally greater than 3 L, which is the volume of the plasma fluid for an average adult. For many polar drugs, an initial volume of 7–10 L may be interpreted as rapid drug distribution within the plasma and some extracellular fluids. For example, the V_p of moxalactam ranges from 0.12 to 0.15 L/kg, corresponding to about 8.4 to 10.5 L for a typical 70-kg patient. In contrast, V_p of hydromorphone is about 24 L, possibly because of its rapid exit from the plasma into tissues even during the initial phase.

Table 5.10: Pharmacokinetic parameters (Mean ± SD) of moxalactam in three groups of patients

Group	A µg/mL	B µg/mL	a hr^{-1}	b hr^{-1}	khr^{-1}
1	138.9 ± 114.9	157.8 ± 87.1	6.8 ± 4.5	0.20 ± 0.12	0.38 ± 0.26
2	115.4 ± 65.9	115.0 ± 40.8	5.3 ± 3.5	0.27 ± 0.08	0.50 ± 0.17
3	102.9 ± 39.4	89.0 ± 36.7	5.6 ± 3.8	0.37 ± 0.09	0.71 ± 0.16
Group	Cl mL/min	VpL/kg	VtL/kg	(VD)ssL/kg	(VD)βL/kg
1	40.5 ± 14.5	0.12 ± 0.05	0.08 ± 0.04	0.20 ± 0.09	0.21 ± 0.09
2	73.7 ± 13.1	0.14 ± 0.06	0.09 ± 0.04	0.23 ± 0.10	0.24 ± 0.12
3	125.9 ± 28.0	0.15 ± 0.05	0.10 ± 0.05	0.25 ± 0.08	0.29 ± 0.09

As in the case of the one-compartment model, V_p may be determined from the dose and the instantaneous plasma–drug concentration, $C^0{}_p$. V_p is also useful in the determination of drug clearance if k is known, as in.

In the two-compartment model, V_p may also be considered as a mass balance factor governed by the mass balance between dose and concentration, ie, drug concentration multiplied by the volume of the fluid must equal to the dose at time zero. At time zero, no drug is eliminated, $D_0 = V_p C_p$. The basic model assumption is that plasma–drug concentration is representative of drug concentration within the distribution fluid. If this statement is true, then the volume of distribution will be 3 L; if it is not, then distribution of drug may also occur outside the vascular pool.

$$V_P = \frac{D_0}{C_P^0} \qquad \qquad ...(5.142)$$

At zero time ($t = 0$), all of the drug in the body is in the central compartment. C_P^0 can be shown to be equal to $A + B$ by the following equation.

$$C_P = Ae^{-at} + Be^{-bt} \qquad \qquad ...(5.143)$$

At $t = 0$, $e^0 = 1$. Therefore,

$$C_P^0 = A + B \qquad \qquad ...(5.144)$$

V_p is determined from equation 5.145 by measuring A and B after feathering the curve, as discussed previously:

$$V_P = \frac{D_0}{A+B} \qquad \dots (5.145)$$

Alternatively, the volume of the central compartment may be calculated from the $[AUC]_0^\infty$ in a manner similar to the calculation for the apparent V_D in the one-compartment model. For a one-compartment model,

$$[AUC]_0^\infty = \frac{D_0}{KV_D} \qquad \dots (5.146)$$

$$[AUC]_0^\infty = \frac{D_0}{KV_D} \qquad \dots (5.146)$$

In contrast, $[AUC]^\circ{}_0$ for the two-compartment model is:

$$[AUC]_0^\infty = \frac{D_0}{KV_P} \qquad \dots (5.147)$$

Rearrangement of this equation yields

$$V_P = \frac{D_0}{K[AUC]_0^\infty} \qquad \dots (5.148)$$

• Apparent volume of distribution at steady state

At steady-state conditions, the rate of drug entry into the tissue compartment from the central compartment is equal to the rate of drug exit from the tissue compartment into the central compartment. These rates of drug transfer are described by the following expressions:

$$D_t K_{21} = D_P K_{12} \qquad \dots (5.149)$$

$$D_t = \frac{K_{12} D_P}{K_{21}} \qquad \dots (5.150)$$

Because the amount of drug in the central compartment, D_p, is equal to $V_p C_p$, by substitution in the above equation,

$$D_t = \frac{K_{12} C_P V_P}{K_{21}} \qquad \qquad ...(5.151)$$

The total amount of drug in the body at steady state is equal to the sum of the amount of drug in the tissue compartment, D_t, and the amount of drug in the central compartment, D_p. Therefore, the apparent volume of drug at steady state $(V_D)_{ss}$ may be calculated by dividing the total amount of drug in the body by the concentration of drug in the central compartment at steady state:

$$(V_D)_{SS} = \frac{D_P + D_t}{C_P} \qquad \qquad ...(5.152)$$

By substitution of equation 5.151 into equation 5.152, and by expressing D_p as $V_p C_p$, a more useful equation for the calculation of $(V_D)_{ss}$ is obtained:

$$(V_D)_{SS} = \frac{C_P V_P + K_{12} V_P C_P / K_{21}}{C_P} \qquad \qquad ...(5.153)$$

This reduces to:

$$(V_D)_{SS} = V_P + \frac{K_{12}}{K_{21}} V_P \qquad \qquad ...(5.154)$$

In practice, equation 5.154 is used to calculate $(V_D)_{ss}$. The $(V_D)_{ss}$ is a function of the transfer constants, k_{12} and k_{21}, which represent the rate constants of drug going into and out of the tissue compartment, respectively. The magnitude of $(V_D)_{ss}$ is dependent on the hemodynamic factors responsible for drug distribution and on the physical properties of the drug, properties which, in turn, determine the relative amount of intra- and extravascular drug remaining in the body.

• Extrapolated volume of distribution

The extrapolated volume of distribution $(V_D)_{exp}$ is calculated by the following equation:

$$(V_D)_{exp} = \frac{D_0}{B} \qquad \text{... (5.155)}$$

Where, B is the y intercept obtained by extrapolation of the b phase of the plasma level curve to the y axis. Because the y intercept is a hybrid constant, as shown by equation 5.141, $(V_D)_{exp}$ may also be calculated by the following expression:

$$(V_D)_{exp} = V_P\left(\frac{a-b}{K_{21}-b}\right) \qquad \text{... (5.156)}$$

This equation shows that a change in the distribution of a drug, which is observed by a change in the value for V_p, will be reflected in a change in $(V_D)_{exp}$.

• Volume of distribution by area

The volume of distribution by area $(V_D)_{area}$, also known as $(V_D)_\beta$, is obtained through calculations similar to those used to find V_p, except that the rate constant b is used instead of the overall elimination rate constant k. $(V_D)_\beta$ is often calculated from total body clearance divided by b and is influenced by drug elimination in the beta, or b phase. Reduced drug clearance from the body may increase AUC, such that $(V_D)_\beta$ is either reduced or unchanged depending on the value of b, as shown by equation 5.156.

$$(V_D)_\beta = (V_D)_{area} = \frac{D_0}{b[AUC]_0^\infty} \qquad \text{... (5.157)}$$

Generally, reduced drug clearance is accompanied by a decrease in the constant b (i.e., an increase in the b elimination half-life). For example, in patients with renal dysfunction, the elimination half-life of the antibiotic amoxicillin is longer because renal clearance is reduced.

Because total body clearance is equal to $D_0 / [AUC]_0^\infty$, $(V_D)\,\beta$ may be expressed in terms of clearance and the rate constant b:

$$(V_D)_\beta = \frac{\text{clearance}}{b} \qquad \ldots (5.158)$$

By substitution of kV_p for clearance in equation 5.158, one obtains:

$$(V_D)_\beta = \frac{KV_P}{b} \qquad \ldots (5.159)$$

Theoretically, the value for b may remain unchanged in patients showing various degrees of moderate renal impairment. In this case, a reduction in $(V_D)\,\beta$ may account for all the decrease in Cl, while b is unchanged in equation 5.159. Within the body, a redistribution of drug between the plasma and the tissue will mask the expected decline in b. The following example in two patients shows that the b elimination rate constant remains the same, while the distributional rate constants change. Interestingly, V_p is unchanged, while $(V_D)\,\beta$ would be greatly changed in the simulated example. An example of a drug showing constant b slope while the renal function as measured by Cl_{cr} decreases from 107 to 56, 34, and 6 mL/min has been observed with the amino glycoside drug gentamicin in various patients after IV bolus dose. Gentamicin follows polyexponential decline with a significant distributive phase. The following simulation problem may help to clarify the situation by changing k and clearance while keeping b constant.

• **Significance of the volumes of distribution**

From equations 5.152 and 5.153 we can observe that $(V_D)_\beta$ is affected by changes in the overall elimination rate (i.e., change in k) and by change in total body clearance of the drug. After the drug is distributed, the total amount of drug in the body during the elimination of b phase is calculated by using $(V_D)_\beta$.

V_p is sometimes called the initial volume of distribution and is useful in the calculation of drug clearance. The magnitudes of the various apparent volumes of distribution have the following relationships to each other:

$$(V_D)_{exp} > (V_D)_\beta > V_P$$

Calculation of another V_D, $(V_D)_{ss}$, is possible in multiple dosing or infusion. $(V_D)_{ss}$ is much larger than V_p; it approximates $(V_D)_\beta$ but differs somewhat in value, depending on the transfer constants.

In a study involving a cardiotonic drug given intravenously to a group of normal and congestive heart failure (CHF) patients, the average AUC for CHF was 40% higher than in the normal subjects. The b elimination constant was 40% less in CHF patients, whereas the average $(V_D)_\beta$ remained essentially the same. In spite of the edematous conditions of these patients, the volume of distribution apparently remained constant. No change was found in the V_p or $(V_D)_\beta$. In this study, a 40% increase in AUC in the CHF subjects was offset by a 40% smaller b elimination constant estimated by using computer methods. Because the dose was the same, the $(V_D)_\beta$ would not change unless the increase in AUC is not accompanied by a change in b elimination constant.

From equation 5.152, the clearance of the drug in CHF patients was reduced by 40% and accompanied by a corresponding decrease in the *b* elimination constant, possibly due to a reduction in renal blood flow as a result of reduced cardiac output in CHF patients. In physiologic pharmacokinetics, clearance (Cl) and volume of distribution (V_D) are assumed to be independent parameters that explain the impact of disease factors on drug disposition. Thus, an increase in AUC of a cardiotonic in a CHF patient was assumed to be due to a reduction in drug clearance, since the volume of distribution was unchanged. The elimination half-life was reduced due to reduction in drug clearance. In reality, pharmacokinetic changes in a complex system are dependent on many factors that interact within the system. Clearance is affected by drug uptake, metabolism, binding, and more; all of these factors can also influence the drug distribution volume. Many parameters are assumed to be constant and independent for simplification of the model. Blood flow is an independent parameter that will affect both clearance and distribution.

However, blood flow is, in turn, affected and regulated by many physiologic compensatory factors.

For drugs that follow two-compartment model kinetics, changes in disease states may not result in different pharmacokinetic parameters. Conversely, changes in pharmacokinetic parameters should not be attributed to physiologic changes without careful consideration of method of curve fitting and intersubject differences. equation 5.159 shows that, unlike a simple one-compartment open model, $(V_D)_\beta$ may be estimated from k, b, and V_p. Errors in fitting are easily carried over to the other parameter estimates even if the calculations are performed by computer. The terms k_{12} and k_{21} often fluctuate due to minor fitting and experimental difference and may affect calculation of other parameters.

• Drug in the tissue compartment

The apparent volume of the tissue compartment (V_t) is a conceptual volume only and does not represent true anatomic volumes. The V_t may be calculated from knowledge of the transfer rate constants and V_p:

$$(V_t) = \frac{K_p K_{12}}{K_{21}} \qquad \qquad \text{... (5.160)}$$

The calculation of the amount of drug in the tissue compartment does not entail the use of V_t. Calculation of the amount of drug in the tissue compartment provides an estimate for drug accumulation in the tissues of the body. This information is vital in estimating chronic toxicity and relating the duration of pharmacologic activity to dose. Tissue compartment drug concentration is an average estimate of the tissue pool and does not mean that all tissues have this concentration. The drug concentration in a tissue biopsy will provide an estimate for drug in that tissue sample. Due to differences in blood flow and drug partitioning into the tissue, and heterogenicity, even a biopsy from the same tissue may have different drug concentrations. Together with V_p and C_p, which calculate the amount of drug in the plasma, the compartment model provides mass balance information. Moreover, the pharmacodynamic activity may correlate better with the tissue drug concentration–time curve.

To calculate the amount of drug in the tissue compartment D_t, the following expression is used:

$$D_t = \frac{K_{12}K_P^0}{a-b}\left(e^{-bt} - e^{-at}\right) \qquad \ldots (5.161)$$

• Drug clearance

The definition of clearance of a drug that follows a two-compartment model is similar to that of the one-compartment model. Clearance is the volume of plasma that is cleared of drug per unit time. Clearance may be calculated without consideration of the compartment model. Thus, clearance may be viewed as a physiologic concept for drug removal, even though the development of clearance is rooted in classical pharmacokinetics.

Clearance is often calculated by a noncompartmental approach, as in equation 5.156, in which the bolus IV dose is divided by the area under the plasma–time concentration curve from zero to infinity, $[AUC]_0^\infty$. In evaluating the $[AUC]_0^\infty$, early time points must be collected frequently to observe the rapid decline in drug concentrations (distribution phase) for drugs with multicompartment pharmacokinetics. In the calculation of clearance using the noncompartmental approach, underestimating the area can inflate the calculated value of clearance.

$$Cl = \frac{D_0}{[AUC]_0^\infty} \qquad \ldots (5.162)$$

Equation 5.162 may be rearranged to equation 5.163 to show that Cl in the two-compartment model is the product of $(V_D)_\beta$ and b.

$$Cl = (V_D)_\beta b \qquad \ldots (5.163)$$

If both parameters are known, then calculation of clearance is simple and more accurate than using the trapezoidal rule to obtain area. Clearance calculations that use the two-compartment model are viewed as model dependent because more assumptions are required, and such calculations cannot be regarded as noncompartmental. However, the assumptions provide additional information and, in some sense, specifically describe the drug concentration–time profile as biphasic.

Clearance is a term that is useful in calculating average drug concentrations. With many drugs, a biphasic profile suggests a rapid tissue distribution phase followed by a slower elimination phase. Multi-compartment pharmacokinetics is an important consideration in understanding drug permeation and toxicity. For example, the plasma–time profiles of aminoglycosides, such as gentamicin, are more useful in explaining toxicity than average plasma or drug concentration taken at peak or trough time.

• Elimination rate constant

In the two-compartment model (IV administration), the elimination rate constant, k, represents the elimination of drug from the central compartment, whereas b represents drug elimination during the beta or elimination phase, when distribution is mostly complete. Because of redistribution of drug out of the tissue compartment, the plasma–drug level curve declines more slowly in the b phase. Hence b is smaller than k; thus k is a true elimination constant, whereas b is a hybrid elimination rate constant that is influenced by the rate of transfer of drug in and out of the tissue compartment. When it is impractical to determine k, b is calculated from the b slope. The $t_{1/2\beta}$ is often used to calculate the drug dose.

Two compartment model: intravenous infusion

Many drugs given by IV infusion follow two-compartment kinetics. For example, the respective distributions of theophylline and lidocaine in humans are described by the two-compartment open model. With two-compartment model drugs, IV infusion requires a distribution and equilibration of the drug before a stable blood level is reached. During a constant IV infusion, drug in the tissue compartment is in distribution equilibrium with the plasma; thus, constant C_{SS} levels also result in constant drug concentrations in the tissue; ie, no net change in the amount of drug in the tissue occurs at steady state. Although some clinicians assume that tissue and plasma concentrations are equal when fully equilibrated, kinetic models predict only that the rates of drug transfer into and out of the compartments are equal at steady state. In other words, drug concentrations in the tissue are also constant, but may differ from plasma concentrations.

The time needed to reach a steady-state blood level depends entirely on the distribution half-life of the drug. The equation describing plasma drug concentration as a function of time is as follows:

$$C_P = \frac{R}{V_P K}\left[1 - \left(\frac{K-b}{a-b}\right)e^{-at} - \left(\frac{a-K}{a-b}\right)e^{-bt}\right] \qquad \dots (5.164)$$

Where, a and b are hybrid rate constants and R is the rate of infusion. At steady state (i.e., $t = \infty$), equation 5.164 reduces to:

$$C_{SS} = \frac{R}{V_P K} \qquad \dots (5.165)$$

By rearranging this equation, the infusion rate for a desired steady-state plasma drug concentration may be calculated.

$$R = C_{SS}V_P K \qquad \dots (5.166)$$

• Loading dose plus iv infusion: two-compartment model

Drugs with long half-lives require a loading dose to more rapidly attain steady-state plasma drug levels. It is clinically desirable to achieve rapid therapeutic drug levels by using a loading dose. However, for drugs that follow the two-compartment pharmacokinetic model, the drug distributes slowly into extravascular tissues (compartment 2). Thus, drug equilibrium is not immediate. The plasma drug concentration of a drug that follows a two-compartment model after various loading doses is shown in. If a loading dose is given too rapidly, the drug may initially give excessively high concentrations in the plasma (central compartment), which then decreases as drug equilibrium is reached. It is not possible to maintain an instantaneous, stable steady-state blood level for a two-compartment model drug with a zero-order rate of infusion. Therefore, a loading dose produces an initial blood level either slightly higher or lower than the steady-state blood level. To overcome this problem, several IV bolus injections given as short intermittent IV infusions may be used as a method for administering a loading dose to the patient.

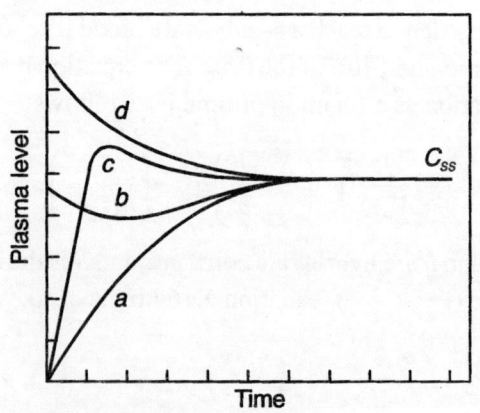

Fig. 5.39: Plasma drug level after various loading doses and rates of infusion for a drug that follows a two-compartment model: a, no loading dose; b, loading dose = R/k (rapid infusion); c, loading dose = R/b (slow infusion); and d, loading dose = R/b (rapid infusion).

- **Apparent volume of distribution at steady state, two-compartment model**

After administration of any drug that follows two-compartment kinetics, plasma drug levels will decline due to elimination, and some redistribution will occur as drug in tissue diffuses back into the plasma fluid. The volume of distribution at steady state, $(V_D)_{SS}$, is the "hypothetical space" in which the drug is assumed to be distributed. The product of the plasma drug concentration with $(V_D)_{SS}$ will give the total amount of drug in the body at that time period, such that $C_{pSS} \times (V_D)_{SS}$ = amount of drug in the body at steady state. At steady-state conditions, the rate of drug entry into the tissue compartment from the central compartment is equal to the rate of drug exit from the tissue compartment into the central compartment. These rates of drug transfer are described by the following expressions:

$$D_t K_{21} = D_P K_{12} \qquad \qquad \text{... (5.167)}$$

$$D_t = \frac{K_{12} D_P}{K_{12}} \qquad \qquad \text{... (5.168)}$$

where D_t is the amount of drug in the tissue compartment. Because the amount of drug in the central compartment, D_p, is equal to $V_p C_p$, by substitution in the above equation,

$$D_t = \frac{K_{12} C_P V_P}{K_{12}} \qquad \qquad \text{... (5.169)}$$

The total amount of drug in the body at steady state is equal to the sum of the amount of drug in the tissue compartment, D_t, and the amount of drug in the central compartment, D_p. Therefore, the apparent volume of drug at steady state $(V_D)_{SS}$ may be calculated by dividing the total amount of drug in the body by the concentration of drug in the central compartment at steady state:

$$(V_D)_{SS} = \frac{D_p + D_t}{C_P} \qquad \qquad \text{... (5.170)}$$

By substitution of equation 5.169 into equation 5.170, and by expressing D_p as $V_p C_p$, a more useful equation for the calculation of $(V_D)_{SS}$ is obtained:

$$(V_D)_{SS} = \frac{C_P V_P + K_{12} V_P C_P / K_{21}}{C_P} \qquad \qquad \text{... (5.171)}$$

This reduces to:

$$(V_D)_{SS} = V_P + \frac{K_{12}}{K_{21}} V_P \qquad \qquad \text{... (5.172)}$$

In practice, equation 5.172 is used to calculate $(V_D)_{SS}$. The $(V_D)_{SS}$ is a function of the transfer constants, k_{12} and k_{21}, which represent the rate constants of drug going into and out of the tissue compartment, respectively. The magnitude of $(V_D)_{SS}$ is dependent on the hemodynamic factors responsible for drug distribution and on the physical properties of the drug, properties which, in turn, determine the relative amount of intra- and extravascular drug.

Another volume term used in two-compartment modeling is $(V_D)_b$ (see). $(V_D)_b$ is often calculated from total body clearance divided by b. Unlike the steady-state volume of distribution, $(V_D)_{SS}$, $(V_D)_b$ is influenced by drug elimination in the beta "b" phase. Reduced drug clearance from the body may increase the area under the curve, AUC, such that $(V_D)_b$ is either reduced or unchanged, depending on the value of b as shown in equation 5.173.

$$(V_D)_b = (V_D)_{\text{area}} = \frac{D_0}{b[AUC]_0^\infty} \qquad \ldots (5.173)$$

Unlike $(V_D)_b$, $(V_D)_{SS}$ is not affected by changes in drug elimination. $(V_D)_{SS}$ reflects the true distributional volume occupied by the plasma and the tissue pool when steady state is reached. Although this volume is not useful in calculating the amount of drug in the body during pre-steady state, $(V_D)_{SS}$ multiplied by the steady-state plasma drug concentration, C_{SS}, yields the amount of drug in the body. This volume is often used to determine the loading drug dose necessary to upload the body to a desired plasma drug concentration. As shown by equation 5.173, $(V_D)_{SS}$ is several times greater than V_p, which represents the volume of the plasma compartment, but differs somewhat in value depending on the transfer constants.

Two Compartment Model: Extravascular Administration

(See zero order and first order absorption rate constant using loo-riegelman method)

Curve Fitting (Method of Residuals) Regression Procedures

(See determination of absorption rate constants from oral absorption data in one compartment model)

Clearance Concept

The clearance concept was first introduced to describe renal excretion of endogenous compounds in order to measure the kidney function. The term is now applied to all organs involved in drug elimination such as liver, lung, the biliary system, etc. and referred to as hepatic clearance, pulmonary clearance, and biliary clearance and so on. The sum of individual clearances by all eliminating organs is called as **total body clearance** or total systemic clearance. It is some time expressed as a sum of renal clearance and non renal clearance.

Clearance is defined as the hypothetical volume of body fluids containing drug from which the drug is removed or cleared completely in a specific period of time. It is expressed in ml/min and is a constant for any given plasma drug concentration. In comparison to apparent volume of distribution which relates plasma drug concentration to the amount of drug in body, clearance relates plasma concentration to the rate of drug elimination.

$$\text{Clearance } (Cl) = \frac{\text{Elimination rate}}{\text{Plasma drug concentration}} \qquad ... (5.174)$$

· Renal clearance (Cl_R)

It can be define as the volume of blood plasma which is completely cleared of the unchanged drug by the kidney per unit time

$$Cl_R = \frac{\text{Rate of urinary excretion}}{\text{Plasma drug concentration}} \qquad ... (5.175)$$

Physiologically speaking, renal clearance is the ratio of "sum of rate of glomerular filtration and active secretion minus rate of reabsorption" to "plasma drug concentration C"

$$Cl_R = \frac{\text{Rate of filtration} + \text{Rate of secretion} - \text{Rate of reabsorption}}{C}$$

$$\dots (5.176)$$

Mechanism of Renal Clearance

Renal excretion is a major route of elimination for many drugs. Drugs that are nonvolatile, water soluble, have a low molecular weight (MW), or are slowly biotransformed by the liver are eliminated by renal excretion. The processes by which a drug is excreted via the kidneys may include any combination of the following:

- **Glomerular filtration**
- **Active tubular secretion**
- **Tubular reabsorption**

Glomerular filtration is a unidirectional process that occurs for most small molecules (MW < 500), including undissociated (nonionized) and dissociated (ionized) drugs. Protein-bound drugs behave as large molecules and do not get filtered at the glomerulus. The major driving force for glomerular filtration is the hydrostatic pressure within the glomerular capillaries. The kidneys receive a large blood supply (approximately 25% of the cardiac output) via the renal artery, with very little decrease in the hydrostatic pressure.

Glomerular filtration rate (GFR) is measured by using a drug that is eliminated by filtration only (ie, the drug is neither reabsorbed nor secreted). Examples of such drugs are inulin and creatinine. Therefore, the clearance of inulin is equal to the GFR, which is equal to 125–130 mL/min. The value for the GFR correlates fairly well with body surface area. Glomerular filtration of drugs is directly related to the free or nonprotein-bound drug concentration in the plasma. As the free drug concentration in the plasma increases, the glomerular filtration for the drug increases proportionately, thus increasing renal drug clearance for some drugs.

Active tubular secretion is an active transport process. As such, active renal secretion is a carrier-mediated system that requires energy input, because the drug is transported against a concentration gradient. The carrier system is capacity limited and may be saturated. Drugs with similar structures may compete for the same carrier system. Two active renal secretion systems have been identified, systems for (1) weak acids and (2) weak bases. For example, probenecid competes with penicillin for the same carrier system (weak acids). Active tubular secretion rate is dependent on renal plasma flow. Drugs commonly used to measure active tubular secretion include p-amino-hippuric acid (PAH) and iodopyracet (Diodrast). These substances are both filtered by the glomeruli and secreted by the tubular cells. Active secretion is extremely rapid for these drugs, and practically all the drug carried to the kidney is eliminated in a single pass. The clearance for these drugs therefore reflects the effective renal plasma flow (ERPF), which varies from 425 to 650 mL/min.

For a drug that is excreted solely by glomerular filtration, the elimination half-life may change markedly in accordance with the binding affinity of the drug for plasma proteins. In contrast, drug protein binding has very little effect on the elimination half-life of the drug excreted mostly by active secretion. Because drug protein binding is reversible, drug bound to plasma protein rapidly dissociates as free drug is secreted by the kidneys. For example, some of the penicillins are extensively protein bound, but their elimination half-lives are short due to rapid elimination by active secretion.

Tubular reabsorption occurs after the drug is filtered through the glomerulus and can be an active or a passive process. If a drug is completely reabsorbed (eg, glucose), then the value for the clearance of the drug is approximately zero. For drugs that are partially reabsorbed, clearance values are less than the GFR of 125–130 mL/min.

The reabsorption of drugs that are acids or weak bases is influenced by the pH of the fluid in the renal tubule (ie, urine pH) and the pK_a of the drug. Both of these factors together determine the percentage of dissociated (ionized) and undissociated (nonionized) drug. Generally, the undissociated species is more lipid soluble (less water soluble) and has greater membrane permeability. The undissociated drug is easily reabsorbed from the renal tubule back into the body. This process of drug reabsorption can significantly reduce the amount of drug excreted, depending on the pH of the urinary fluid and the pK_a of the drug. The pK_a of the drug is a constant, but the normal urinary pH may vary from 4.5 to 8.0, depending on diet, pathophysiology, and drug intake. Vegetable and fruit diets or diets rich in carbohydrates result in higher urinary pH, whereas diets rich in protein result in lower urinary pH. Drugs such as ascorbic acid and antacids such as sodium carbonate may decrease (acidify) or increase (alkalinize) the urinary pH, respectively, when administered in large quantities. By far the most important changes in urinary pH are caused by fluids administered intravenously. Intravenous fluids, such as solutions of bicarbonate or ammonium chloride, are used in acid–base therapy. Excretion of these solutions may drastically change urinary pH and alter drug reabsorption and drug excretion by the kidney.

The percentage of ionized weak acid drug corresponding to a given pH can be obtained from the **Henderson–Hesselbalch equation**.

$$P^H = P^{K_a} + \log\frac{[\text{ionized}]}{[\text{nonionized}]} \qquad \dots (5.177)$$

Rearrangement of this equation yields

$$\frac{[\text{ionized}]}{[\text{nonionized}]} = 10^{P^H - PK_a} \qquad \dots (5.178)$$

$$\text{Fraction of drug ionized } = \frac{[\text{ionized}]}{[\text{ionized}]+[\text{nonionized}]} \qquad \dots (5.179)$$

$$= \frac{10^{P^H - PK_2}[\text{nonionized}]}{[\text{ionized}]+[\text{nonionized}]}$$

$$= \frac{10^{P^H - PK_2}}{1+10^{P^H - PK_2}}$$

The fraction or percent of weak acid drug ionized in any pH environment may be calculated with equation 5.179. For acidic drugs with pK_a values from 3 to 8, a change in urinary pH affects the extent of dissociation. The extent of dissociation is more greatly affected by changes in urinary pH for drugs with a pK_a of 5 than with a pK_a of 3. Weak acids with pK_a values of less than 2 are highly ionized at all urinary pH values and are only slightly affected by pH variations.

Table 5.11: Effect of urinary pH and pK_a on the ionization of drugs

pH of Urine	Percent of Drug Ionized: $pK_a = 3$	Percent of Drug Ionized: $pK_a = 5$
7.4	100	99.6
5	99	50.0
4	91	9.1
3	50	0.99

For a weak base drug, the Henderson–Hasselbalch equation is given as:

$$P^H = P^{K_a} + \log\frac{[\text{nonionized}]}{[\text{ionized}]} \qquad ... (5.180)$$

and

$$\text{Percent of drug ionized} = \frac{1 + 10^{P^H - PK_a}}{10^{P^H - PK_a}} \qquad ... (5.181)$$

The greatest effect of urinary pH on reabsorption occurs with weak base drugs with pK_a values of 7.5–10.5.

From the Henderson–Hesselbalch relationship, a concentration ratio for the distribution of a weak acid or basic drug between urine and plasma may be derived. The urine–plasma (U/P) ratios for these drugs are as follows.

For weak acids,

$$\frac{U}{P} = \frac{1 + 10^{pH_{urine} - pK_a}}{1 + 10^{pH_{plasma} - pK_a}} \qquad \text{... (5.182)}$$

For weak bases,

$$\frac{U}{P} = \frac{1 + 10^{pK_a - pH_{urine}}}{1 + 10^{pK_a - pH_{plasma}}} \qquad \text{... (5.183)}$$

For example, amphetamine, a weak base, will be reabsorbed if the urine pH is made alkaline and more lipid-soluble nonionized species are formed. In contrast, acidification of the urine will cause the amphetamine to become more ionized (form a salt). The salt form is more water soluble and less likely to be reabsorbed and has a tendency to be excreted into the urine more quickly. In the case of weak acids (such as salicylic acid), acidification of the urine causes greater reabsorption of the drug and alkalinization of the urine causes more rapid excretion of the drug.

Clearance ratio

Clearance ratio is defined as ratio of renal clearance of drug to renal clearance of creatinine.

$$\text{Renal clearance ratio} = \frac{Cl_R \text{ of drug}}{Cl_R \text{ of creatinine}} \qquad \text{... (5.184)}$$

Depending upon whether the drug is only filtered, filtered and secreted or filtered and reabsorbed, the clearance ratio will vary. The renal clearance values range from zero to 650ml/min and the clearance ratio from zero to five.

Determination of Renal Clearance

Graphical methods

The clearance is given by the slope of the curve obtained by plotting the rate of drug excretion in urine (dD_u/dt) against C_p (eq. 5.186). For a drug that is excreted rapidly, dD_u/dt is large, the slope is steeper, and clearance is greater (, line *A*). For a drug that is excreted slowly through the kidney, the slope is smaller (, line *B*).

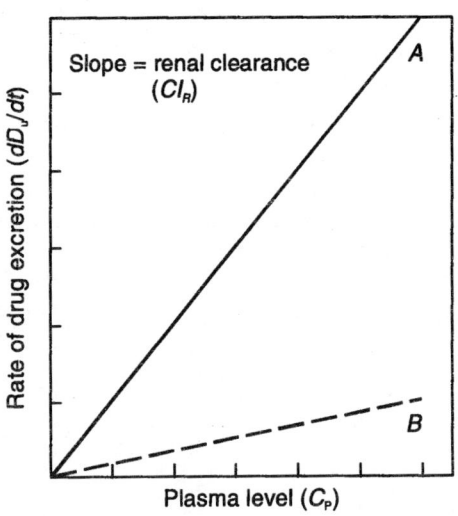

Fig. 5.40: Rate of drug excretion versus concentration of drug in the plasma. Drug *A* has a higher clearance than drug *B*, as shown by the slopes of line *A* and line *B*.

$$Cl_R = \frac{dD_u / dt}{C_P} \qquad \qquad ... (5.185)$$

Multiplying both sides by C_p gives

$$Cl_R C_P = \frac{dD_u}{dt} \qquad \qquad ... (5.186)$$

By rearranging Equation 6.28 and integrating, one obtains

$$\int_0^{dD_u} dD_u = Cl_R \int_0^t C_P dt \qquad \qquad ... (5.187)$$

$$[D_u]_0^t = Cl_R [AUC]_0^t \qquad \qquad ... (5.188)$$

A graph is then plotted of cumulative drug excreted in the urine versus the area under the concentration–time curve. Renal clearance is obtained from the slope of the curve. The area under the curve can be estimated by the trapezoidal rule or by other measurement methods. The disadvantage of this method is that if a data point is missing, the cumulative amount of drug excreted in the urine is difficult to obtain. However, if the data are complete, then the determination of clearance is more accurate by this method.

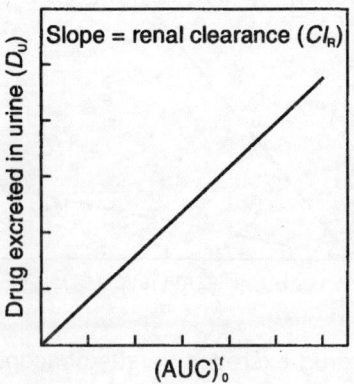

Fig. 5.41: Cumulative drug excretion versus *AUC*. The slope is equal to Cl_R.

By plotting cumulative drug excreted in the urine from t_1 to t_2, $[D_u]_{0t1}^t$ versus $[AUC]_{2t}^t$, one obtains an equation similar to that presented previously:

$$\int_{D_u^1}^{D_u^2} dD_u = Cl_R \int_{t_1}^{t_2} C_p dt \qquad \qquad \text{... (5.189)}$$

$$[D_u]_{t_1}^{t_2} = Cl_R [AUC]_{t_1}^{t_2} \qquad \qquad \text{... (5.190)}$$

The slope is equal to the renal clearance.

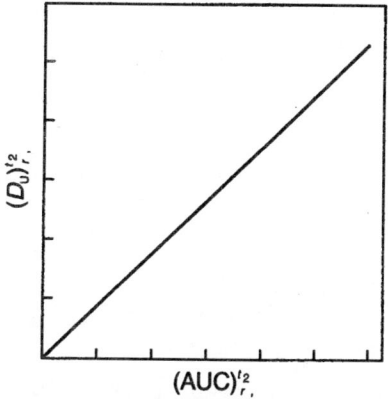

Fig. 5.42: Drug excreted versus $(AUC)^t{}_{2t1}$. The slope is equal to Cl_R.

Model-independent methods

Clearance rates may also be estimated by a single (nongraphical) calculation from knowledge of the $[AUC]_0^\infty$, the total amount of drug absorbed, FD_0, and the total amount of drug excreted in the urine, D_u^∞.. For example, if a single IV bolus drug injection is given to a patient and the $[AUC]_0^\infty$ is obtained from the plasma drug level–time curve, then total body clearance is estimated by

$$Cl_T = \frac{D_0}{[AUC]_0^\infty} \qquad \dots (5.191)$$

If the total amount of drug excreted in the urine, D_u^∞ has been obtained, then renal clearance is calculated by

$$Cl_R = \frac{D_0^\infty}{[AUC]_0^\infty} \qquad \dots (5.192)$$

The calculations using equations 5.191 and 5.192 allow for rapid and easily obtainable estimates of drug clearance. However, only a single dose estimate is obtained; therefore, the calculations do not reflect nonlinear changes in the clearance rates, as indicated in.

Clearance can also be calculated from fitted parameters. If the volumes of distribution and elimination constants are known, body clearance (Cl_T), renal clearance (Cl_R), and hepatic clearance (Cl_h) can be calculated according to the following expressions:

$$Cl_T = KV_D \qquad \qquad \text{... (5.193)}$$

$$Cl_R = K_C V_D \qquad \qquad \text{... (5.194)}$$

$$Cl_h = K_m V_D \qquad \qquad \text{... (5.195)}$$

Total body clearance (Cl_T) is equal to the sum of renal clearance and hepatic clearance and is based on the concept that the entire body acts as a drug-eliminating system.

$$Cl_T = Cl_R + Cl_h \qquad \qquad \text{... (5.196)}$$

By substitution of equations 5.193 and 5.194 into equation 5.196,

$$Cl_T = Cl_R + Cl_h \qquad \qquad \text{... (5.196)}$$

$$KV_D = K_c V_D + K_m V_D \qquad \qquad \text{... (5.197)}$$

Dividing by V_D on both sides of Equation 6.39,

$$K = K_c + K_m \qquad \qquad \text{... (5.198)}$$

Nonlinear Pharmacokinetics: Introduction

Linear pharmacokinetic models using simple first-order kinetics were introduced to describe the course of drug disposition and action. These linear models assumed that the pharmacokinetic parameters for a drug would not change when different doses or multiple doses of a drug were given. With some drugs, increased doses or chronic medication can cause deviations from the linear pharmacokinetic profile previously observed with single low doses of the same drug. This nonlinear pharmacokinetic behavior is also termed **dose-dependent pharmacokinetics.**

Many of the processes of drug absorption, distribution, biotransformation, and excretion involve enzymes or carrier-mediated systems. For some drugs given at therapeutic levels, one of these specialized processes may become saturated. As shown in, various causes of nonlinear pharmacokinetic behavior are theoretically possible. Besides saturation of plasma protein-binding or carrier-mediated systems, drugs may demonstrate nonlinear pharmacokinetics due to a pathologic alteration in drug absorption, distribution, and elimination. For example, aminoglycosides may cause renal nephrotoxicity, thereby altering renal drug excretion. In addition, gallstone obstruction of the bile duct will alter biliary drug excretion. In most cases, the main pharmacokinetic outcome is a change in the apparent elimination rate constant.

Table 5.12: Examples of drugs showing nonlinear kinetics

Cause	Drug
Saturable transport in gut wall	**GI Absorption** Riboflavin, gebapentin, L-dopa, baclofen, ceftibuten
Intestinal metabolism	Salicylamide, propranolol
Drugs with low solubility in GI but relatively high dose	Chorothiazide, griseofulvin, danazol
Saturable gastric or GI decomposition	Penicillin G, omeprazole, saquinavir
Saturable plasma protein binding	**Distribution** Phenylbutazone, lidocaine, salicylic acid, ceftriaxone, diazoxide, phenytoin, warfarin, disopyramide
Cellular uptake	Methicillin (rabbit)
Tissue binding	Imiprimine (rat)
CSF transport	Benzylpenicillins
Saturable transport into or out of tissues	Methotrexate
Active secretion	**Renal Elimination** Mezlocillin, para-aminohippuric acid
Tubular reabsorption	Riboflavin, ascorbic acid, cephapirin
Change in urine pH	Salicylic acid, dextroamphetamine

Saturable metabolism	**Metabolism** Phenytoin, salicyclic acid, theophylline, valproic acid[b]
Cofactor or enzyme limitation	Acetaminophen, alcohol
Enzyme induction	Carbamazepine
Altered hepatic blood flow	Propranolol, verapamil
Metabolite inhibition	Diazepam
Biliary secretion Enterohepatic recycling	**Biliary Excretion** Iodipamide, sulfobromophthalein sodium Cimetidine, isotretinoin

Non-linear Pharmacokinetics with Special Reference to one Compartment Model After I.V. Drug Administration

• (See estimation of K_m and V_{max} in michaelis menten equation).

Detection of Nonlinearity (Saturation Mechanism)

A number of drugs demonstrate saturation or capacity-limited metabolism in humans. Examples of these saturable metabolic processes include glycine conjugation of salicylate, sulfate conjugation of salicylamide, acetylation of p-aminobenzoic acid, and the elimination of phenytoin. Drugs that demonstrate saturation kinetics usually show the following characteristics.

1. Elimination of drug does not follow simple first-order kinetics—that is, elimination kinetics is nonlinear.

2. The elimination half-life changes as dose is increased. Usually, the elimination half-life increases with increased dose due to saturation of an enzyme system. However, the elimination half-life might decrease due to "self"-induction of liver biotransformation enzymes, as is observed for carbamazepine.

3. The area under the curve (AUC) is not proportional to the amount of bioavailable drug.

4. The saturation of capacity-limited processes may be affected by other drugs that require the same enzyme or carrier-mediated system (ie, competition effects).

5. The composition and/or ratio of the metabolites of a drug may be affected by a change in the dose.

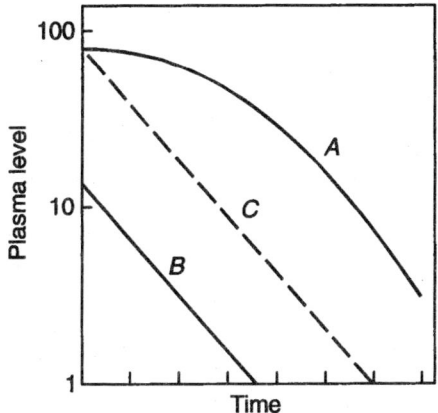

Fig. 5.43: Plasma level–time curves for a drug that exhibits a saturable elimination process. Curves *A* and *B* represent high and low doses of drug, respectively, given in a single IV bolus. The terminal slopes of curves *A* and *B* are the same. Curve *C* represents the normal first-order elimination of a different drug.

Because these drugs have a changing apparent elimination constant with larger doses, prediction of drug concentration in the blood based on a single small dose is difficult. Drug concentrations in the blood can increase rapidly once an elimination process is saturated. In general, metabolism (biotransformation) and active tubular secretion of drugs by the kidney are the processes most usually saturated. Shows plasma level–time curves for a drug that exhibits saturable kinetics. When a large dose is given, a curve is obtained with an initial slow elimination phase followed by a much more rapid elimination at lower blood concentrations (curve *A*). With a small dose of the drug, apparent first-order kinetics is observed, because no saturation kinetics occur (curve *B*). If the pharmacokinetic data were estimated only from the blood levels described by curve *B*, then a twofold increase in the dose would give the blood profile presented in curve *C*, which considerably underestimates the drug concentration as well as the duration of action.

In order to determine whether a drug is following dose-dependent kinetics, the drug is given at various dosage levels and a plasma level–time curve is obtained for each dose. The curves should exhibit parallel slopes if the drug follows dose-independent kinetics. Alternatively, a plot of the areas under the plasma level–time curves at various doses should be linear.

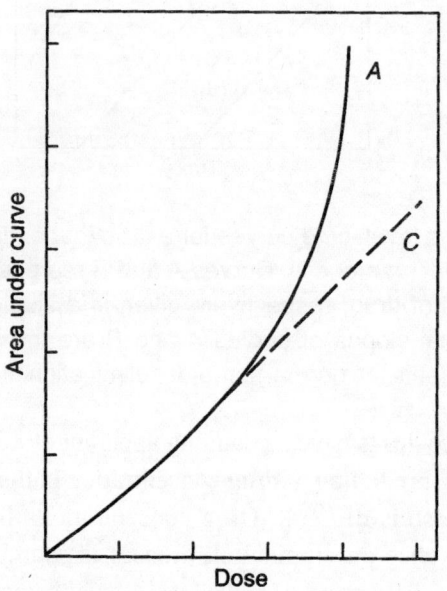

Fig. 5.44: Area under the plasma level–time curve versus dose for a drug that exhibits a saturable elimination process. Curve *A* represents dose-dependent or saturable elimination kinetics. Curve *C* represents dose-independent kinetics.

• Saturable enzymatic elimination processes

The elimination of drug by a saturable enzymatic process is described by

Michaelis–Menten kinetics. If C_p is the concentration of drug in the plasma, then

$$\text{Elimination rate} = \frac{dC_P}{dt} = \frac{V_{max} C_P}{K_M + C_P} \qquad \text{... (5.199)}$$

Where V_{max} is the maximum elimination rate and K_M is the Michaelis constant that reflects the capacity of the enzyme system.

It is important to note that K_M is not an elimination constant, but is actually a hybrid rate constant in enzyme kinetics, representing both the forward and backward reaction rates and equal to the drug concentration or amount of drug in the body at $0.5 V_{max}$. The values for K_M and V_{max} are dependent on the nature of the drug and the enzymatic process involved.

The elimination rate of a hypothetical drug with a K_M of 0.1 µg/mL and a V_{max} of 0.5 µg/mL per hour is calculated in by means of equation 5.199. Because the ratio of the elimination rate to drug concentration

Table 5.13: Effect of drug concentration on the elimination rate and rate constant

Drug Concentration (µg/mL)	Elimination Rate (µg/mL per hr)	Elimination Rate/ Concentration (hr⁻¹)
0.4	0.400	1.000
0.8	0.444	0.556
1.2	0.462	0.385
1.6	0.472	0.294
2.0	0.476	0.238
2.4	0.480	0.200
2.8	0.483	0.172
3.2	0.485	0.152
10.0	0.495	0.0495
10.4	0.495	0.0476
10.8	0.495	0.0459
11.2	0.496	0.0442
11.6	0.496	0.0427

changes as the drug concentration changes (i.e., dC_p/dt is not constant, eq. 5.199), the rate of drug elimination also changes and is not a first-order or linear process. In contrast, a first-order elimination process would yield the same elimination rate constant at all plasma drug concentrations. At drug concentrations of 0.4–10 μg/mL, the enzyme system is not saturated and the rate of elimination is a mixed or nonlinear process. At higher drug concentrations, 11.2 μg/mL and above, the elimination rate approaches the maximum velocity (V_{max}) of approximately 0.5 μg/mL per hour. At V_{max}, the elimination rate is a constant and is considered a zero-order process.

Equation 5.199 describes a nonlinear enzyme process that encompasses a broad range of drug concentrations. When the drug concentration C_p is large in relation to K_M ($C_p >> K_m$), saturation of the enzymes occurs and the value for K_M is negligible. The rate of elimination proceeds at a fixed or constant rate equal to V_{max}. Thus, elimination of drug becomes a zero-order process and equation 5.199 becomes:

$$-\frac{dC_P}{dt} = \frac{V_{max} C_P}{C_P} = V_{max} \qquad \text{... (5.200)}$$

Michaelis Menten Equation

The kinetics of capacity limited or a saturable process is best described by michaelis – menten equation:

$$-\frac{dC}{dt} = \frac{V_{max} C}{K_m + C} \qquad \text{... (5.201)}$$

Where,

$-dc/dt$ = rate of decline of drug concentration with time,

V_{max} = theoretical maximum rate of the process,

K_m = Michaelis constant.

Three situations can now be considered depending upon the values of Km and C.

(1) When $K_m = C$: Under this situation Michaelis menten equation reduces to:

$$-\frac{dC}{dt} = \frac{V_{max}}{2} \qquad \ldots (5.202)$$

i.e., the rate of process is equal to one-half its maximum rate.

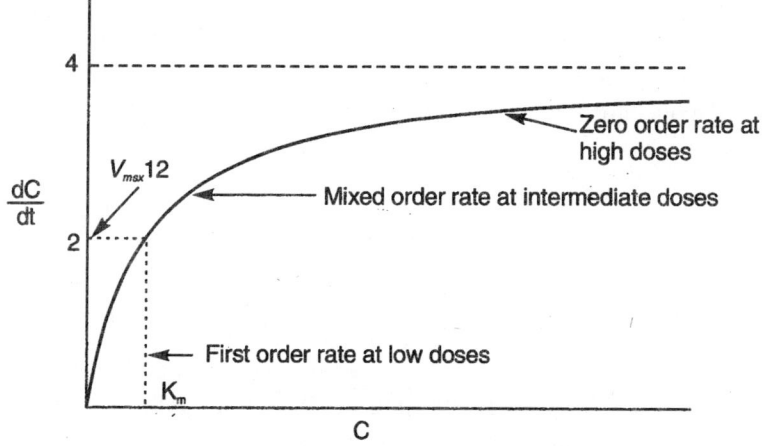

Fig. 5.45: A plot of Michaelis Menten equation (elimination rate dC/dt Versus Concentration C). Initially, the rate increases linearly (first order) with concentration, becomes mixed order at higher concentration and then reaches maximum (V_{max}) beyond which it proceeds at a constant rate (Zero-order).

2. When $K_m \gg C$: Here $Km + C = Km$ and the Michaelis Menten equation reduces to:

$$-\frac{dC}{dt} = \frac{V_{max}}{K_m} \qquad \ldots (5.203)$$

The above equation is identical to the one that describes first-order elimination of a drug where $V_{max}/k_m = K_E$. This means that the drug concentration in the body that results from usual dosage regimen of most drugs is well below the k_m of the elimination process with certain exceptions such as phenytoin and alcohol.

3. When $K_m << C$: under this condition, $K_m + C = C$ and the Michaelis Menten equation will become:

$$-\frac{dC}{dt} = V_{max} \qquad \qquad ... (5.204)$$

The above equation is identical to the one that describes a zero order process *i.e.*, the rate process occurs at a constant rate and is independent of drug concentration e.g., metabolism of ethanol.

• **Estimation of K_m and V_{max}**

The parameters of capacity – limited processes like metabolism, renal tubular secretion and biliary excretion can be easily defined by assuming one-compartment kinetics for the drug and that elimination involves only a single capacity –limited process.

Equation 5.199 relates the rate of drug biotransformation to the concentration of the drug in the body. The same equation may be applied to determine the rate of enzymatic reaction of a drug in vitro. When an experiment is performed with solutions of various concentration of drug C, a series of reaction rates (v) may be measured for each concentration. Special plots may then be used to determine K_M and V_{max}.

Equation 5.205 may be rearranged into equation 5.206.

$$V = \frac{V_{max} C}{K_M + C} \qquad \qquad ... (5.205)$$

$$\frac{1}{V} = \frac{K_M}{V_{max}} \frac{1}{C} + \frac{1}{V_{max}} \qquad \qquad ... (5.206)$$

Equation 5.206 is a linear equation when 1/v is plotted against 1/C. The *y*-intercept for the line is $1/V_{max}$, and the slope is K_M/V_{max}. An example of a drug reacting enzymatically with rate (v) at various concentrations

C is shown in. A plot of $1/v$ versus $1/C$ is shown in. A plot of $1/v$ versus $1/C$ is linear with an intercept of 0.33 mmol. Therefore,

$$\frac{1}{V_{max}} = 033 \text{ min mL/}\mu\text{mol}$$

$$\frac{1}{V_{max}} = 3 \ \mu\text{mol/mLmin}$$

Because the slope = $1.65 = K_M/V_{max} = K_M/3$ or $K_M = 3 \times 1.65 \ \mu\text{mol/}$ mL = 5 μmol/mL. Alternatively, K_M may be found from the x intercept, where $-1/K_M$ is equal to the x intercept. (This may be seen by extending the graph to intercept the x axis in the negative region.)

Table 5.14: Information necessary for graphic determination of v_{max} and k_m

Observation Number	C (µM/mL)	V (µM/mL per min)	1/V (mL per min/µM)	1/C (mL/µM)
1	1	0.500	2.000	1.000
2	6	1.636	0.611	0.166
3	11	2.062	0.484	0.090
4	16	2.285	0.437	0.062
5	21	2.423	0.412	0.047
6	26	2.516	0.397	0.038
7	31	2.583	0.337	0.032
8	36	2.504	0.379	0.027
9	41	2.673	0.373	0.024
10	46	2.705	0.369	0.021

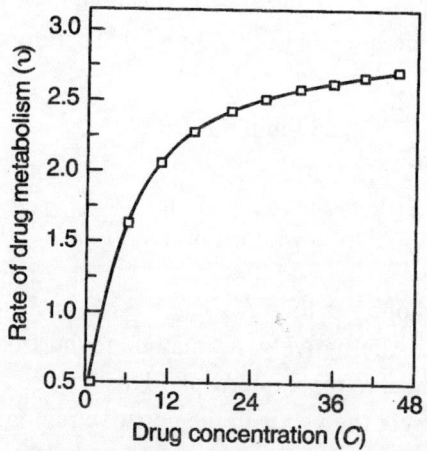

Fig. 5.46: Plot of rate of drug metabolism at various drug concentrations. (K_M = 0.5 µmol/mL, V_{max} = 3 µmol/mL per minute.)

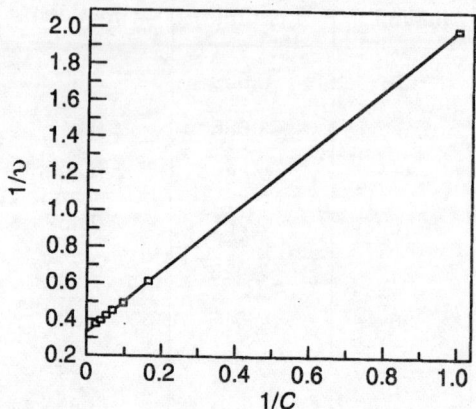

Fig. 5.47: Plot of $1/v$ versus $1/C$ for determining K_M and V_{max}.

With this plot, the points are clustered. Other methods are available that may spread the points more evenly. These methods are derived from rearranging equation 5.206 into equations 5.207 and 5.208.

$$\frac{C}{V} = \frac{1}{V_{max}}C + \frac{K_M}{V_{max}} \qquad \ldots (5.207)$$

$$V = -K_M\frac{V}{C} + V_{max} \qquad \ldots (5.208)$$

A plot of C/v versus C would yield a straight line with $1/V_{max}$ as slope and K_M/V_{max} as intercept (eq. 5.207). A plot of v versus v/C would yield a slope of $-K_M$ and an intercept of V_{max} (eq. 5.208). The necessary calculations for making the above plots are shown in. The plots are shown in. It should be noted that the data are spread out better by the two latter plots. Calculations from the slope show that the same K_M and V_{max} are obtained as in. When the data are more scattered, one method may be more accurate than the other. A simple approach is to graph the data and examine the linearity of the graphs. The same basic type of plot is used in the clinical literature to determine K_M and V_{max} for individual patients for drugs that undergo capacity-limited kinetics.

Table 5.15: Calculations Necessary for Graphic Determination of K_M and V_{max}

C (µM/mL)	v (µM/mL per min)	C/v (min)	v/C (1/min)
1	0.500	2.000	0.500
6	1.636	3.666	0.272
11	2.062	5.333	0.187
16	2.285	7.000	0.142
21	2.423	8.666	0.115
26	2.516	10.333	0.096
31	2.583	12.000	0.083
36	2.634	13.666	0.073
41	2.673	15.333	0.065
46	2.705	17.000	0.058

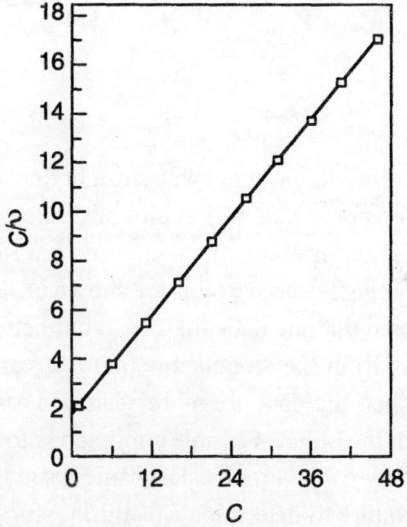

Fig. 5.48: Plot of C/v versus C for determining K_M and V_{max}.

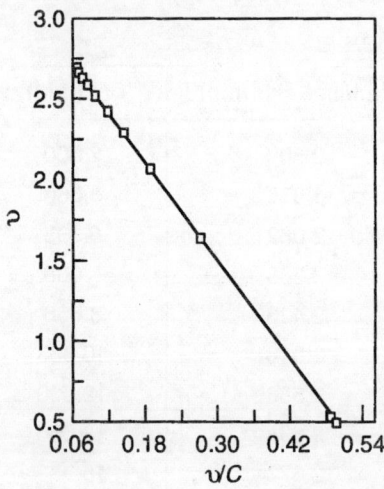

Fig. 5.49: Plot of v versus v/C for determining K_M and V_{max}.

• Determination of k_m and v_{max} in patients

Equation 5.205 shows that the rate of drug metabolism (v) is dependent on the concentration of the drug (C). This same basic concept may be applied to the rate of drug metabolism of a capacity-limited drug in the body. The body may be regarded as a single compartment in which the drug is dissolved. The rate of drug metabolism will vary depending on the concentration of drug C_p as well as on the metabolic rate constants K_M and V_{max} of the drug in each individual.

An example for the determination of K_M and V_{max} is given for the drug phenytoin. Phenytoin undergoes capacity-limited kinetics at therapeutic drug concentrations in the body. To determine K_M and V_{max}, two different dose regimens are given at different times, until steady state is reached. The steady-state drug concentrations are then measured by assay. At steady state, the rate of drug metabolism (v) is assumed to be the same as the rate of drug input R (dose/day). Therefore equation 5.209 may be written for drug metabolism in the body similar to the way drugs are metabolized in vitro (eq. 5.205). However, steady state will not be reached if the drug input rate, R, is greater than the V_{max}; instead, drug accumulation will continue to occur without reaching a steady-state plateau.

$$R = \frac{V_{max} C_{SS}}{K_M + C_{SS}} \quad \ldots (5.209)$$

where R = dose/day or dosing rate; C_{ss} = steady-state plasma drug concentration, V_{max} = maximum metabolic rate constant in the body, and K_M = Michaelis–Menten constant of the drug in the body.

• Determination of k_m and v_{max} by direct method

When steady-state concentrations of phenytoin are known at only two dose levels, there is no advantage in using the graphic method. K_M and V_{max} may be calculated by solving two simultaneous equations formed by substituting C_{SS} and R (eq. 5.209) with C_1, R_1, C_2, and R_2. The equations contain two unknowns, K_M and V_{max}, and may be solved easily.

$$R_1 = \frac{V_{max} C_1}{K_M + C_1} \qquad \text{... (5.210)}$$

$$R_2 = \frac{V_{max} C_2}{K_M + C_2} \qquad \text{... (5.211)}$$

Combining the two equations yields equation 5.212.

$$K_M = \frac{R_2 - R_1}{(R_1/C_1) - (R_2/C_2)} \qquad \text{... (5.212)}$$

Where C_1 is steady-state plasma drug concentration after dose 1, C_2 is steady-state plasma drug concentration after dose 2, R_1 is the first dosing rate, and R_2 is the second dosing rate. To calculate K_M and V_{max}, use Equation 9.15 with the values $C_1 = 8.6$ mg/L, $C_2 = 25.1$ mg/L, $R_1 = 150$ mg/day, and $R_2 = 300$ mg/day. The results are

$$K_M = \frac{300 - 150}{(150/8.6) - (300/25.1)} = 27.3 \, mg/L$$

Substitute K_M into either of the two simultaneous equations to solve for V_{max}.

$$150 = \frac{V_{max}(8.6)}{27.3 + 8.6}$$

$$V_{max} = 626 \text{ mg/day}$$

• **Interpretation of k_m and v_{max}**

An understanding of Michaelis–Menten kinetics provides insight into the nonlinear kinetics and helps to avoid dosing a drug at a concentration near enzyme saturation. For example, in the above phenytoin dosing example, since K_M occurs at $0.5 V_{max}$, $K_M = 27.3$ mg/L, the implication is that at a plasma concentration of 27.3 mg/L, enzymes responsible for phenytoin metabolism are eliminating the drug at 50% V_{max}, i.e., 0.5 x 626 mg/day or 313 mg/day. When the subject is receiving 300 mg of phenytoin per day, the plasma drug concentration of phenytoin is 8.6 mg/L, which is considerably below the K_M of 27.3mg/L. In practice, the K_M in patients can range from 1 to 15 mg/L, V_{max} can range from 100 to 1000 mg/day. Patients with a low K_M tend to have greater changes in plasma concentrations during dosing adjustments. Patients with a smaller K_M (same V_{max}) will show a greater change in the rate of elimination when plasma drug concentration changes compared to subjects with a higher K_M. A subject with the same V_{max}, but different K_M, is shown in. (For another example, see the slopes of the two curves generated in).

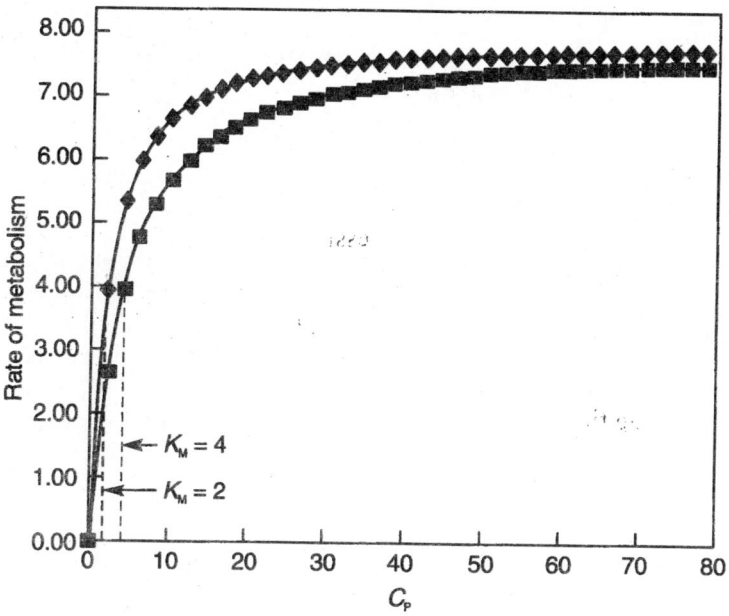

Fig. 5.50: Diagram showing the rate of metabolism when V_{max} is constant (8 µg/mL/hr) and K_M is changed (K_M = 2 µg/mL for top curve and K_M = 4 µg/mL for bottom curve). Note the rate of metabolism is faster for the lower K_M, but saturation starts at lower concentration.

Questions

Essay questions

1. Describe the zero order and first order absorption rate constant using wagner- nelson and loo-riegelman methods.

2. Determine the pharmacokinetic parameter from plasma and urine data after drug administration by oral, parenteral and other route.

3. Explain clearance concept, mechanism of renal clearance, clearance ratio. How to determine the renal clearance.

Short questions

1. What is the significance of plasma drug concentration measurement? Explain.

2. What is compartment model? Describe mammillary model and caternary model.

3. Write a note on curve fitting regression procedures

4. Explain saturation mechanism.

5. Explain michaelis menten equation and estimate K_m and V_{max}.

6. What is flip-flop phenomenon? Explain.

7. What is lag time? Explain.

Chapter—6

CLINICAL PHARMACOKINETICS

Definition and Scope

During the drug development process, large numbers of patients are tested to determine optimum dosing regimens, which are then recommended by the manufacturer to produce the desired pharmacologic response in the majority of the anticipated patient population. However, intra- and interindividual variations will frequently result in either a subtherapeutic (drug concentration below the MEC) or toxic response (drug concentrations above the minimum toxic concentration, MTC), which may then require adjustment to the dosing regimen. **Clinical pharmacokinetics** is the application of pharmacokinetic methods to drug therapy. Clinical pharmacokinetics involves a multidisciplinary approach to individually optimized dosing strategies based on the patient's disease state and patient-specific considerations. The study of clinical pharmacokinetics of drugs in disease states requires input from medical and pharmaceutical research is a list of 10 age-adjusted rates of death from 10 leading causes of death in the United States, 2003. The influence of many diseases on drug disposition is not adequately studied. Age, gender, genetic, and ethnic differences can also result in pharmacokinetic differences that may affect the outcome of drug therapy. The study of pharmacokinetic differences of drugs in various population groups is termed population pharmacokinetics.

Table 6.1: Ratio of age-adjusted death rates, by male/female ratio from the 10 leading causes of death in the USA, 2003

Disease	Rank	Male: Female
Disease of heart	1	1.5
Malignant neoplasms	2	1.5
Cerebrovascular diseases	3	4.0
Chronic lower respiration diseases	4	1.4
Accidents and others*	5	2.2
Diabetes mellitus	6	1.2
Pneumonia and influenza	7	1.4
Alzheimers	8	0.8
Nephrotis, nephrotic syndrome and nephrosis	9	1.5
Septicemia	10	1.2

Pharmacokinetics is also applied to therapeutic drug monitoring (TDM) for very potent drugs such as those with a narrow therapeutic range, in order to optimize efficacy and to prevent any adverse toxicity. For these drugs, it is necessary to monitor the patient, either by monitoring plasma drug concentrations (eg, theophylline) or by monitoring a specific pharmacodynamic endpoint such as prothrombin clotting time (eg, warfarin). Pharmacokinetic and drug analysis services necessary for safe drug monitoring are generally provided by the clinical pharmacokinetic service (CPKS). Some drugs frequently monitored are the aminoglycosides and anticonvulsants. Other drugs closely monitored are those used in cancer chemotherapy, in order to minimize adverse side effects.

Dosage Adjustment in Patient with and Without Renal and Hepatic Failure

❖ Effect of Renal Impairment on Pharmacokinetics

The kidney is an important organ in regulating body fluids, electrolyte balance, removal of metabolic waste, and drug excretion from the body. Impairment or degeneration of kidney function affects the pharmacokinetics of drugs. Some of the more common causes of kidney failure include disease, injury, and drug intoxication. List some of the conditions that may lead to chronic or acute renal failure. Acute diseases or trauma to the kidney can cause uremia, in which glomerular filtration is impaired or reduced, leading to accumulation of excessive fluid and blood nitrogenous products in the body. Uremia generally reduces glomerular filtration and/or active secretion, which leads to a decrease in renal drug excretion resulting in a longer elimination half-life of the administered drug.

PyelonephritisInflammation and deterioration of the pyelonephrons due to infection, antigens, or other idiopathic causes.HypertensionChronic overloading of the kidney with fluid and electrolytes may lead to kidney insufficiency.Diabetes mellitusThe disturbance of sugar metabolism and acid-base balance may lead to or predispose a patient to degenerative renal disease.Nephrotoxic drugs/metalsCertain drugs taken chronically may cause irreversible kidney damage—eg, the aminoglycosides, phenacetin, and heavy metals, such as mercury and lead.HypovolemiaAny condition that causes a reduction in renal blood flow will eventually lead to renal ischemia and damage.NeophroallergensCertain compounds may produce an immune type of sensitivity reaction with nephritic syndrome—eg, quartan malaria nephrotoxic serum.

In addition to changing renal elimination directly, uremia can affect drug pharmacokinetics in unexpected ways. For example, declining renal function leads to disturbances in electrolyte and fluid balance, resulting in physiologic and metabolic changes that may alter the pharmacokinetics and pharmacodynamics of a drug. Pharmacokinetic processes such as drug distribution (including both the volume of distribution and protein binding) and elimination (including both biotransformation and renal excretion) may also be altered by renal impairment. Both therapeutic and toxic responses may be altered as a result of changes in drug sensitivity at the receptor site. Overall, uremic patients have special dosing considerations to account for such pharmacokinetic and pharmacodynamic alterations.

Table 6.2: Common causes of kidney failure

Pyelonephritis	Inflammation and deterioration of the pyelonephrons due to infection, antigens, or other idiopathic causes.
Hypertension	Chronic overloading of the kidney with fluid and electrolytes may lead to kidney insufficiency.
Diabetes mellitus	The disturbance of sugar metabolism and acid-base balance may lead to or pre-dispose a patient to degenerative renal disease.
Nephrotoxic drugs/metals	Certain drugs taken chronically may cause irreversible kidney damage—eg, the aminoglycosides, phenacetin, and heavy metals, such as mercury and lead.
Hypovolemia	Any condition that causes a reduction in renal blood flow will eventually lead to renal ischemia and damage.
Neophroallergens	Certain compounds may produce an immune type of sensitivity reaction with nephritic syndrome—eg, quartan malaria nephrotoxic serum.

Pharmacokinetic considerations

Uremic patients may exhibit pharmacokinetic changes in bioavailability, volume of distribution, and clearance. The oral bioavailability of a drug in severe uremia may be decreased as a result of disease-related changes in gastrointestinal motility and pH caused by nausea, vomiting, and diarrhea. Mesenteric blood flow may also be altered. However, the oral bioavailability of a drug such as propranolol (which has a high first-pass effect) may be increased in patients with renal impairment as a result of the decrease in first-pass hepatic metabolism.The apparent volume of distribution depends largely on drug protein binding in plasma or tissues and total body water. Renal impairment may alter the distribution of the drug as a result of changes in fluid balance, drug protein binding, or other factors that may cause changes in the apparent volume of distribution. The plasma protein binding of weak acidic drugs in uremic patients is decreased, whereas the protein binding of weak basic drugs is less affected. The decrease in drug protein binding results in a larger fraction of free drug and an increase in the volume of distribution. However, the net elimination half-life is generally increased as a result of the dominant effect of reduced glomerular filtration. Protein binding of the drug may be further compromised due to the accumulation of metabolites of the drug and accumulation of various biochemical metabolites, such as free fatty acids and urea, which may compete for the protein-binding sites for the active drug.Total body clearance of drugs in uremic patients is also reduced by either a decrease in the glomerular filtration rate and possibly active tubular secretion or reduced hepatic clearance resulting from a decrease in intrinsic hepatic clearance.In clinical practice, estimation of the appropriate drug dosage regimen in patients with impaired renal function is based on an estimate of the remaining renal function of the patient and a prediction of the total body clearance. A complete pharmacokinetic analysis of the drug in the uremic patient is not possible. Moreover, the patient's uremic condition may not be stable and may be changing too rapidly for pharmacokinetic analysis. Each of the approaches for the calculation of a dosage regimen has certain assumptions and limitations that must be carefully assessed by the clinician before any approach is taken. Dosing guidelines for individual drugs in patients with renal impairment may be found in various reference books, such as the Physicians' Desk Reference, and in the medical literature.

General approaches for dose adjustment in renal disease

Several approaches are available for estimating the appropriate dosage regimen for a patient with renal impairment. Each of these approaches has similar assumptions, as listed in. Most of these methods assume that the required therapeutic plasma drug concentration in uremic patients is similar to that required in patients with normal renal function. Uremic patients are maintained on the same C^{∞}_{av} after multiple oral doses or multiple IV bolus injections. For IV infusions, the same C_{SS} is maintained. (C_{SS} is the same as C^{∞}_{av} after the plasma drug concentration reaches steady state.

The design of dosage regimens for uremic patients is based on the pharmacokinetic changes that have occurred as a result of the uremic condition. Generally, drugs in patients with uremia or kidney impairment have prolonged elimination half-lives and a change in the apparent volume of distribution. In less severe uremic conditions there may be neither edema nor a significant change in the apparent volume of distribution. Consequently, the methods for dose adjustment in uremic patients are based on an accurate estimation of the drug clearance in these patients.

Several specific clinical approaches for the calculation of drug clearance based on monitoring kidney function are presented later in this chapter. Two general pharmacokinetic approaches for dose adjustment include methods based on drug clearance and methods based on the elimination half-life.

Dose Adjustment Based on Drug Clearance

Methods based on drug clearance try to maintain the desired C^{∞}_{av} after multiple oral doses or multiple IV bolus injections as total body clearance, Cl_T, changes. The calculation for C^{∞}_{av} is,

Table 6.3 Common assumptions in dosing renal-impaired patient

Assumption	Comment
Creatinine clearance accurately measures the degree of renal impairment	Creatinine clearance estimates may be biased. Renal impairment should also be verified by physical diagnosis and other clinical tests.
Drug follows dose-independent pharmacokinetics	Pharmacokinetics should not be dose-dependent (nonlinear).
Nonrenal drug elimination remains constant	Renal disease may also affect the liver and cause a change in nonrenal drug elimination (drug metabolism).
Drug absorption remains constant	Unchanged drug absorption from gastrointestinal tract.
Drug clearance, Cl_u, declines linearly with creatinine clearance, Cl_{cr}	Normal drug clearance may include active secretion and passive filtration and may not decline linearly.
Unaltered drug protein binding	Drug protein binding may be altered due to accumulation of urea, nitrogenous wastes, and drug metabolites.
Target drug concentration remains constant	Changes in electrolyte composition such as potassium may affect sensitivity to the effect of digoxin. Accumulation of active metabolities may cause more intense pharmacodynamic response compared to parent drug alone.

$$C_{av}^{\infty} = FD_0 / CL_T \tau \qquad \ldots (6.1)$$

For patients with a uremic condition or renal impairment, total body clearance of the uremic patient will change to a new value, Cl_T^U. Therefore, to maintain the same desired C_{av}^{∞}, the dose must be changed to a uremic dose D_0^U, or the dosage interval must be changed to τ^u, as shown in the following equation:

$$C_{av}^\infty = \frac{D_0^N}{CL_T^N \tau^N} = \frac{D_0^U}{Cl_T^U \tau^U} \qquad \text{... (6.2)}$$

Where, the superscripts N and u represent normal and uremic conditions, respectively.

Rearranging Equation 6.2 and solving for D_0^U.

$$D_0^U = \frac{D_0^N CL_T^U \tau^U}{CL_T^N \tau^N} \qquad \text{... (6.3)}$$

If the dosage interval is kept constant, then the uremic dose D_0^U is equal to a fraction $\left(Cl_\perp T^\dagger U / Cl_\perp T^\dagger N\right)$ of the normal dose, as shown in the equation.

$$D_0^U = \frac{D_0^N CL_T^U}{CL_T^N} \qquad \text{... (6.4)}$$

For IV infusions the same desired C_{SS} is C_{av}^∞ maintained both for patients with normal renal function and for patients with renal impairment. Therefore, the rate of infusion, R, must be changed to a new value, R^U, for the uremic patient, as described by the equation.

$$C_{SS} = \frac{R}{CL_T^N} = \frac{R^U}{CL_T^U} \qquad \text{... (6.5)}$$
$$\text{(Normal) \quad (Uremic)}$$

Dose Adjustment Based on Changes in the Elimination Rate Constant

The overall elimination rate constant for many drugs is reduced in the uremic patient. A dosage regimen may be designed for the uremic patient either by reducing the normal dose of the drug and keeping the frequency of dosing (dosage interval) constant, or by decreasing the frequency of dosing (prolonging the dosage interval) and keeping the dose constant. Doses of drugs with a narrow therapeutic range should be reduced—

particularly if the drug has accumulated in the patient prior to deterioration of kidney function.

The usual approach to estimating a multiple-dosage regimen in the normal patient is to maintain a desired C^∞_{av}, as shown in Equation 6.1. Assuming the V_D is the same in both normal and uremic patients and is constant, and then the uremic dose D_0^U is a fraction (k^U/k^N) of the normal dose:

$$D_0^U = \frac{D_0^N K^U}{K^N} \qquad \ldots (6.6)$$

When the elimination rate constant for a drug in the uremic patient cannot be determined directly, indirect methods are available to calculate the predicted elimination rate constant based on the renal function of the patient. The assumptions on which these dosage regimens are calculated include the following.

1. The renal elimination rate constant (k_R) decreases proportionately as renal function decreases. (Note that k_R is the same as k_e as used in previous chapters.)

2. The nonrenal routes of elimination (primarily, the rate constant for metabolism) remain unchanged.

3. Changes in the renal clearance of the drug are reflected by changes in the creatinine clearance.

The overall elimination rate constant is the sum total of all the routes of elimination in the body, including the renal rate and the nonrenal rate constants:

$$K^U = K_{nr} + K_R^U \qquad \ldots (6.7)$$

Where, K_{nr} is the nonrenal elimination rate constant and K_R is the renal excretion rate constant.

Renal clearance is the product of the apparent volume of distribution and the rate constant for renal excretion:

$$Cl_R^U = K_R^U V_D^U \qquad \ldots (6.8)$$

Rearrangement of Equation 6.8 gives

$$K_R^U = Cl_R^U \cdot \frac{1}{V_D^U} \qquad \qquad ... (6.9)$$

Assuming that the apparent volume of distribution and nonrenal routes of elimination do not change in uremia, then $K_{nr}^U = K_{nr}^N$ and $V_D^U = V_D^N$.

Substitution of Equation 6.9 into Equation 6.7 gives

$$K^U = K_{nr} + \frac{1}{V_D} \cdot Cl_R^U \qquad \qquad ... (6.10)$$

From Equation 6.10, a change in the renal clearance, Cl_R^U, due to renal impairment will be reflected in a change in the overall elimination rate constant K_u. Because changes in the renal drug clearance cannot be accessed directly in the uremic patient, Cl_R^U is usually related to a measurement of kidney function by the glomerular filtration rate (GFR), which in turn is estimated by changes in the patient's creatinine clearance.

Dose Adjustment for Uremic Patients

Dose adjustment for drugs in uremic or renally impaired patients should be made in accordance with changes in pharmacodynamics and pharmacokinetics of the drug in the individual patient. Active metabolites of the drug may also be formed and must be considered for additional pharmacologic effects when adjusting dose. The following methods may be used to estimate an initial and maintenance dose regimen. After initiating the dosage, the clinician should continue to monitor the pharmacodynamics and pharmacokinetics of the drug. He or she should also evaluate the patient's renal function, which may be changing.

• Basis for dose Adjustment in Uremia

The loading drug dose is based on the apparent volume of distribution of the patient. It is generally assumed that the apparent volume of distribution is not altered significantly and therefore that the loading dose of the drug is the same in uremic patients as in subjects with normal renal function.

The maintenance dose is based on clearance of the drug in the patient. In the uremic patient, the rate of renal drug excretion has decreased, leading to a decrease in total body clearance. Most methods for dose adjustment assume nonrenal drug clearance to be unchanged. The fraction of normal renal function remaining in the uremic patient is estimated from creatinine clearance.

After the remaining total body clearance in the uremic patient is estimated, a dosage regimen may be developed by (1) decreasing the maintenance dose, (2) increasing the dosage interval, or (3) changing both maintenance dose and dosage interval.

Although total body clearance is a more accurate index of drug dosing, the elimination half-life of the drug is more commonly used for dose adjustment because of its convenience. Clearance allows for the prediction of steady-state drug concentrations, while elimination half-life yields information on the time it takes to reach steady-state concentration.

• Nomograms

Nomograms are charts available for use in estimating dosage regimens in uremic patients. The nomograms may be based on serum creatinine concentrations, patient data (height, weight, age, gender), and the pharmacokinetics of the drug. As discussed by, each nomogram has errors in its assumptions and drug database.

Most methods for dose adjustment in renal disease assume that non-renal elimination of the drug is not affected by renal impairment and that the remaining renal excretion rate constant in the uremic patient is proportional to the product of a constant and the creatinine clearance, Cl_{Cr}.

$$K_U = K_{nr} + \alpha \, Cl_{Cr} \qquad \ldots (6.11)$$

Where, k_{nr} is the nonrenal elimination rate constant and α is a constant. Equation 6.11 is similar to Equation 6.10, where $\alpha = 1/V_D$, and can be used for the construction of a nomogram. Shows a graphical representation of Equation 6.11 for four different drugs, each with a different renal excretion rate constant. The fractions of drug excreted in the urine unchanged, fe, for drugs A, B, C, and D are 5%, 50%, 75%, and 90%, respectively. A creatinine clearance of ≥ 80 mL/min is considered an adequate glomerular filtration rate in subjects with normal renal function. The uremic elimination rate constant (k_u) is the sum of the nonrenal elimination rate constant and the renal elimination rate constant, which is decreased due to renal impairment. If the patient has complete renal shutdown (i.e.creatinine clearance = 0 mL/min), then the intercept on the y axis represents the percent of drug elimination due to nonrenal drug elimination routes. Drug D, which is excreted 90% unchanged in the urine, has the steepest slope (equivalent to á in Eq. 6.11) and is most affected by small changes in creatinine clearance; whereas drug A, which is excreted only 5% unchanged in the urine (i.e. 95% eliminated by nonrenal routes), is least affected by a decrease in creatinine clearance.

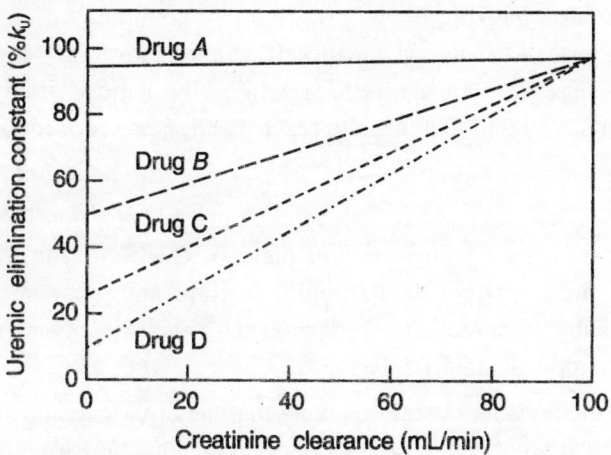

Fig. 6.1: Relationship between creatinine clearance and the drug elimination rate constant.

The nomogram method of provides an estimate of the ratio of the uremic elimination rate constant (k_u) to the normal elimination rate constant (k_N) on the basis of creatinine clearance. For this method, provided a list of drugs grouped according to the amount of drug excreted unchanged in the urine. From the k_u/k_N ratio, the uremic dose can be estimated according to Equation 6.12:

$$\text{Uremic dose} = \frac{K_U}{K_N} \times \text{normal dose} \qquad ...(6.12)$$

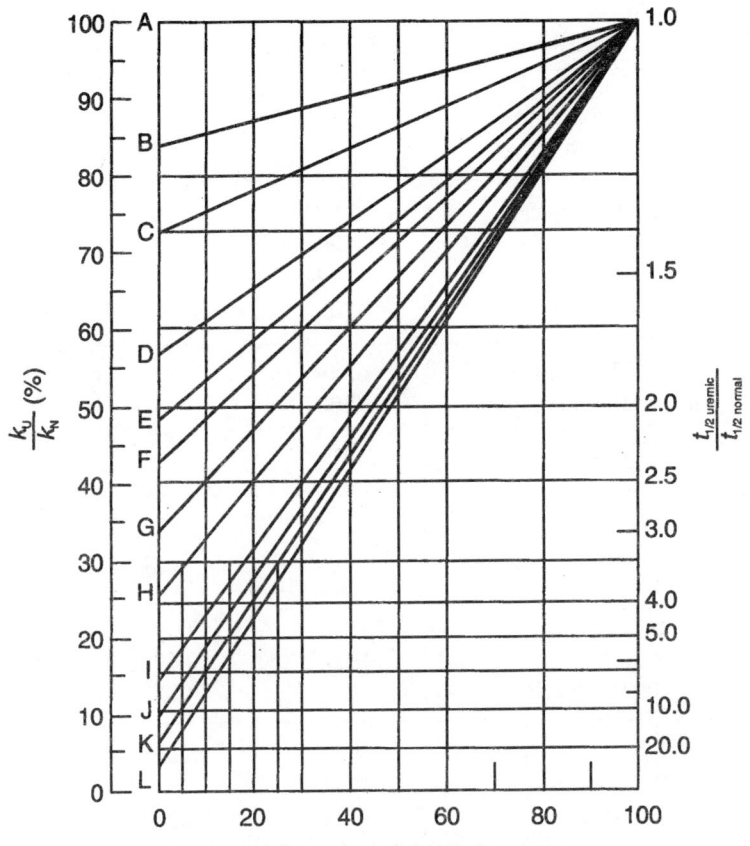

Fig. 6.2: Nomograph describes the changes in the percentage of normal elimination rate constant (left ordinate) and the consequent geometric increase in elimination half-life (right ordinate) as a function of creatinine clearance.

Table 6.4: Elimination Rate Constants for Various Drugs

Group	Drug	k_N (hr⁻¹)	k_{nr} (hr⁻¹)	k_{nr}/k_N%
A	Minocycline	0.04	0.04	100.0
	Rifampicin	0.25	0.25	100.0
	Lidocaine	0.39	0.36	92.3
	Digitoxin	0.114	0.10	87.7

Group	Drug	k_N (hr^{-1})	k_{nr} (hr^{-1})	k_{nr}/k_N%
B	Doxycycline	0.037	0.031	83.8
	Chlortetracycline	0.12	0.095	79.2
C	Clindamycin	0.16	0.12	75.0
	Chloramphenicol	0.26	0.19	73.1
	Propranolol	0.22	0.16	72.8
	Erythromycin	0.39	0.28	71.8
D	Trimethoprim	0.054	0.031	57.4
	Isoniazid (fast)	0.53	0.30	56.6
	Isoniazid (slow)	0.23	0.13	56.5
E	Dicloxacillin	1.20	0.60	50.0
	Sulfadiazine	0.069	0.032	46.4
	Sulfamethoxazole	0.084	0.037	44.0
F	Nafcillin	1.26	0.54	42.8
	Chlorpropamide	0.020	0.008	40.0
	Lincomycin	0.15	0.06	40.0
G	Colistimethate	0.154	0.054	35.1
	Oxacillin	1.73	0.58	33.6
	Digoxin	0.021	0.007	33.3
H	Tetracycline	0.120	0.033	27.5
	Cloxacillin	1.21	0.31	25.6
	Oxytetracycline	0.075	0.014	18.7
I	Amoxicillin	0.70	0.10	14.3
	Methicillin	1.40	0.19	13.6
J	Ticarcillin	0.58	0.066	11.4
	Penicillin G	1.24	0.13	10.5
	Ampicillin	0.53	0.05	9.4
	Carbenicillin	0.55	0.05	9.1

Group	Drug	k_N (hr^{-1})	k_{nr} (hr^{-1})	$k_{nr}/k_N\%$
K	Cefazolin	0.32	0.02	6.2
	Cephaloridine	0.51	0.03	5.9
	Cephalothin	1.20	0.06	5.0
	Gentamicin	0.30	0.015	5.0
L	Flucytosine	0.18	0.007	3.9
	Kanamycin	0.28	0.01	3.6
	Vancomycin	0.12	0.004	3.3
	Tobramycin	0.32	0.010	3.1
	Cephalexin	1.54	0.032	2.1

(k_N is for patients with normal renal function, k_{nr} is for patients with severe renal impairment, and $k_{nr}/k_N\%$ = percent of normal elimination in severe renal impairment).

When the dosage interval is kept constant, the uremic dose is always a smaller fraction of the normal dose. Instead of reducing the dose for a uremic patient, the usual dose is kept constant and the dosage interval is prolonged according to the following equation:

$$\text{Dosage interval in uremia, } \tau_U = \frac{K_N}{K_U} \times \tau_N \qquad \text{... (6.13)}$$

Where, τ is the dosage interval for the dose in uremic patients and τ_N is the dosage interval for the dose in patients with normal renal function.

• Fraction of drug excreted unchanged (*fe*) methods

For many drugs, the fraction of drug excreted unchanged (*fe*) is available in the literature. Lists various drugs with their *fe* value and elimination half-life. The *fe* method for estimating a dosage regimen in the uremic patient is a general method that may be applied to any drug whose *fe* is known.

Table 6.5: Fraction of drug excreted unchanged (*fe*) and elimination half-life values

Drug	Fe	$t_{1/2 \text{ normal}}$ (hr)[a]
Acebutolol	0.44 ± 0.11	2.7 ± 0.4
Acetaminophen	0.03 ± 0.01	2.0 ± 0.4
Acetohexamide	0.4	1.3
Allopurinol	0.1	2–8
Active metabolite		16–30
Alprenolol	0.005	3.1 ± 1.2
Amantadine	0.85	10
Amikacin	0.98	2.3 ± 0.4
Amiloride	0.5	8 ± 2
Amoxicillin	0.52 ± 0.15	1.0 ± 0.1
Amphetamine	0.4–0.45	12
Amphotericin B	0.03	360
Ampicillin	0.90 ± 0.08	1.3 ± 0.2
Atenolol	0.85	6.3 ± 1.8
Azlocillin	0.6	1.0
Bacampicillin	0.88	0.9
Baclofen	0.75	3–4
Bleomycin	0.55	1.5–8.9
Bretylium	0.8 ± 0.1	4–17
Bumetanide	0.33	3.5
Carbenicillin	0.82 ± 0.09	1.1 ± 0.2
Cefalothin	0.52	0.6 ± 0.3
Cefamandole	0.96 ± 0.03	0.77
Cefazolin	0.80 ± 0.13	1.8 ± 0.4
Cefoperazone	0.2–0.3	2.0
Cefotaxime	0.5–0.6	1–1.5
Cefoxitin	0.88 ± 0.08	0.7 ± 0.13
Cefuroxime	0.92	1.1
Cephalexin	0.96	0.9 ± 0.18
Chloramphenicol	0.05	2.7 ± 0.8
Chlorphentermine	0.2	120
Chlorpropamide	0.2	36
Chlorthalidone	0.65 ± 0.09	44 ± 10
Cimetidine	0.77 ± 0.06	2.1 ± 1.1

Drug	Fe	$t_{1/2\,normal}$ (hr)[a]
Clindamycin	0.09—0.14	2.7 ± 0.4
Clofibrate	0.11–0.32	13 ± 3
Clonidine	0.62 ± 0.11	8.5 ± 2.0
Colistin	0.9	3
Cytarabine	0.1	2
Cyclophosphamide	0.3	5
Dapsone	0.1	20
Dicloxacillin	0.60 ± 0.07	0.7 ± 0.07
Digitoxin	0.33 ± 0.15	166 ± 65
Digoxin	0.72 ± 0.09	42 ± 19
Disopyramide	0.55 ± 0.06	7.8 ± 1.6
Doxycycline	0.40 ± 0.04	20 ± 4
Erythromycin	0.15	1.1–3.5
Ethambutol	0.79 ± 0.03	3.1 ± 0.4
Ethosuximide	0.19	33 ± 6
Flucytosine	0.63–0.84	5.3 ± 0.7
Flunitrazepam	0.01	15 ± 5
Furosemide	0.74 ± 0.07	0.85 ± 0.17
Gentamicin	0.98	2–3
Griseofulvin	0	15
Hydralazine	0.12–0.14	2.2–2.6
Hydrochlorothiazide	0.95	2.5 ± 0.2
Indomethacin	0.15 ± 0.08	2.6–11.2
Isoniazid		
Rapid acetylators	0.07 ± 0.02	1.1 ± 0.2
Slow acetylators	0.29 ± 0.05	3.0 ± 0.8
Isosorbide dinitrate	0.05	0.5
Kanamycin	0.9	2.1 ± 0.2
Lidocaine	0.02 ± 0.01	1.8 ± 0.4
Lincomycin	0.6	5
Lithium	0.95 ± 0.15	22 ± 8
Lorazepam	0.01	14 ± 5
Meperidine	0.04–0.22	3.2 ± 0.8
Methadone	0.2	22
Methicillin	0.88 ± 0.17	0.85 ± 0.23
Methotrexate	0.94	8.4

Drug	Fe	$t_{1/2 \text{ normal}}$ (hr)[a]
Methyldopa	0.63 ± 0.10	1.8 ± 0.2
Metronidazole	0.25	8.2
Mexiletine	0.1	12
Mezlocillin	0.75	0.8
Minocycline	0.1 ± 0.02	18 ± 4
Minoxidil	0.1	4
Moxalactam	0.82–0.96	2.5–3.0
Nadolol	0.73 ± 0.04	16 ± 2
Nafcillin	0.27 ± 0.05	0.9–1.0
Nalidixic acid	0.2	1.0
Netilmicin	0.98	2.2
Neostigmine	0.67	1.3 ± 0.8
Nitrazepam	0.01	29 ± 7
Nitrofuraniton	0.5	0.3
Nomifensine	0.15–0.22	3.0 ± 1.0
Oxacillin	0.75	0.5
Oxprenolol	0.05	1.5
Pancuronium	0.5	3.0
Pentazocine	0.2	2.5
Phenobarbital	0.2 ± 0.05	86 ± 7
Pindolol	0.41	3.4 ± 0.2
Pivampicillin	0.9	0.9
Polymyxin B	0.88	4.5
Prazosin	0.01	2.9 ± 0.8
Primidone	0.42 ± 0.15	8.0 ± 4.8
Procainamide	0.67 ± 0.08	2.9 ± 0.6
Propranolol	0.005	3.9 ± 0.4
Quinidine	0.18 ± 0.05	6.2 ± 1.8
Rifampin	0.16 ± 0.04	2.1 ± 0.3
Salicylic acid	0.2	3
Sisomicin	0.98	2.8
Sotalol	0.6	6.5–13
Streptomycin	0.96	2.8
Sulfisoxazole	0.53 ± 0.09	5.9 ± 0.9
Sulfinpyrazone	0.45	2.3
Tetracycline	0.48	9.9 ± 1.5

Drug	Fe	$t_{1/2\ normal}$ (hr)[a]
Thiamphenicol	0.9	3
Thiazinamium	0.41	
Theophylline	0.08	9 ± 2.1
Ticarcillin	0.86	1.2
Timolol	0.2	3–5
Tobramycin	0.98	2.2 ± 0.1
Tocainide	0.20-0.70 (0.40 mean)	1.6–3
Tolbutamide	0	5.9 ± 1.4
Triamterene	0.04 ± 0.01	2.8 ± 0.9
Trimethoprim	0.53 ± 0.02	11 ± 1.4
Tubocurarine	0.43 ± 0.08	2 ± 1.1
Valproic acid	0.02 ± 0.02	16 ± 3

Half-life is a derived parameter that changes as a function of both clearance and volume of distribution. It is independent of body size, because it is a function of these two parameters (Cl, V_D), each of which is proportional to body size. It is important to consider that half-life is the time to eliminate 50% of the "drug" from the body (plasma), not the time in which 50% of the effect is lost.

The Giusti–Hayton (1973) method assumes that the effect of reduced kidney function on the renal portion of the elimination constant can be estimated from the ratio of the uremic creatinine clearance, Cl_{Cr}^U, to the normal creatinine clearance, Cl_{Cr}^N:

$$\frac{K_T^U}{K^N} = \frac{Cl_{Cr}^U}{Cl_{Cr}^U} \qquad \ldots (6.14)$$

Where, K_r^U is the uremic renal excretion rate constant and K_r^N is the normal renal excretion rate constant.

$$K_r^U = K_r^U \cdot \frac{Cl_{Cr}^U}{Cl_{Cr}^N} \qquad \ldots (6.15)$$

Because the overall uremic elimination rate constant, k_U, is the sum of renal and nonrenal elimination,

$$K_U = K_{nr}^U + K_r^U \qquad \text{... (6.16)}$$

$$K_U = K_{nr}^U + K_r^N \left(\frac{Cl_{Cr}^U}{Cl_{Cr}^N} \right)$$

Dividing Equation 6.16 by k_N on both sides yields

$$\frac{K_U}{K_N} = \frac{K_{nr}^U}{K_N} + \frac{K_r^N}{K_N} \left(\frac{Cl_{Cr}^U}{Cl_{Cr}^N} \right) \qquad \text{... (6.17)}$$

Let $fe = K_r^N / K_N$ = fraction of drug excreted unchanged in the urine and $1 - fe = K_{nr}^U / K_N$ = fraction of drug excreted by nonrenal routes. Substitution into Equation 6.17 yields the Giusti–Hayton equation, where G is the Giusti–Hayton factor, which can be calculated from the *fe* and the ratio of uremic to normal clearance:

$$\frac{K_U}{K_N} = (1 - fe) + fe \left(\frac{Cl_{Cr}^U}{Cl_{Cr}^N} \right)$$

or,

$$\frac{K_U}{K_N} = 1 - fe \left(1 - \frac{Cl_{Cr}^U}{Cl_{Cr}^N} \right) = G \qquad \text{... (6.18)}$$

The Giusti–Hayton equation is useful for most drugs for which the fraction of drug excreted by renal routes has been reported in the literature. The ratio K_{nr}^U / k_N can be calculated from the fraction of drug excreted by the kidney, normal creatinine clearance, and the creatinine clearance in the uremic patient.

- **Comparison of the Various Methods for dose Adjustment in Uremic Patients**

All of the methods mentioned previously have similar limitations. For example, the drug must follow dose-independent kinetics and the volume of distribution of the drug must remain relatively constant in the uremic patient. As mentioned, it is usually assumed that the nonrenal routes of elimination, such as hepatic clearance, do not change. Because no correction for metabolites is made, any drug having an active pharmacologic metabolite must be additionally modified. Another assumption in the use of these methods is that pharmacologic response is unchanged in the uremic patient. This assumption may be unrealistic for drugs that act differently in the disease state. For example, the pharmacologic response with digoxin is dependent on the potassium level in the body, and the potassium level in the uremic patient may be rather different from that of the normal individual. In a patient undergoing dialysis, loss of potassium may increase the potential of toxic effect of the drug digoxin. For many drugs, studies have shown that the incidence of adverse effects is increased in uremic patients. It is often impossible to distinguish whether the increase in adverse effect is due to a pharmacokinetic change or to a pharmacodynamic change in the receptor sensitivity to the drug. In any event, these observations point out the fact that dose adjustment must be regarded as a preliminary estimation to be followed with further adjustments in accordance with the observed clinical response.

• General clearance method

The general clearance method is based on the methods discussed above. This method is popular in clinical settings because of its simplicity. The method assumes that creatinine clearance, Cl_{Cr}, is a good indicator of renal function and that the renal clearance of a drug, Cl_R, is proportional to Cl_{Cr}. Therefore, renal drug clearance, Cl_R^U, in the uremic patient is,

$$Cl_R^U = \frac{Cl_{Cr}^U}{Cl_{Cr}^N} \times Cl_R \qquad \text{... (6.19)}$$

$$Cl_u = Cl_{nr} + Cl_R \cdot \frac{Cl_{Cr}^U}{Cl_{Cr}^N} \qquad \text{... (6.20)}$$

Where, Cl_u is the total body clearance in the uremic patient.

If the ratio $\dfrac{Cl_{Cr}^U}{Cl_{Cr}^N}$, Cl_{nr}, and Cl_R are known, the total body clearance in the uremic patient may be estimated using Equation 6.20. Alternatively, if the normal total body clearance, Cl, and *fe* are known, Equation 6.21 may be obtained by substitution in Equation 6.20:

$$Cl_u = Cl(1 - fe) + fe\, Cl \cdot \frac{Cl_{Cr}^U}{Cl_{Cr}^N} \qquad \text{... (6.21)}$$

Equation 6.21 calculates drug clearance in the uremic patient using the fraction of drug excreted unchanged (*fe*), total body clearance of the drug (Cl) in the normal subject, and the ratio of creatinine clearance of the uremic to that of the normal patient.

Dividing Equation 6.21 on both sides by Cl yields the ratio Cl_u/Cl, reflecting the fraction of the uremic/normal drug dose.

$$\frac{Cl_U}{Cl} = (1 - fe) + fe \cdot \frac{Cl_{Cr}^U}{Cl_{Cr}^N} \qquad \text{... (6.22)}$$

• **The wagner method**

The methods for renal dose adjustment discussed in the previous sections all assume that the volume of distribution and the fraction of drug excreted by nonrenal routes are unchanged. These assumptions are convenient and hold true for many drugs. However, in the absence of reliable information assuring the validity of these assumptions, the equations should be demonstrated as statistically reliable in practice. A statistical approach was used by, who established a linear relationship between creatinine concentration and the first-order elimination constant of the drug in patients. The Wagner method is described in greater detail in the previous edition.

This method takes advantage of the fact that the elimination constant for a patient can be obtained from the creatinine clearance, as follows:

$$K\% = a + b \, Cl_{Cr} \qquad \qquad ...(6.23)$$

The values of a and b are determined statistically for each drug from pooled data on uremic patients. The method is simple to use and should provide accurate determination of elimination constants for patients when a good linear relationship exists between elimination constant and creatinine concentration. The theoretical derivation of this approach is as follows:

$K\%$ = total elimination rate constant

K_{nr} = nonrenal elimination rate constant (%)

K_R = renal excretion rate constant

Cl = total body clearance of drug

$$R = \frac{Cl}{Cl_{Cr}} \qquad \qquad ...(6.24)$$

$$Cl = R \, Cl_{Cr}$$

$$K = K_{nr} + \frac{R}{V_D} \, Cl_{Cr}$$

$$100K = 100 \, K_{nr} + \frac{100R}{V_D} \, Cl_{Cr}$$

$$K\% = a + b \, Cl_{Cr} \qquad \qquad ...(6.25)$$

Equation 6.25 can also be used with drugs that follow the two-compartment model. In such cases the terminal half-life is used and b, the terminal slope of elimination curve, is substituted for the elimination rate constant, k. Since the equation assumes a constant nonrenal elimination constant (k_{nr}) and volume of distribution, any change in these two parameters will result in an error in the estimated elimination constant.

❖ Effect of Hepatic Disease on Pharmacokinetics

Drugs are often metabolized by one or more enzymes located in cellular membranes in different parts of the liver. Drugs and metabolites may also be excreted by biliary secretion. Hepatic disease may lead to drug accumulation, failure to form an active or inactive metabolite, increased bioavailability after oral administration, and other effects including possible alteration in drug protein binding, and kidney function.

The major difficulty in estimating hepatic clearance in patients with hepatic disease is the complexity and stratification of the liver enzyme systems. In contrast, creatinine clearance has been used successfully to measure kidney function and renal clearance of drugs. Clinical laboratory tests measure only a limited number of liver functions. Some clinical laboratory tests, such as the aspartate aminotransferase (AST) and alanine aminotransferases (ALT) are common serum enzyme tests that detect liver cell damage rather than liver function. Other laboratory tests, such as serum bilirubin, are used to measure biliary obstruction or interference with bile flow. Presently, no single test accurately assesses the total liver function. Usually, a series of clinical laboratory tests are used in clinical practice to detect the presence of liver disease, distinguish among different types of liver disorders, gauge the extent of known liver damage, and follow the response to treatment. A few tests have been used to relate the severity of hepatic impairment to predicted changes in the pharmacokinetic profile of the drug (FDA Guidance for Industry, 2003). Examples of these tests include the ability of the liver to eliminate marker drugs such as antipyrine, indocyanine green, monoethylglycine-xylidide, and galactose. Furthermore, endogenous substrates such as albumin or bilirubin, or a functional measure such as prothrombin time, have been used for the evaluation of liver impairment.

Dosage considerations in hepatic disease

Several physiologic and pharmacokinetic factors are relevant in considering dosage of a drug in patients with hepatic disease. Chronic disease or tissue injury may change the accessibility of some enzymes as a result of redirection or detour of hepatic blood circulation. Liver disease affects the quantitative and qualitative synthesis of albumin, globulins, and other circulating plasma proteins that subsequently affect drug plasma protein binding and distribution. As mentioned, most liver function tests indicate only that the liver has been damaged; they do not assess the function of the cytochrome P-450 enzymes or intrinsic clearance by the liver.

Table 6.6: Considerations in dosing patients with hepatic impairment

Item	Comments
Nature and severity of liver disease	Not all liver diseases affect the pharmacokinetics of the drugs to the same extent.
Drug elimination	Drugs eliminated by the liver >20% are less likely to be affected by liver disease. Drugs that are eliminated mainly via renal route will be least affected by liver disease
Route of drug administration	Oral drug bioavailability may be increased by liver disease due to decrease first-pass effects
Protein binding	Drug protein binding may be altered due to alteration in hepatic synthesis of albumin
Hepatic blood flow	Drugs with flow dependent hepatic clearance will be more affected by change in hepatic blood flow
Intrinsic clearance	Metabolism of drugs with high intrinsic clearance may be impaired
Biliary obstruction	Biliary excretion of some drugs and metabolites, particularly glucuronide metabolites, may be impaired
Pharmacodynamic changes	Tissue sensitivity to drug may be altered
Therapeutic range	Drugs with a wide therapeutic range will be less affected by moderate hepatic impairment

Because there is no readily available measure of hepatic function that can be applied to calculate appropriate doses, enzyme-dependent drugs are usually given to patients with hepatic failure in half-doses, or less. Response or plasma levels then must be monitored. Drugs with flow-dependent clearance are avoided if possible in patients with liver failure. When necessary, doses of these drugs may need to be reduced to as low as one-tenth of the conventional dose, for an orally administered agent. Starting therapy with low doses and monitoring response or plasma levels provides the best opportunity for safe, efficacious treatment.

Fraction of drug metabolized

Drug elimination in the body may be divided into: (1) fraction of drug excretion unchanged, *fe*, and (2) fraction of drug metabolized. The latter is usually estimated from $1 - fe$; alternatively, the fraction of drug metabolized may be estimated from the ratio of Cl_h/Cl, where Cl_h is hepatic clearance and Cl is total body clearance. Knowing the fraction of drug eliminated by the liver allows estimation of total body clearance when hepatic clearance is reduced. Drugs with low *fe* values (or, conversely, drugs with a higher fraction of metabolized drug) are more affected by a change in liver function due to hepatic disease.

$$Cl_h = Cl(1 - fe) \qquad \qquad ...(6.26)$$

Equation 6.26 assumes that all metabolisms occur in the liver, and all the unchanged drug is excreted in the urine.

Active drug and the metabolite

For many drugs, both the drug and the metabolite contribute to the overall therapeutic response of the patient to the drug. The concentration of both the drug and the metabolite in the body should be known. When the pharmacokinetic parameters of the metabolite and the drug are similar, the overall activity of the drug can become more or less potent as a result of a change in liver function; that is, (1) when the drug is more potent than the metabolite, the overall pharmacologic activity will increase in the hepatic-impaired patient because the parent drug concentration will be higher; (2) when the drug is less potent than the metabolite, the overall pharmacologic activity in the hepatic patient will decrease because less of the active metabolite is formed.

Changes in pharmacologic activity due to hepatic disease may be much more complex when both the pharmacokinetic parameters as well as the pharmacodynamics of the drug change as a result of the disease process. In such cases, the overall pharmacodynamic response may be greatly modified, making it necessary to monitor the response change with the aid of a pharmacodynamic model.

Table 6.7: Pugh's Modification of Child's Classification (Total points: 5–6 = mild dysfunction; 7–9 = moderate dysfunction; >9 = severe dysfunction

	1 Point	2 Points	3 Points
Encephalopathy (grade)	None	1 or 2	3 or 4
Ascites	Absent	Slight	Moderate
Bilirubin (mg/dL)	1–2	2–3	>3
Albumin (gm/dL)	>3.5	2.8–3.5	<2.8
Prothrombin time (sec > control)	1–4	4–10	>10

Hepatic Blood Flow and Intrinsic Clearance

Blood flow changes can occur in patients with chronic liver disease (often due to viral hepatitis or chronic alcohol use). In some patients with severe liver cirrhosis, fibrosis of liver tissue may occur, resulting in intra- or extrahepatic shunt. Hepatic arterial-venous shunts may lead to reduced drug fraction of drug extracted and an increase in the bioavailability of drug. In other patients, resistance to blood flow may be increased as a result of tissue damage and fibrosis, causing a reduction in intrisic hepatic clearance.

The following equation may be applied to estimate hepatic clearance of a drug after assessing changes in blood flow and intrinsic clearance (Cl_{int}):

$$Cl_h = \frac{QCl_{int}}{Q+Cl_{int}} \qquad \text{... (6.27)}$$

Alternatively, when both Q and the extraction ratio, ER, are known in the patient, Cl may also be estimated:

$$Cl = Q\,(ER) \qquad \text{... (6.28)}$$

Unlike changes in renal disease, in which serum creatinine concentration may be used to monitor changes in renal function such as glomerular filtration (GFR), the above physiologic model equation may not be adequate to account for accurate prediction of changes in hepatic clearance. Calculations based on model equations must be corroborated by clinical assessment.

Pathophysiologic assessment

In practice, patient information about changes in hepatic blood flow may not be available, because special electromagnetic or ultrasound techniques are required to measure blood flow and are not routinely available. The clinician/pharmacist may have to make an empirical estimate of the blood flow change after examining the patient and reviewing the available liver function tests.

Table 6.8: Severity Classification Schemes for Liver Disease

	Child–Turcotte Classification		
	Grade A	**Grade B**	**Grade C**
Bilirubin (mg/dL)	<2.0	2.0–3.0	>3.0
Albumin (gm/dL)	>3.5	3.0–3.5	<3.0
Ascites	None	Easily controlled	Poorly controlled
Neurological disorder	None	Minimal	Advanced
Nutrition	Excellent	Good	Poor

While chronic hepatic disease is more likely to change the metabolism of a drug, acute hepatitis due to hepatotoxin or viral inflammation is often associated with marginal or less severe changes in metabolic drug clearance. The clinician may make an assessment based on acceptable risk criteria on a case-by-case basis. List useful endpoints for assessing the extent of hepatic dysfunction.

In general, basic pharmacokinetics treats the body globally and more readily applies to dosing estimation. However, drug clearance based on individual eliminating organs is more informative and provides more insight into the pharmacokinetic changes in the disease process. A practical method for dosing hepatic-impaired patients is still in its early stages of development. While the hepatic blood flow model is useful for predicting changes in hepatic clearance resulting from alterations in hepatic blood flow, Q_a and Q_v, extrahepatic changes can also influence pharmacokinetics in hepatic-impaired patients. Global changes in distribution may occur outside the liver. Extrahepatic metabolism and other hemodynamic changes may also occur and can be accounted for more completely by monitoring total body clearance of the drug using basic pharmacokinetics. For example, lack of local change in hepatic drug clearance should not be prematurely interpreted as "no change" in overall drug clearance. Reduced albumin and á-acid glycoprotein (AAG), for example, may change the volume of distribution of the drug and therefore alter total body clearance on a global basis.

Hormonal Influence

Hormones can also affect the rate of metabolism. In hyperthyroid patients, the rate of metabolism of many drugs is increased, as are, for example, the rates for theophylline, digoxin, and propranolol. In hypothyroid disease, the rate of metabolism of these drugs may be decreased. In children with human growth hormone (HGH) deficiency, administration of HGH decreases the half-life of theophylline.

Table 6.9: Drugs with significantly decreased metabolism in chronic liver disease

Antipyrine	Caffeine
Cefoperazone	Chlordiazepoxide
Chloramphenicol	Diazepam
Erythromycin	Hexobarbital
Metronidazole	Lidocaine
Meperidine	Metoprolol
Pentazocine	Propranolol
Tocainide	Theophylline
Verapamil	Promazine

Example

After IV bolus administration of 1 g of cefoperazone to normal and chronic hepatitis patients, urinary excretion of cefoperazone was significantly increased in cirrhosis patients, from 23.95 ± 5.06% for normal patients to 51.09 ± 11.50% in cirrhosis patients. Explain **(a)** why there is a change in the percent of unchanged cefoperazone excreted in the urine of patients with cirrhosis, and **(b)** suggest a quantitative test to monitor the hepatic elimination of cefoperazone.

Liver function tests and hepatic metabolic markers

Drug markers used to measure residual hepatic function may correlate well with hepatic clearance of one drug but correlate poorly with substrate metabolized by a different enzyme within the same cytochrome P-450 subfamily. Some useful marker compounds are listed below.

1. Aminotransferase (normal ALT, male, 10–55 U/L; female, 7–30 U/L; normal AST, male, 10–40, U/L; female, 9–25 U/L). Aminotransferases are enzymes found in many tissues that include serum glutamic oxaloacetic transaminase (AST, formerly

SGOT) and alanine aminotransferase (ALT, formerly SGPT). ALT is liver-specific, but AST is found in liver and many other tissues, including cardiac and skeletal muscle. Leakage of aminotransferases into the plasma is used as an indicator of many types of hepatic disease and hepatitis. The AST/ALT ratio is used in differential diagnosis. In acute liver injury, AST/ALT is d"1, whereas in alcoholic hepatitis the AST/ALT > 2.

2. Alkaline phosphatase (male, 45–115 U/L; female, 30–100 U/L). Like aminotransferase, alkaline phosphatase (AP) is normally present in many tissues, and is present on the canalicular domain of the hepatocyte plasma membrane. Plasma AP may be elevated in hepatic disease because of increased AP production and released into the serum. In cholestasis, or bile flow obstruction, AP release is facilitated by bile acid solubilization of the membranes. Marked AP elevations may indicate hepatic tumors or biliary obstruction in the liver, or disease in other tissues such as bone, placenta, or intestine.

3. Bilirubin (normal total = 0–1.0 mg/dL, direct = 0–0.4 mg/dL). Bilirubin consists of both a water-soluble, conjugated, "direct" fraction and a lipid-soluble, unconjugated, "indirect" fraction. The unconjugated form is bound to albumin and is therefore not filtered by the kidney. Since impaired biliary excretion results in increases in conjugated (filtered) bilirubin, hepatobiliary disease can result in increases in urinary bilirubin. Unconjugated hyperbilirubinemia results from either increased bilirubin production or defects in hepatic uptake or conjugation. Conjugated hyperbilirubinemia results from defects in hepatic excretion.

4. Prothrombin time (PT; normal, 11.2–13.2 sec). With the exception of Factor VIII, all coagulation factors are synthesized by the liver. Therefore, hepatic disease can alter coagulation. Decreases in PT (the rate of conversion of prothrombin to thrombin) therefore are suggestive of acute or chronic liver failure or biliary

obstruction. Vitamin K is also important in coagulation, so vitamin K deficiency can also decrease PT.

Example

Paclitaxel, an anticancer agent for solid tumors and leukemia, has extensive tissue distribution, high plasma protein binding (approximately 90–95%), and variable systemic clearance. Average paclitaxel clearance ranges from 87 to 503 mL/min/m² (5.2–30.2 L/h/m²) with minimal renal excretion of parent drug, 10%. Paclitaxel is extensively metabolized by the liver to three primary metabolites. Cytochrome P-450 enzymes of the CYP3A and CYP2C subfamilies appear to be involved in hepatic metabolism of paclitaxel. What are the precautions in administering paclitaxel to patients with liver disease?

Solution

Although paclitaxel has first-order pharmacokinetics at normal doses, its elimination may be saturable in some patients with genetically reduced intrinsic clearance due to CYP3A or CYP2C. The clinical importance of saturable elimination will be greatest when large dosages are infused over a shorter period of time. In these situations, achievable plasma concentrations are likely to cause saturation of binding. Thus, small changes in dosage or infusion duration may result in disproportionately large alterations in paclitaxel systemic exposure, potentially influencing patient response and toxicity.

❖ Dosing of Drugs in the Elderly

Defining "elderly" is difficult. The geriatric population is often arbitrarily defined as patients who are older than 65 years, and many of these people live active and healthy lives. In addition, there is an increasing number of people who are living more than 85 years, who are often considered as the "older elderly" population. The aging process is more often associated with physiologic changes during aging rather than purely chronological age. Chronologically, the elderly have been classified as the young old (ages 65–75 years), the old (ages 75–85 years), and the old old (age > 85 years). Performance capacity and the loss of homeostatic reserve decreases with advanced age but occurs to a different degree in each organ and in each patient. Physiologic and cognitive functions tend to change with the aging process and can affect compliance and the therapeutic safety and efficacy of a prescribed drug. The elderly also tend to be on multiple drug therapy due to concomitant illness. Decreased cognitive function in some geriatric patients, complicated drug dosage schedules, and/or the high cost of drug therapy may result in poor drug compliance, resulting in lack of drug efficacy, possible drug interactions, and/or drug intoxication.

Several vital physiologic functions related to age as measured by markers show that renal plasma flow, glomerular filtration, cardiac output, and breathing capacity can drop from 10% to 30% in elderly subjects compared to those at age 30. The physiologic changes due to aging may necessitate special considerations in administering drugs in the elderly. For some drugs, an age-dependent increase in adverse drug reactions or toxicity may be observed. This apparent increased drug sensitivity in the elderly may be due to pharmacodynamic and/or pharmacokinetic changes. The pharmacodynamic hypothesis assumes that age causes alterations in the quantity and quality of target drug receptors, leading to enhanced drug response. Quantitatively, the number of drug receptors may decline with age, whereas qualitatively, a change in the affinity for the drug may occur. Alternatively, the pharmacokinetic hypothesis assumes that age-dependent increases in adverse drug reactions are due to physiologic changes in drug absorption, distribution, and elimination, including renal excretion and hepatic clearance.

In the elderly, age-dependent alterations in drug absorption may include a decline in the splanchnic blood flow, altered gastrointestinal motility, increase in gastric pH, and alteration in the gastrointestinal absorptive surface. The incidence of achlorhydria in the elderly may have an effect on the dissolution of certain drugs such as weak bases and certain dosage forms that require an acid environment for disintegration and release. From a distribution consideration, drug protein binding in the plasma may decrease as a result of decrease in the albumin concentration, and the apparent volume of distribution may change due to a decrease in muscle mass and an increase in body fat. Renal drug excretion generally declines with age as a result of decrease in the glomerular filtration rate and/or active tubular secretion. Moreover, the activity of the enzymes responsible for drug biotransformation may decrease with age, leading to a decline in hepatic drug clearance.

Elderly patients may have several different pathophysiologic conditions that require multiple drug therapy that increases the likelihood for a drug interaction. Moreover, increased adverse drug reactions and toxicity may result from poor patient compliance. Both penicillin and kanamycin show prolonged $t_{1/2}$ in the aged patient, as a consequence of an age-related gradual reduction in the kidney size and function. The Gault–Cockroft rule for calculating creatinine clearance clearly quantitates a reduction in clearance with increased age. Age-related changes in plasma albumin and α_1-acid glycoprotein may also be a factor in the binding of drugs in the body.

A general equation that allows calculation of maintenance dose for a patient of any age (except neonates and infants) when maintenance of same Css, av is desired is:

$$\text{Patient's dose} = \frac{(\text{Weight in kg})^{0.7} \ (140 - \text{age in years})}{1660} \times \text{adult dose}$$

$$\text{... (6.29)}$$

❖ Dosing of Drugs in the Obese Patient

Obesity is a major problem in the United States and is also becoming a problem in other countries. Obesity has been associated with increased mortality resulting from increases in the incidence of hypertension, atherosclerosis, coronary artery disease, diabetes, and other conditions compared to nonobese patients. A patient is considered obese if actual body weight exceeds ideal or desirable body weight by 20%, according to Metropolitan Life Insurance Company data (latest published tables). Ideal or desirable body weights are based on average body weights and heights for males and for females considering age. Athletes who have a greater body weight due to greater muscle mass are not considered obese. Obesity often is defined by body mass index (BMI), a value that normalizes body weight based on height. BMI is expressed as body weight (kg) divided by the square of the person's height (meters) or kg/m². BMI is calculated according to the following two equations:

$$BMI = \left[weight \frac{lb}{height(in)^2} \right] \times 703 \qquad \text{... (6.30)}$$

$$BMI = \left[weight \frac{kg}{height(cm)^2} \right] \times 10,000 \qquad \text{... (6.30)}$$

Table 6.10 Five weight classifications based on BMI

	BMI
Underweight	<18.5
Normal body weight	18.5–24.9
Overweight	25–29.9
Obese	30–39.9
Extreme obesity	>40

The obese patient (BMI > 30) has a greater accumulation of fat tissue than is necessary for normal body functions. Adipose (fat) tissue has a smaller proportion of water compared to muscle tissue. Thus, the obese patient has a smaller proportion of total body water to total body weight compared to the patient of ideal body weight, which could affect the apparent volume of distribution of the drug. For example, showed a significant difference in the apparent volume of distribution of antipyrine in obese patients (0.46 L/kg) compared to ideal-body-weight patients (0.62 L/kg) based on actual total body weight. Ideal body weight (IBW) refers to the appropriate or normal weight for a male or female based on age, height, weight, and frame size; ideal body weights are generally obtained from the latest table of desirable weights for men and women compiled by the Metropolitan Life Insurance Company.

In addition to differences in total body water per kilogram body weight in the obese patient, the greatest proportion of body fat in these patients could lead to distributional changes in the drug's pharmacokinetics due to partitioning of the drug between lipid and aqueous environments. Drugs such as digoxin and gentamicin are very polar and tend to distribute into water rather than into fat tissue. Although lipophilic drugs are associated with larger volumes of distribution in obese patients compared to hydrophilic drugs, there are exceptions and the effect of obesity on specific drugs must be considered for accurate dosing strategy.

Other pharmacokinetic parameters may be altered in the obese patient as a result of physiologic alterations, such as fatty infiltration of the liver affecting biotransformation and cardiovascular changes that may affect renal blood flow and renal excretion.

Dosing by actual body weight may result in overdosing of drugs such as aminoglycosides (eg, gentamicin), which are very polar and are distributed in extracellular fluids. Dosing of these drugs is based on ideal body weight. Lean body weight has been estimated by several empirical equations based on the patient's height and actual (total) body weight. The following equations have been used for estimating lean body weight, particularly for adjustment of dosage in renally impaired patients:

$$\text{LBW (males)} = 50 \text{ kg} + 2.3 \text{ kg for each inch over 5 ft} \quad ... \text{ (6.32)}$$
$$\text{LBW (females)} = 45.5 \text{ kg} + 2.3 \text{ kg for each inch over 5 ft} ... \text{ (6.33)}$$

Where, LBW is lean body weight.

❖ Dosing of Drugs in Infants and Children

Infants and children have different dosing requirements than adults. Dosing of drugs in this population requires a thorough consideration of the differences in the pharmacokinetics and pharmacology of a specific drug in the preterm newborn infant, newborn infant (birth to 28 days), infant (28 days to 23 months), young child (2 to 5 years), older child (6 to 11 years), adolescent (12 to 18 years), and the adult (FDA Guidance for Industry, 2000). Unfortunately, the pharmacokinetics and pharmacodynamics of most drugs are not well known in children under 12 years of age. The variation in body composition and the maturity of liver and kidney function are potential sources of differences in pharmacokinetics with respect to age. For convenience, "infants" are here arbitrarily defined as children 0 to 2 years of age. However, within this group, special consideration is necessary for infants less than 4 weeks (1 month) old, because their ability to handle drugs often differs from that of more mature infants.

In addition to different dosing requirements for the pediatric population, there is a need to consider the use of pediatric dosage forms that permit more accurate dosing and patient compliance. For example, liquid pediatric drug products may come with a calibrated dropper or a premeasured teaspoon (5 mL) for accurate dosing and have a cherry flavor for pediatric patient compliance. Pediatric drug formulations may also contain different drug concentrations compared to the adult drug formulation. Furthermore, alternative drug delivery such as an intramuscular antibiotic drug injection into the gluteus medius may be considered for a pediatric patient, as opposed to the deltoid muscle for an adult patient.

Table 6.11: Comparison of newborn and adult renal clearances

	Average Infant	Average Adult
Body weight (kg)	3.5	70
Body water		
(%)	77	58
(L)	2.7	41
Inulin clearance		
(mL/min)	Approx 3	130
k (min^{-1})	3/2700 = 0.0011	130/41,000 = 0.0032
t $_{1/2}$ (min)	630	220
PAH clearance		
(mL/min)	Approx 12	650
k (min^{-1})	12/2800 = 0.0043	650/41,000 = 0.016
t $_{1/2}$ (min)	160	43

In general, complete hepatic function is not attained until the third week of life. Oxidative processes are fairly well developed in infants, but there is a deficiency of conjugative enzymes. In addition, many drugs exhibit reduced binding to plasma albumin in infants. Newborns show only 30–50% of the renal activity of adults on the basis of activity per unit of body weight. Drugs that are heavily dependent on renal excretion will have a sharply decreased elimination half-life. For example, the penicillins are excreted for the most part through the kidney. The elimination half-lives of such drugs are much reduced in infants, as shown in Table 6.11.

Computations are for a drug distributed in the whole body water, but any other V_D would give the same relative values.

Table 6.12: Elimination half-lives of drugs in infants and adults

Drug	Half-Life in Neonates (hr)	Half-Life in Adults (hr)
Penicillin G	3.2	0.5
Ampicillin	4	1–1.5
Methicillin	3.3/1.3	0.5
Carbenicillin	5–6	1–1.5
Kanamycin	5–5.7	3–5
Gentamicin	5	2–3

A simple formula in comparison to DuBois and DuBois for computing surface area (SA) in square meters is **Mosteller's equation**:

$$SA \text{ (in m}^2) = \frac{(\text{height} \times \text{weight})^{1/2}}{60} \qquad \dots (6.34)$$

Infants and children require larger mg/kg doses than adults because:

1. their body surface area per kg body weight is larger, and hence
2. larger volume of distribution (particularly TBW and ECF).

The child's maintenance dose can be calculated from adult dose by using the following equation:

$$\text{Child's dose} = \frac{\text{SA of child (in m}^2) \times \text{adult dose}}{1.73} \quad \text{... (6.35)}$$

Where, 1.73 is surface area in m^2 of an average 70 kg adult. Since the surface area of a child is in proportion to the body weight according to equation 6.36,

$$\text{SA (in m}^2) = \text{body weight (in kg)}^{0.7} \quad \text{... (6.36)}$$

The following relationship can also be written for child's dose:

$$\text{Child's dose} = [\text{weight of child in kg} / 70]^{0.7} \times \text{adult dose} \quad \text{... (6.37)}$$

As the TBW in neonates is 30% more than that in adults,

1. the Vd for most water soluble drugs is larger in infants, and

2. the Vd for most lipid soluble drugs is smaller.

Pharmacokinetic Drug Interaction and its Significance in Combination Therapy

Drug interaction generally refers to a modification of the expected drug response in the patient as a result of exposure of the patient to another drug or substance. Some unintentional drug interactions produce adverse reactions in the patient, whereas some drug interactions may be intentional, to provide an improved therapeutic response or to decrease adverse drug effects. Drug interactions may include drug–drug interactions, food–drug interactions, or chemical–drug interactions, such as the interaction of a drug with alcohol or tobacco. A listing of food interactions is given in. A drug–laboratory test interaction pertains to an alteration in a diagnostic laboratory test result because of the drug.

The risk of a drug interaction increases with multiple drug therapy, multiple prescribers, poor patient compliance, and patient risk factors, such as predisposing illness (diabetes, hypertension, etc) or advancing age. Multiple drug therapy has become routine in most acute and chronic care settings. Elderly patients and patients with various predisposing illnesses tend to be a population using multiple drug therapy. A recent student survey found an average of 8 to 12 drugs per patient used in a group of hospital patients. Screening for drug interactions should be performed whenever multiple drug uses are involved. Many computer programs will "flag" a potential drug interaction. However, the pharmacist needs to determine the clinical significance of the interaction. The determination of the clinical significance of a potential drug interaction should be documented in the literature. The likelihood of a drug interaction may be classified as an established drug interaction, probable drug interaction, possible drug interaction, or unlikely drug interaction. The size of the dose and the duration of therapy, the onset (rapid, delayed), the severity (major, minor) of the potential interaction, and extrapolation to related drugs should also be considered.

Preferably, drugs that interact should be avoided or given sufficiently far apart so that the interaction is minimized. In situations involving two drugs of choice that may interact, dose adjustment based on pharmacokinetic and therapeutic considerations of one or both of the drugs may be necessary. Dose adjustment may be based on clearance or elimination half-life of the drug. Assessment of the patient's renal function, such as serum creatinine concentration, and liver function indicators, such as alkaline phosphatase, alanine aminotransferase (ALT), aspartate aminotransferase (AST), or other markers of hepatic metabolism, should be undertaken. In general, if the therapeutic response is predictable from serum drug concentration, dosing at regular intervals may be based on a steady-state concentration. When the elimination half-life is changed by drug interaction, the dosing interval may be extended or the dose reduced. Some examples of pharmacokinetic drug interactions are listed in. A more complete discussion of pharmacologic and therapeutic drug interactions of drugs is available in standard textbooks on clinical pharmacology.

Table 6.13: Pharmacokinetic drug interactions

Drug Interaction	Examples (Precipitant Drugs)	Effect (Object Drugs)
Bioavailability		
Complexation/ chelation	Calcium, magnesium, or aluminum and iron salts	Tetracycline complexes with divalent cations, causing a decreased bioavailability
Adsorption binding/ ionic interaction	Cholestyramine resin (anion-exchange resin binding)	Decreased bioavailability of thyroxine, and digoxin; binds anionic drugs and reduces absorption
Adsorption	Antacids (adsorption)	Decreased bioavailability of antibiotics
	Charcoal, antidiarrheals	Decreased bioavailability of many drugs
increased GI motility	Laxatives, cathartics	Increases GI motility, decreases bioavailability for drugs which are absorbed slowly; may also affect the bioavailability of drugs from controlled release products
Decreased GI motility	Anticholinergic agents	Propantheline decreases the gastric emptying of acetaminophen (APAP), delaying APAP absorption from the small intestine

Drug Interaction	Examples (Precipitant Drugs)	Effect (Object Drugs)
Alteration of gastric pH	H-2 blockers, antacids	Both H-2 blockers and antacids increase gastric pH; the dissolution of ketoconazole is reduced, causing decreased drug absorption
Alteration of intestinal flora	Antibiotics (eg, tetracyclines, penicillin)	Digoxin has better bioavailability after erythromycin; erythromycin administration reduces bacterial inactivation of digoxin
Inhibition of drug metabolism in intestinal cells	Monoamine oxidase inhibitors (MAO-I) (eg, tranylcypromine, phenelzine)	Hypertensive crisis may occur in patients treated with MAO-I and foods containing tyramine
Distribution		
Protein binding	Warfarin-phenylbutazone	Displacement of warfarin from binding
	Phenytoin–valproic acid	Displacement of phenytoin from binding
Hepatic elimination		
Enzyme induction	Smoking (polycyclic aromatic hydrocarbons)	Smoking increases theophylline clearance

Drug Interaction	Examples (Precipitant Drugs)	Effect (Object Drugs)
	Barbiturates	Phenobarbital increases the metabolism of warfarin
Enzyme inhibition	Cimetidine	Decreased theophylline, diazepam metabolism
Mixed-function oxidase		
	Fluvoxamine	Diazepam $t_{1/2}$ longer
	Quinidine	Decreased nifedipine metabolism
	Fluconazole	Increased levels of phenytoin, warfarin
Other enzymes	Monoamine oxidase inhibitors, MAO-I (eg, pargyline, tranylcypromine)	Serious hypertensive crisis may occur following ingestion of foods with a high content of tyramine or other pressor substances (eg, cheddar cheese, red wines)
Inhibition of biliary secretion	Verapamil	Decreased biliary secretion of digoxin causing increased digoxin levels

Drug Interaction	Examples (Precipitant Drugs)	Effect (Object Drugs)
Renal clearance		
Glomerular filtration rate (GFR) and renal blood flow	Methylxanthines (eg, caffeine, theobromine)	Increased renal blood flow and GFR will decrease time for reabsorption of various drugs, leading to more rapid urinary drug excretion
Active tubular secretion	Probenecid	Probenecid blocks the active tubular secretion of penicillin and some cephalosporin antibiotics
Tubular reabsorption and urine pH	Antacids, sodium bicarbonate	Alkalinization of the urine increases the reabsorption of amphetamine and decreases its clearance
		Alkalinization of urine pH increases the ionization of salicylates, decreases reabsorption and increases its clearance
Diet		
Charcoal hamburgers	Theophylline	Elimination half-life of theophylline decreases due to increased metabolism

Drug Interaction	Examples (Precipitant Drugs)	Effect (Object Drugs)
Grapefruit	Terfenadine, cyclosporin	Blood levels of terfenadine and cyclosporine increase due to decreased metabolism
Virus drug interactions Reye's syndrome	Aspirin	Aspirin in children exposed to certain viral infections such as influenza B virus leads to Reye's syndrome

Many drugs affect the cytochrome P-450 (CYP) family of hemoprotein enzymes that catalyze drug biotransformation. Some examples of substrates of CYPs are:

Table 6.14: Some examples of substrates of CYPs

CYP1A2	Amitriptyline, fluvoxamine
CYP2B6	Cyclophosphamide
CYP2C9	Ibuprofen, fluoxetine, tolbutamide, amitriptyline
CYP2C19	Omeprazole, S-methenytoin, amitriptyline
CYP2D6	Propanolol, amitriptyline, fluoxetine, paroxetine
CYP2E1	Halothane
CYP3A4	Erythromycin, clarithromycin, midazolam, diazapam
CYP3A5	Clarithromycin, simvastatin, indinavir
CYP3A6	Erythromycin, clarithromycin, diltiazam

Many calcium channel blockers, macrolides, and protease inhibitors are substrates of CYP3A4, CYP3A5, or CYP3A6. An enzyme substrate may competitively interfere with other substrates metabolism if co-administered. Drug inducers of CYPs may also result in drug interactions by accelerating the rate of drug metabolism. When an unusually high plasma level is observed as a result of co-administration of a second drug, pharmacists should check whether the two drugs share a common CYP substrate. New substrates are still being discovered. For example, many proton inhibitors share the common CYP2C19 substrate, and many calcium channel blockers are CYP3A4 substrates. It is important to assess the clinical significance with the clinician before alarming the patient. It is also important to suggest an alternative drug therapy to the clinician if a clinically significant drug interaction is likely to be occurring.

Some examples of pharmacokinetic drug interactions are discussed in more detail below and in. Many side effects occur as a result of impaired or induced (stimulated) drug metabolism. Changes in pharmacokinetics due to impaired drug metabolism should be evaluated quantitatively. For example, acetaminophen is an OTC drug that has been used safely for decades, but incidences of severe hepatic toxicity leading to coma have occurred in some subjects with impaired liver function because of chronic alcohol use. Drugs that have reactive intermediates, active metabolites, and or metabolites with a longer half-life than the parent drug need to be considered carefully if there is a potential for a drug interaction. A polar metabolite may also distribute to a smaller fluid volume, leading to high concentration in some tissues. Drug interactions involving metabolism may be temporal, observed as a delayed effect. Temporal drug interactions are more difficult to detect in a clinical situation.

All pharmacokinetic interactions result due to alteration in the rate of absorption, distribution, metabolism or excretion of drugs (and therefore also called as **ADME interaction**). Such a change is reflected in the altered duration and intensity of pharmacologic action of the drug due to variation in plasma concentration precipitated by altered ADME. All factors which influence the ADME of a drug affect its pharmacokinetics.

Interaction affecting absorption of drugs

Altered absorption after oral administration is very common. The interaction may result in a change in the rate of absorption (an increase or decrease), a change in the amount of drug absorbed (an increased or decreased) or both. Several mechanisms may be involved in the alteration of drug absorption from the GIT. In general, drugs that are not absorbed completely/rapidly are more susceptible to changes in GI absorption. A decreased in the rate of absorption is clinically significant in acute condition such as pain where the drug is administered in a single dose but is of little importance for drugs used in chronic therapy.

An alteration in parenteral drug absorption is rare but can occur when an adrenergic agent such as adrenaline or a cholinergic drug such as methacholine is extravascularly injected concomitantly with another drug. The systemic absorption of the drug latter is altered due to vasoconstriction or vasodilation by these agents.

Interactions affecting distribution of drugs

Though several factors govern the distribution of drugs to various tissues, clinically significant interactions result due to competition between drugs for binding to proteins/tissues and displacement of one drug by the other. Competitive displacement which results when two drugs are capable of binding to the same site on the protein causes the most significant interactions. Greater risk of interactions exists when the displaced drug is highly protein bound (more then 95%) has small volume of distribution and has narrow therapeutic index (e.g. tolbutamide, warfarin and phenytoin), and when the displacer drug has a higher degree of affinity than the drug to be displaced. In such situations, displacement of even a small percent of drug result in a tremendous increase in the free form of the drug which precipitates increased therapeutic or toxic effects.

Drugs may also be displaced from binding sites in tissues. An interesting example of this are oral hypoglycemic such as the sulfonyl ureas (tolbutamide, glibenclamide, etc,) These agents exert their therapeutics effect by displacing insulin from protein binding sites in pancreas, plasma and other regions resulting in its elevated levels.

Interactions affecting metabolism of drugs

The most important and the most common cause of pharmacokinetic interactions is alteration in the rate of biotransformation of drugs. Major problems arise when one drug either induces or inhibits the metabolism of another drug. Even the environmental chemicals can bring about such an effect. The influences of enzyme inducers and inhibitors become more pronounced when drugs susceptible to first – pass hepatic metabolism are given concurrently. The metabolic pathway usually affected is phase I oxidation. Enzyme inducers reduce the blood level and clinical efficacy of co-administered drugs but may also enhance the toxicity of drugs having active metabolites. In contrast to enzyme induction which is usually not hazardous, enzyme inhibition leads to accumulation of drug to toxic levels and serious adverse effect may be precipitated.

Interaction affecting excretion of drugs

Clinically significant renal excretion interactions occur when an appreciable amount of drug or its active metabolite(s) are eliminated in the urine. Excretion pattern can be affected by alteration in GFR, renal blood flow, passive tubular reabsorption, active tubular secretion and urine pH. An interesting pharmacokinetic interaction that results due to the pharmacodynamic drug effect is between thiazide diuretics and lithium. Owing to the influence of former on the renal tubular transport of sodium, the lithium ions are retained in the body resulting in its toxicity.

Biliary excretion, the other major mechanism of drug excretion, is altered by agents that inhibit biliary transport or modify bile flow rate.

Questions

Essay questions

1. Define clinical pharmacokinetics. Explain dosage adjustment in patient with renal failure.

2. What is drug interaction? Write its significance in combination therapy.

Short questions

1. Explain dosage adjustment in patient with hepatic failure.
2. Write a note on dosing of drugs in elderly.
3. Explain dosing of drugs in obese patient.
4. Write a note on dosing of drugs in infant and children.
5. What is the scope of clinical pharmacokinetics? Explain.

Chapter—7

BIOAVAILABILITY AND BIOEQUIVALENCE

Bioavailability Studies

Therapeutic effectiveness of the drug depends on ability of dosage form to release/deliver the medicament to its site of action, at rate and amount sufficient to elicit desired pharmacologic response. This attribute of the dosage form is referred to as physiologic availability, biologic availability or simply bioavailability.

Rate and extent of absorption of unchanged drug from its dosage form is known as **bioavailability**. If the size of dose to be administered is same, bioavailability of drug from dosage form depends upon three major factors:

(1) Pharmaceutic factors related to physicochemical properties of drug and characteristics of dosage form.

(2) Patient related factors.

(3) Route of administration.

The influence of route of administration on drugs bioavailability is generally in following order: Parenteral > oral > rectal > topical.

The dose available to patient is called **bioavailable dose**. IV injection of drug result in 100% bioavailability as absorption process is bypassed. In orally administered drug, bioavailable dose is often less than administered dose. Amount of drug that reaches systemic circulation (i.e., extent of bioavailability) is called as **systemic availability or simply availability**. The term **bioavailable fraction F** refers to the fraction of administered dose that enters the systemic circulation.

$$F = \frac{\text{Bioavailable dose}}{\text{Administered dose}} \qquad \text{... (7.1)}$$

Why bioavailability studies?

1. Bioavailability studies performed for both approved active drug ingredients and not yet approved for marketing by FDA. New formulation of active drug ingredient or therapeutic moieties must be approved prior to marketing by FDA. FDA must ensure that drug product is safe and effective, and meet all applicable standards of identity, strength, quality and purity. To ensure these standards are met, FDA requires bioavailability / pharmacokinetic studies and where necessary bioequivalence studies for all drug products.

2. For unmarketed drugs which do not have full NDA approval by FDA, in vitro / in vivo bioequivalence studies must be performed on drug formulation proposed for marketing as generic drug product. Essential pharmacokinetic parameters including rate and extent of systemic absorption, elimination half life and rate of excretion and metabolism should be established after single and multiple dose administration. Data from these in vivo bioavailability studies are important to establish recommended dosage regimens and to support drug labeling.

3. In vivo bioavailability studies are also performed for new formulations of active ingredients that have full NDA approval and are approved for marketing. Purpose of these studies is to determine bioavailability and to characterize pharmacokinetics of new formulations, new dosage forms or new salt or ester relative to reference formulation.

4. These studies are useful in determining safety and efficacy of drug products.

Bioavailability studies are used to define the effect of changes in physicochemical property of drug substances and effect of drug product on pharmacokinetics of drug.

Objectives of Bioavailability Studies

1. Primary stage of development of suitable dosage form for a new drug entity.
2. Development of new formulations of existing drugs.
3. Determination of influence of excipients, patient related factors and possible interactions with other drugs on efficiency of absorption.
4. Control of quality of drug product during early stages of marketing in order to determine the influence of processing factors, storage and stability on drug absorption.

Considerations in Bioavailability Studies

• Selection of Subjects

A number of factors such as health, age, weight, enzyme status and number are concern. It is better to have the subjects of similar kinetics to avoid major variations.

(1)**Health:** Subjects should be of great health that is ascertained by various biochemical and medical examination.

(2) **Age:** Elderly and children have different kinetics to adults. Subjects between 18 – 35 years are preferred.

(3) **Number:** Number of participants should be kept minimum required for carrying out a reliable, well designed study.

(4) **Weight:** The apparent volume of distribution is usually proportional to weight in subjects of normal weight and height. However, in overweight and underweight V_d may be different. Hence, to better match the subject, normal weights are preferred. Usually 140-200 lb.

(5) **Enzyme status:** Enzyme activity can be altered by altered kinetics

of the drug in case of smokers or subjects taking other drugs leading to drug-drug interaction.

● **Study Design**

Usually, a complete cross over study design is used. With this design each subject receives all products with a washout period between each dose administration. This is a Latin square crossover design where each subject receives each drug product only once. Here each subject act as his own control and subject to subject variation is reduced.

● **Washout Period:**

The time interval between two treatments is called **"washout period"**. It is required for the elimination of the administered dose of a drug so as to avoid a carryover effect. Usually, a period of 10 half-lives should be allowed between two treatments ensuring elimination of 99.9% of the administered dose. The number of washout period depends upon the type of crossover study design used and number of formulations to be evaluated.

In case of Digitoxin,

✓ **Half –life:** 6 to 9 days

✓ **Study design:** Latin square crossover design for four formulations.

✓ **Duration:** 1 year

● **Relative and Absolute Availability**

The area under the drug concentration–time curve (AUC) is used as a measure of the total amount of unaltered drug that reaches the systemic circulation. The AUC is dependent on the total quantity of available drug, FD_0, divided by the elimination rate constant, k, and the apparent volume of distribution; V_D. F is the fraction of the dose absorbed. After IV administration, F is equal to unity, because the entire dose enters the systemic circulation. Therefore, the drug is considered to be completely available after IV administration. After oral administration of a drug, F

may vary from a value of 0 (no drug absorption) to 1 (complete drug absorption).

Relative availability

Relative (apparent) availability is the availability of the drug from a drug product as compared to a recognized standard. The fraction of dose systemically available from an oral drug product is difficult to ascertain. The availability of drug in the formulation is compared to the availability of drug in a standard dosage formulation, usually a solution of the pure drug evaluated in a crossover study. The relative availability of two drug products given at the same dosage level and by the same route of administration can be obtained using the following equation:

$$\text{Realative availability} = \frac{[\text{AUC}]_A}{[\text{AUC}]_B} \qquad \ldots (7.2)$$

Where, drug product B is the recognized reference standard. This fraction may be multiplied by 100 to give percent relative availability.

When different doses are administered, a correction for the size of the dose is made, as in the following equation:

$$\text{Realative availability} = \frac{[\text{AUC}]_A / dose\,A}{[\text{AUC}]_B / dose\,B} \qquad \ldots (7.3)$$

Urinary drug excretion data may also be used to measure relative availability, as long as the total amount of intact drug excreted in the urine is collected. The percent relative availability using urinary excretion data can be determined as follows:

$$\text{Precent realative availability} = \frac{[Du]_A^\infty}{[Du]_B^\infty} \times 100 \qquad \ldots (7.4)$$

Where, $[D_u]^\infty$ is the total amount of drug excreted in the urine.

Absolute availability

The absolute availability of drug is the systemic availability of a drug after extravascular administration (eg, oral, rectal, transdermal, subcutaneous) compared to IV dosing. The absolute availability of a drug is generally measured by comparing the respective AUCs after extravascular and IV administration. This measurement may be performed as long as V_D and k are independent of the route of administration. Absolute availability after oral drug administration using plasma data can be determined as follows:

$$\text{Absolute availability} = F = \frac{[AUC]_{PO} / dose_{PO}}{[AUC]_{IV} / dose_{IV}} \quad \text{... (7.5)}$$

Absolute availability, F, may be expressed as a fraction or as a percent by multiplying $F \times 100$. Absolute availability using urinary drug excretion data can be determined by the following:

$$\text{Absolute availability} = \frac{[Du]_{PO}^{\infty} / dose_{PO}}{[Du]_{IV}^{\infty} / dose_{IV}} \quad \text{... (7.6)}$$

The absolute bioavailability is also equal to F, the fraction of the dose that is bioavailable. Absolute availability is sometimes expressed as a percent, i.e., $F = 1$, or 100%. For drugs given intravascularly, such as by IV bolus injection, $F = 1$ because the entire drug is completely absorbed. For all extravascular routes of administration, such as the oral route (PO), the absolute bioavailability F may not exceed 100% ($F > 1$). F is usually determined by Equation 7.5 or 7.6, where PO is the oral route or any other extravascular route of drug administration.

• Single-dose Studies

Single-dose studies recommended for:

1. Dosage forms that are to be evaluated only for bioequivalence purpose.

2. Dosage forms meant for a single dose administration for a therapeutic benefit such as analgesic for relief of headache.

● **Multiple dose studies**

Multiple dose studies recommended for:

1. Dosage forms designed to achieve special release profiles. E.g. time-release products, enteric-coated preparations.
2. Drugs undergoing first pass metabolism.
3. Special dosage regimens such as loading dose.

● **Study Conditions**

1. Subject should be maintained on a uniform diet and none of them should have taken any drug at least one week prior to the study.
2. Before the commencement of study it is necessary to define the study condition such as fasting period before the administration, time period after drug product administration, during which fasting is continued.
3. In general studies are carried out on subjects fasted overnight.

● **Pharmacological effects of metabolites**

1. Bioavailability measurement is based on the unchanged drug.
2. Drugs having biologically active metabolites, their concentration in systemic circulation can influence greatly the therapeutic efficacy of the drug.
3. It was found especially significant for drugs which exhibits first pass metabolism during pre-absorptive phase.
4. Phenacetin has more side effects than, its metabolite acetaminophen, which is also pharmacologically active form.
5. In case of aspirin its metabolite salicylic acid is pharmacologically inactive and exhibits serious toxicity.
6. Based on above findings, it is good practice in bioavailability

studies to examine the presence of major metabolites in blood and urine, to determine their concentration and, if possible, pharmacological activity of each.

- **Assay method**
  1. The analytical method used to quantitates the levels of drug and/ or its metabolites must be selective e.g., for the unchanged drug in presence of its metabolites.
  2. It must be sensitive enough to measure the expected low drug levels in the samples collected last.

Bioequivalence Studies

Differences in the predicted clinical response or an adverse event may be due to differences in the pharmacokinetic and/or pharmacodynamic behavior of the drug among individuals or to differences in the bioavailability of the drug from the drug product. Bioequivalent drug products that have the same systemic drug bioavailability will have the same predictable drug response. However, variable clinical responses among individuals that are unrelated to bioavailability may be due to differences in the pharmacodynamics of the drug. Differences in pharmacodynamics, ie, the relationship between the drug and the receptor site, may be due to differences in receptor sensitivity to the drug. Various factors affecting pharmacodynamic drug behavior may include age, drug tolerance, drug interactions, and unknown pathophysiologic factors.

The bioavailability of a drug may be more reproducible among fasted individuals in controlled studies who take the drug on an empty stomach. When the drug is used on a daily basis, however, the nature of an individual's diet and lifestyle may affect the plasma drug levels because of variable absorption in the presence of food or even a change in the metabolic clearance of the drug. reported that patients on a high-carbohydrate diet have a much longer elimination half-life of theophylline, due to the reduced metabolic clearance of the drug ($t_{1/2}$, 18.1 hours), compared to patients on normal diets ($t_{1/2} = 6.76$ hours). Previous studies demonstrated that the theophylline drug product was completely bioavailable. The higher plasma drug concentration resulting from a carbohydrate diet may subject the patient to a higher risk of drug intoxication with theophylline. The effect of food on the availability of theophylline has been reported by the FDA concerning the risk of higher theophylline plasma concentrations from a 24-hour sustained-release drug product taken with food. Although most bioavailability drug studies use fasted volunteers, the diet of patients actually using the drug product may increase, decrease, or have no affect on the bioavailability of the drug.

Equivalence: This term compares the drug products to the characters or functions to the set of standards.

Bioequivalence: It refers that the drug substance in two or more identical dosage forms, reaches systemic circulation at the same rate and to the same relative extent. i.e. their plasma conc.- time profiles will be identical without significant statistical differences.

Pharmaceutical equivalence: Drug products in identical dosage forms that contains the same active ingredients, use the same route of administration, and are identical in strength or conc., quality, purity, content uniformity; however they may differ in containing excipients

Pharmaceutical alternatives: Drug products that contain the same therapeutic moiety but as different salt, ester or complex. For example, tetracycline phosphate or tetracycline- hydrochloride equivalent to 250 mg tetracycline.

Therapeutic Equivalence

It indicates that two or more drug products that contain same therapeutically active ingredients elicit identical pharmacologic effect and can control the disease to the same extent.

Bio-inequivalence: When statistically significant differences are observed in the bioavailability of two or more drug products called as bio-inequivalence.

Reference standard: It is a formulation marketed with fully approved data by the FDA. It is the global innovators or original manufacturer's brand name product.

Example: NICE (Nimesulide), DICLOGESIC (Diclofenac)

Test/Generic: It contains the same active ingredient in same formulation gives same efficacy but cheaper. It may be a new formulation or new dosage form of existing form.

Example: NICIP, DICLOVEROL. It decreases consumers cost. It is used in 44% of all prescriptions.

Bases for Determining Bioequivalence

Bioequivalence is established if the *in-vivo* bioavailability of a test drug product (usually the generic product) does not differ significantly (i.e., statistically insignificant) in the product's rate and extent of drug absorption, as determined by comparison of measured parameters (e.g., concentration of the active drug ingredient in the blood, urinary excretion rates, or pharmacodynamic effects), from that of the reference listed drug (usually the brand-name product) when administered at the same molar dose of the active moiety under similar experimental conditions, either single dose or multiple dose.

In a few cases, a drug product that differs from the reference listed drug in its rate of absorption, but not in its extent of absorption, may be considered bioequivalent if the difference in the rate of absorption is intentional and appropriately reflected in the labeling and/or the rate of absorption is not detrimental to the safety and effectiveness of the drug product.

Drug Products with Possible Bioavailability and Bioequivalence Problems

Lack of bioavailability or bioequivalence may be suspected when evidence from well-controlled clinical trials or controlled observations in patients of various marketed drug products do not give comparable therapeutic effects. These drug products need to be evaluated either *in- vitro* (eg, drug dissolution/release test) or *in vivo* (eg, bioequivalence study) to determine if the drug product has a bioavailability problem.

In addition, during the development of a drug product, certain biopharmaceutical properties of the active drug substance or the formulation of the drug product may indicate that the drug may have variable bioavailability and/or a bioequivalence problem. Some of these biopharmaceutic properties include:

- The active drug ingredient has low solubility in water (eg, less than 5 mg/mL).

- The dissolution rate of one or more such products is slow (eg, less than 50% in 30 minutes when tested with a general method specified by the FDA).

- The particle size and/or surface area of the active drug ingredient are critical in determining its bioavailability.

- Certain structural forms of the active drug ingredient (eg, polymorphic forms, solvates, complexes, and crystal modifications) dissolve poorly, thus affecting absorption.

- Drug products that have a high ratio of excipients to active ingredients (eg, greater than 5:1).

- Specific inactive ingredients (eg, hydrophilic or hydrophobic excipients and lubricants) either may be required for absorption of the active drug ingredient or therapeutic moiety or may interfere with such absorption.

- The active drug ingredient, therapeutic moiety, or its precursor is absorbed in large part in a particular segment of the GI tract or is absorbed from a localized site.

- The degree of absorption of the active drug ingredient, therapeutic moiety, or its precursor is poor (eg, less than 50%, ordinarily in comparison to an intravenous dose), even when it is administered in pure form (eg, in solution).

- There is rapid metabolism of the therapeutic moiety in the intestinal wall or liver during the absorption process (first-order metabolism), so that the rate of absorption is unusually important in the therapeutic effect and/or toxicity of the drug product.

- The therapeutic moiety is rapidly metabolized or excreted, so that rapid dissolution and absorption are required for effectiveness.

- The active drug ingredient or therapeutic moiety is unstable in specific portions of the GI tract and requires special coatings or formulations (eg, buffers, enteric coatings, and film coatings) to ensure adequate absorption.

- The drug product is subject to dose-dependent kinetics in or near the therapeutic range, and the rate and extent of absorption are important to bioequivalence.

Bioequivalence Example

A simulated example of the results for a single-dose, fasting study is shown in and in. As shown by the *ANOVA*, no statistical differences for the pharmacokinetic parameters AUC_{0-t}, $AUC_{0-\infty}$, and C_{max} were observed between the Test product and the brand-name product. The 90% confidence limits for the mean pharmacokinetic parameters of the Test product were within $0.80 - 1.25$ ($80 - 125\%$) of the reference product means based on log transformation of the data. The power test for the AUC measures were above 99%, showing good precision of the data. The power test for the C_{max} values was 87.9%, showing that this parameter was more variable.

The results were obtained from a two-way, crossover, single-dose study in 36 fasted, healthy, adult male and female volunteers. No statistical differences were observed for the mean values between Test and Reference products.

Shows the results for a hypothetical bioavailability study in which three different tablet formulations were compared to a solution of the drug given in the same dose. As shown in the table, the bioavailability from all three tablet formulations was greater than 80% of that of the solution. According to the ANOVA, the mean AUC values were neither

Table 7.1: Bioavailability comparison of a generic (test) and brand-name (reference) drug products (log-normal transformed data)

Variable	Units	Geometric Mean		% Ratio	90% Confidence Interval (Lower Limit, Upper Limit)	P Values for Product Effects	Power of ANOVA	ANOVA % CV
		Test	Reference					
C_{max}	ng/mL	344.79	356.81	96.6	(89.5, 112)	0.3586	0.8791	17.90%
AUC_{0-t}	ng hr/mL	2659.12	2674.92	99.4	(95.1, 104)	0.8172	1.0000	12.60%
AUC		2708.63	2718.52	99.6	(95.4, 103)	0.8865	1.0000	12.20%
T_{max}	Hr	4.29	4.24	101				
K_{elim}	1/hr	0.0961	0.0980	98.1				
$t_{1/2}$	Hr	8.47	8.33	101.7				

statistically different from each other nor different from that of the solution. However, the 90% confidence interval for the AUC showed that for tablet A, the bioavailability was less than 80% (i.e., 74%), compared to the solution at the low-range estimate and would not be considered bioequivalent based on AUC.

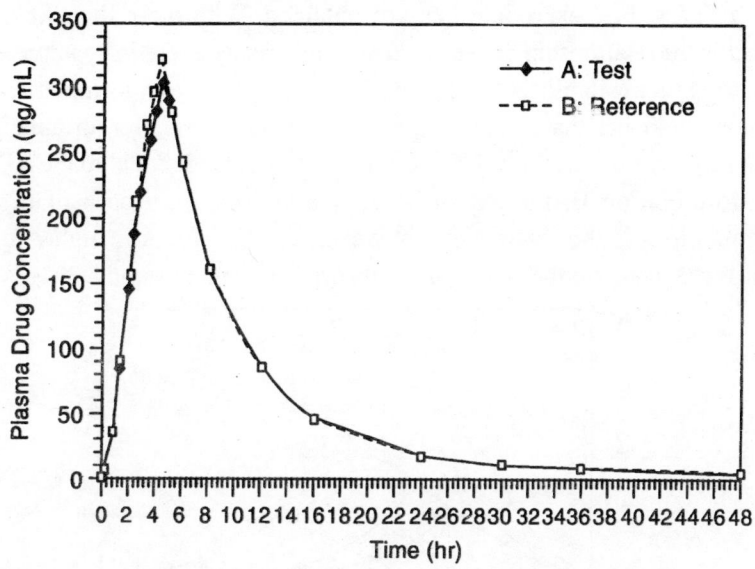

Fig. 7.1: Bioequivalence of test and reference drug products: mean plasma drug concentrations.

Table 7.2: Summary of the results of a bioavailability study

Dosage Form	c_{max} (µg/mL)	t_{max} (hr)	AUC_{0-24} (µg hr/ mL)	F	90% Confidence Interval for AUC
Solution	16.1 ± 2.5	1.5 ± 0.85	1835 ± 235		
Tablet A	10.5 ± 3.2	2.5 ± 1.0	1523 ± 381	81	74–90%
Tablet B	13.7 ± 4.1	2.1 ± 0.98	1707 ± 317	93	88–98%
Tablet C	14.8 ± 3.6	1.8 ± 0.95	1762 ± 295	96	91–103%

For illustrative purposes, consider a drug that has been prepared at the same dosage level in three formulations, A, B, and C. These formulations are given to a group of volunteers using a three-way, randomized crossover design. In this experimental design, all subjects receive each formulation once. From each subject, plasma drug level and urinary drug excretion data are obtained. With these data we can observe the relationship between plasma and urinary excretion parameters and drug bioavailability. The rate of drug absorption from formulation A is more rapid than that from formulation B, because the t_{max} for formulation A is shorter. Because the AUC for formulation A is identical to the AUC for formulation B, the extent of bioavailability from both of these formulations is the same. Note, however, the C_{max} for A is higher than that for B, because the rate of drug absorption is more rapid.

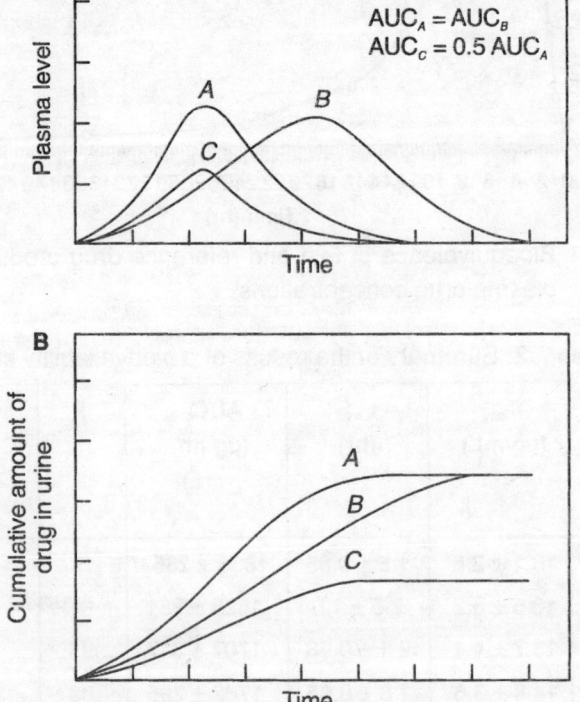

Fig. 7.2: Corresponding plots relating plasma concentration and urinary excretion data.

The C_{max} is generally higher when the extent of drug bioavailability is greater. The rate of drug absorption from formulation C is the same as that from formulation A, but the extent of drug available is less. The C_{max} for formulation C is less than that for formulation A. The decrease in C_{max} for formulation C is proportional to the decrease in AUC in comparison to the drug plasma level data for formulation A. The corresponding urinary excretion data confirm these observations. These relationships are summarized in. The table illustrates how bioavailability parameters for plasma and urine change when only the extent and rate of bioavailability are changed, respectively. Formulation changes in a drug product may affect both the rate and extent of drug bioavailability.

Table 7.3: Relationship of plasma level and urinary excretion parameters to drug bioavailability

Extent of Drug Bioavailability Decreases		Rate of Drug Bioavailability Decreases	
Parameter	Change	Parameter	Change
Plasma data			
t_{max}	Same	t_{max}	Increase
C_{max}	Decrease	C_{max}	Decrease
AUC	Decrease	AUC	Same
Urine data			
t^{∞}	Same	t^{∞}	Increase
$[dD_u / dt]_{max}$	Decrease	$[dD_u / dt]_{max}$	Decrease
D^{∞}_u	Decrease	D^{∞}_u	Same

Clinical Significance of Bioequivalence Studies

Bioequivalence of different formulations of the same drug substance involves equivalence with respect to rate and extent of systemic drug absorption. Clinical interpretation is important in evaluating the results of a bioequivalence study. A small difference between drug products, even if statistically significant, may produce very little difference in therapeutic response. Generally, two formulations whose rate and extent of absorption differ by 20% or less are considered bioequivalent. The considered that differences of less than 20% in AUC and C_{max} between drug products are "unlikely to be clinically significant in patients." The Task Force further stated that "clinical studies of effectiveness have difficulty detecting differences in doses of even 50–100%." Therefore, normal variation is observed in medical practice and plasma drug levels may vary among individuals greater than 20%.

According to, a small, statistically significant difference in drug bioavailability from two or more dosage forms may be detected if the study is well controlled and the number of subjects is sufficiently large. When the therapeutic objectives of the drug are considered, an equivalent clinical response should be obtained from the comparison dosage forms if the plasma drug concentrations remain above the minimum effective concentration (MEC) for an appropriate interval and do not reach the minimum toxic concentration (MTC). Therefore, the investigator must consider whether any statistical difference in bioavailability would alter clinical efficiency.

Special populations, such as the elderly or patients on drug therapy, are generally not used for bioequivalence studies. Normal, healthy volunteers are preferred for bioequivalence studies, because these subjects are less at risk and may more easily endure the discomforts of the study, such as blood sampling. Furthermore, the objective of these studies is to evaluate the bioavailability of the drug from the dosage form, and use of healthy subjects should minimize both inter- and intrasubject variability. It is theoretically possible that the excipients in one of the dosage forms tested may pose a problem in a patient who uses the generic dosage form.

For the manufacture of a dosage form, specifications are set to provide uniformity of dosage forms. With proper specifications, quality control procedures should minimize product-to-product variability by different manufacturers and lot-to-lot variability with a single manufacturer.

Special Concerns in Bioavailability and Bioequivalence Studies

The general bioequivalence study designs and evaluation, such as the comparison of AUC, C_{max}, and t_{max}, may be used for systemically absorbed drugs and conventional oral dosage forms. However, for certain drugs and dosage forms, systemic bioavailability and bioequivalence are difficult to ascertain. Drugs and drug products (e.g., cyclosporine, chlorpromazine, verapamil, isosorbide dinitrate, sulindac) are considered to be highly variable if the intrasubject variability in bioavailability parameters is greater than 30% by analysis of variance coefficient of variation. The number of subjects required to demonstrate bioequivalence for these drug products may be excessive, requiring more than 60 subjects to meet current FDA bioequivalence criteria. The intrasubject variability may be due to the drug itself or to the drug formulation or to both. The FDA has held public forums to determine whether the current bioequivalence guidelines need to be changed for these highly variable drugs.

Table 7.4: Problems in bioavailability and bioequivalence

Drugs with high intrasubject variability	Inhalation
Drugs with long elimination half-life	Ophthalmic
Biotransformation of drugs	Intranasal
Stereoselective drug metabolism	Bioavailable drugs that should not produce peak drug levels
Drugs with active metabolites	Potassium supplements
Drugs with polymorphic metabolism	Endogeneous drug levels
Nonbioavailable drugs (drugs intended for local effect)	Hormone replacement therapy
Antacids	Biotechnology-derived drugs
Local anesthetics	Erythropoietin interferon
Anti-infectives	Protease inhibitors
Anti-inflammatory steroids	Complex drug substances
Dosage forms for nonoral administration Transdermal	Conjugated estrogens

For drugs with very long elimination half-lives or a complex elimination phase, a complete plasma drug concentration–time curve (i.e., three elimination half-lives or an AUC representing 90% of the total AUC) may be difficult to obtain for a bioequivalence study using a crossover design. For these drugs, a truncated (shortened) plasma drug concentration–time curve (0 – 72 hr) may be more practical. The use of a truncated plasma drug concentration–time curve allows for the measurement of peak absorption and decreases the time and cost for performing the bioequivalence study.

Many drugs are stereoisomers, and each isomer may give a different pharmacodynamic response and may have a different rate of biotransformation. The bioavailability of the individual isomers may be difficult to measure because of problems in analysis. Some drugs have active metabolites, which should be quantitated as well as the parent drug. Drugs such as thioridazine and selegilene have two active metabolites. The question for such drugs is whether bio-equivalence should be proven by matching the bioavailability of both metabolites and the parent drug. Assuming both biotransformation pathways follow first-order reaction kinetics, then the metabolites should be in constant ratio to the parent drug. Genetic variation in metabolism may present a bioequivalence problem. For example, the acetylation of procainamide to N-acetylprocainamide demonstrates genetic polymorphism, with two groups of subjects consisting of rapid acetylators and slow acetylators. To decrease intersubject variability, a bioequivalence study may be performed on only one phenotype, such as the rapid acetylators.

Some drugs (eg, benzocaine, hydrocortisone, anti-infectives, and antacids) are intended for local effect and formulated as topical ointments, oral suspensions, or rectal suppositories. These drugs should not have significant systemic bioavailability from the site of administration. The bioequivalence determination for drugs that are not absorbed systemically from the site of application can be difficult to assess. For these nonsystemic-absorbable drugs, a "surrogate" marker is needed for bioequivalence determination. For example, the acid-neutralizing capacity of an oral antacid and the binding of bile acids to cholestyramine resin have been used as surrogate markers in lieu of *in-vivo* bioequivalence studies.

Table 7.5: Possible surrogate markers for bioequivalence studies

Drug Product	Drug	Possible Surrogate Marker for Bioequivalence
Metered-dose inhaler (FEV$_1$)	Albuterol	Forced expiratory volume
Topical steroid	Hydrocortisone	Skin blanching
Anion-exchange resin	Cholestyramine	Binding to bile acids
Antacid	Magnesium and aluminum hydroxide gel	Neutralization of acid
Topical antifungal	Ketoconazole	Drug uptake into stratum corneum

Various drug delivery systems and newer dosage forms are designed to deliver the drug by a nonoral route, which may produce only partial systemic bioavailability. For the treatment of asthma, inhalation of the drug (e.g., albuterol, beclomethasone dipropionate) has been used to maximize drug in the respiratory passages and to decrease systemic side effects. Drugs such as nitroglycerin given transdermally may differ in release rates, in the amount of drug in the transdermal delivery system, and in the surface area of the skin to which the transdermal delivery system is applied. Thus, the determination of bioequivalence among different manufacturers of transdermal delivery systems for the same active drug is difficult. Dermatokinetics are pharmacokinetic studies that investigate drug uptake into skin layers after topical drug administration.

The drug is applied topically, the skin is peeled at various time periods after the dose, using transparent tape, and the drug concentrations are measured in the skin.

Drugs such as potassium supplements are given orally and may not produce the usual bioavailability parameters of AUC, C_{max}, and t_{max}. For these drugs, more indirect methods must be used to ascertain bioequivalence. For example, urinary potassium excretion parameters are more appropriate for the measurement of bioavailability of potassium supplements. However, for certain hormonal replacement drugs (eg, levothyroxine), the steady-state hormone concentration in hypothyroid individuals, the thyroidal-stimulating hormone level, and pharmacodynamic endpoints may also be appropriate to measure.

Measures of Bioavailability, C_{max}, T_{max} and Area under the Curve (Auc)

Direct and indirect methods may be used to assess drug bioavailability. The *in-vivo* bioavailability of a drug product is demonstrated by the rate and extent of drug absorption, as determined by comparison of measured parameters, eg, concentration of the active drug ingredient in the blood, cumulative urinary excretion rates, or pharmacological effects. For drug products that are not intended to be absorbed into the bloodstream, bioavailability may be assessed by measurements intended to reflect the rate and extent to which the active ingredient or active moiety becomes available at the site of action. The design of the bioavailability study depends on the objectives of the study, the ability to analyze the drug (and metabolites) in biological fluids, the pharmacodynamics of the drug substance, the route of drug administration, and the nature of the drug product. Pharmacokinetic and/or pharmacodynamic parameters as well as clinical observations and *in-vitro* studies may be used to determine drug bioavailability from a drug product.

Table 7.6: Methods for assessing bioavailability

Plasma drug concentration Time for peak plasma (blood) concentration (t_{max}) Peak plasma drug concentration (C_{max}) Area under the plasma drug concentration–time curve (AUC)
Urinary drug excretion Cumulative amount of drug excreted in the urine (D_u) Rate of drug excretion in the urine (dD_u / dt) Time for maximum urinary excretion (t)
Acute pharmacodynamic effect Maximum pharmacodynamic effect (E_{max}) Time for maximum pharmacodynamic effect Area under the pharmacodynamic effect–time curve Onset time for pharmacodynamic effect
Clinical observations Well-controlled clinical trials

Measurement of drug concentrations in blood, plasma, or serum after drug administration is the most direct and objective way to determine systemic drug bioavailability. By appropriate blood sampling, an accurate description of the plasma drug concentration–time profile of the therapeutically active drug substance(s) can be obtained using a validated drug assay.

(t_{max}): **The time of peak plasma concentration, t_{max},** corresponds to the time required to reach maximum drug concentration after drug administration. At t_{max}, peak drug absorption occurs and the rate of drug absorption exactly equals the rate of drug elimination. Drug absorption still continues after t_{max} is reached, but at a slower rate. When comparing drug products, t_{max} can be used as an approximate indication of drug absorption rate. The value for t_{max} will become smaller (indicating less time required to reach peak plasma concentration) as the absorption rate for the drug becomes more rapid. Units for t_{max} are units of time (e.g., hours, minutes).

C_{max}: **The peak plasma drug concentration,** C_{max}, represents the maximum plasma drug concentration obtained after oral administration of drug. For many drugs, a relationship is found between the pharmacodynamic drug effect and the plasma drug concentration. C_{max} provides indications that the drug is sufficiently systemically absorbed to provide a therapeutic response. In addition, C_{max} provides warning of possibly toxic levels of drug. The units of C_{max} are concentration units (eg, mg/mL, ng/mL). Although not a unit for rate, C_{max} is often used in bioequivalence studies as a surrogate measure for the rate of drug bioavailability.

AUC: **The area under the plasma level–time curve,** AUC, is a measurement of the extent of drug bioavailability. The AUC reflects the total amount of active drug that reaches the systemic circulation. The AUC is the area under the drug plasma level–time curve from $t = 0$ to $t = \infty$, and is equal to the amount of unchanged drug reaching the general circulation divided by the clearance.

$$[AUC]_0^\infty = \int_0^\infty C_p \, dt \qquad \text{... (7.7)}$$

$$[AUC]_0^\infty = \frac{FD_0}{\text{clearance}} = \frac{FD_0}{KV_D} \qquad \text{... (7.8)}$$

Where, F = fraction of dose absorbed, D_0 = dose, k = elimination rate constant, and V_D = volume of distribution. The AUC is independent of the route of administration and processes of drug elimination as long as the elimination processes do not change. The AUC can be determined by a numerical integration procedure, such as the trapezoidal rule method. The units for AUC are concentration time (eg, μg hr/mL).

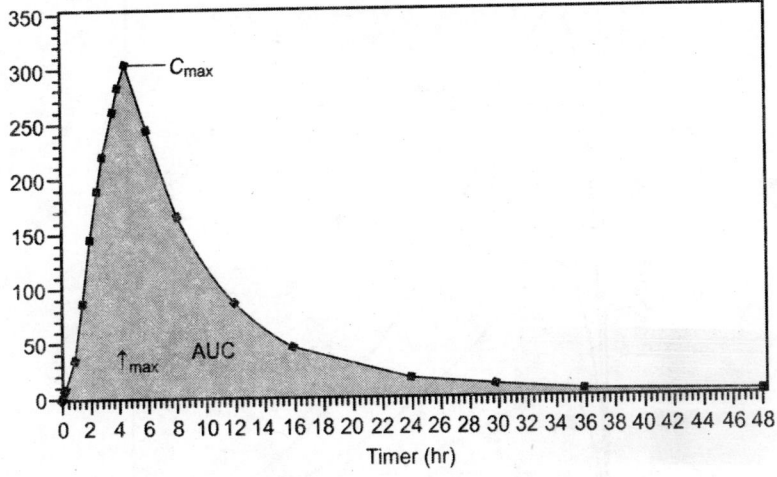

Fig. 7.3: Plasma drug concentration–time curve.

For many drugs, the AUC is directly proportional to dose. For example, if a single dose of a drug is increased from 250 to 1000 mg, the AUC will also show a fourfold increase.

In some cases, the AUC is not directly proportional to the administered dose for all dosage levels. For example, as the dosage of drug is increased, one of the pathways for drug elimination may become saturated. Drug elimination includes the processes of metabolism and excretion. Drug metabolism is an enzyme-dependent process. For drugs such as salicylate and phenytoin, continued increase of the dose causes saturation of one of the enzyme pathways for drug metabolism and consequent prolongation of the elimination half-life. The AUC thus increases disproportionally to the increase in dose, because a smaller amount of drug is being eliminated (ie, more drug is retained). When the AUC is not directly proportional to the dose, bioavailability of the drug is difficult to evaluate because drug kinetics may be dose dependent.

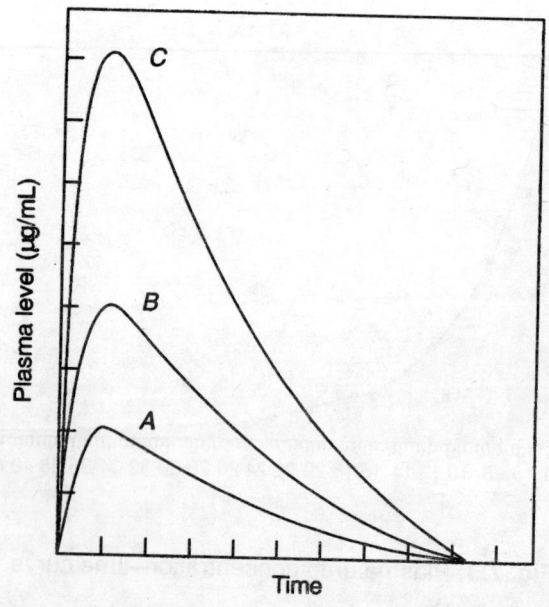

Fig. 7.4: Plasma level–time curve following administration of single doses of **(A)** 250 mg, **(B)** 500 mg, and **(C)** 1000 mg of drug.

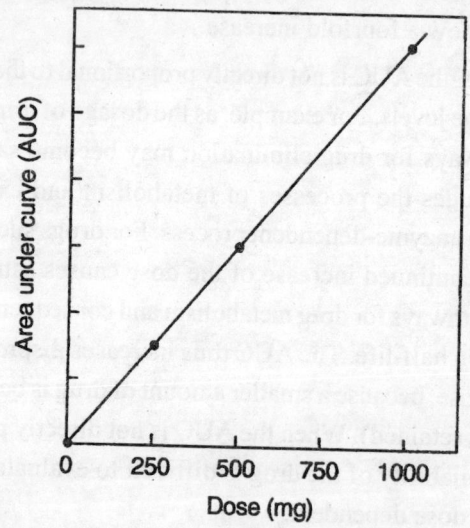

Fig. 7.5: Linear relationship between AUC and dose (data from).

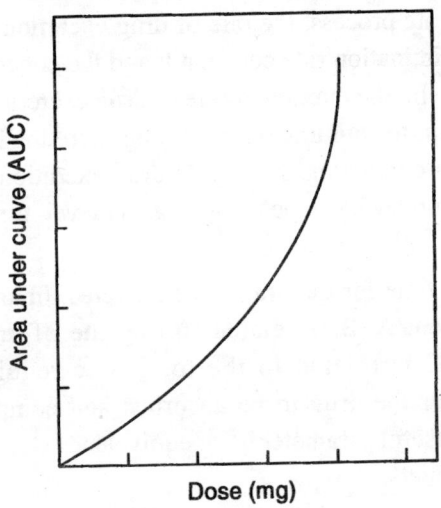

Fig. 7.6: Relationship between AUC and dose when metabolism is saturable.

Urinary drug excretion data

Urinary drug excretion data is an indirect method for estimating bioavailability. The drug must be excreted in significant quantities as unchanged drug in the urine. In addition, timely urine samples must be collected and the total amount of urinary drug excretion must be obtained.

D^∞_u: The cumulative amount of drug excreted in the urine, D^∞_u, is related directly to the total amount of drug absorbed. Experimentally, urine samples are collected periodically after administration of a drug product. Each urine specimen is analyzed for free drug using a specific assay. A graph is constructed that relates the cumulative drug excreted to the collection-time interval. The relationship between the cumulative amount of drug excreted in the urine and the plasma level–time curve is shown in. When the drug is almost completely eliminated (point C), the plasma concentration approaches zero and the maximum amount of drug excreted in the urine, D^∞_u, is obtained.

dD_u/dt: The rate of drug excretion. Because most drugs are eliminated by a first-order rate process, the rate of drug excretion is dependent on the first-order elimination rate constant k and the concentration of drug in the plasma C_p. In, the maximum rate of drug excretion, $(dD_u/dt)_{max}$, is at point B, whereas the minimum rate of drug excretion is at points A and C. Thus, a graph comparing the rate of drug excretion with respect to time should be similar in shape as the plasma level–time curve for that drug.

$t^∞$: The total time for the drug to be excreted. In and , the slope of the curve segment A–B is related to the rate of drug absorption, whereas point C is related to the total time required after drug administration for the drug to be absorbed and completely excreted $t = ∞$. The $t^∞$ is a useful parameter in bioequivalence studies that compare several drug products.

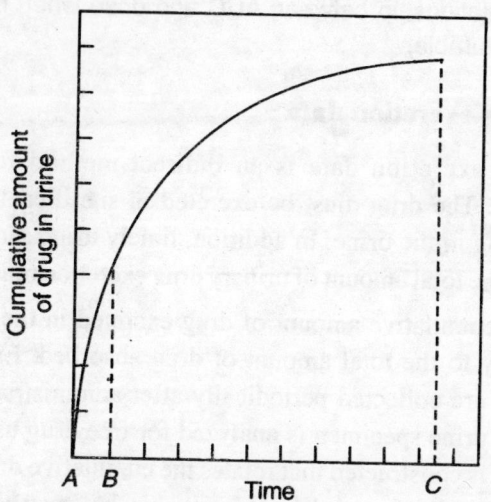

Fig. 7.7: Corresponding plots relating the plasma level–time curve and the cumulative urinary drug excretion

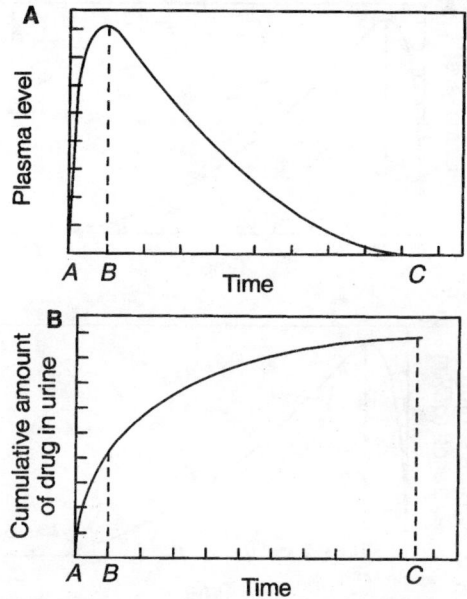

Fig. 7.8: Corresponding plots relating the plasma level–time curve and the cumulative urinary drug excretion.

Acute pharmacodynamic effect

In some cases, the quantitative measurement of a drug in plasma or urine lacks an assay with sufficient accuracy and/or reproducibility. For locally acting, nonsystemically absorbed drug products, such as topical corticosteroids, plasma drug concentrations may not reflect the bioavailability of the drug at the site of action. An acute pharmacodynamic effect, such as an effect on forced expiratory volume, FEV_1 (inhaled bronchodilators) or skin blanching (topical corticosteroids) can be used as an index of drug bioavailability. In this case, the acute pharmacodynamic effect is measured over a period of time after administration of the drug product. Measurements of the pharmacodynamic effect should be made with sufficient frequency to permit a reasonable estimate for a time period at least three times the half-life of the drug. This approach may be particularly applicable to

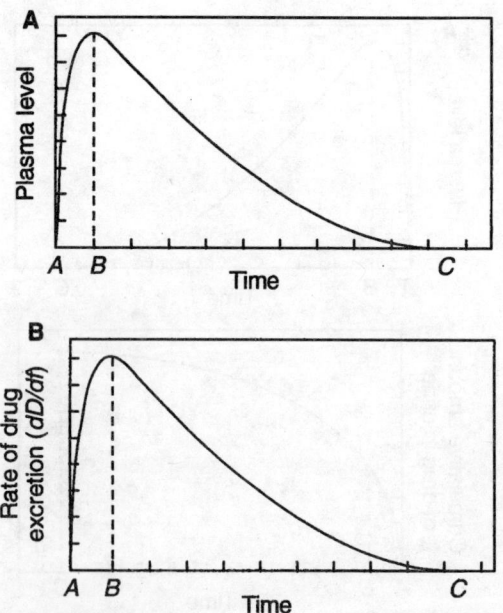

Fig. 7.9: Corresponding plots relating the plasma level–time curve and the rate of urinary drug excretion.

dosage forms that are not intended to deliver the active moiety to the bloodstream for systemic distribution.

The use of an acute pharmacodynamic effect to determine bioavailability generally requires demonstration of a dose–response curve. Bioavailability is determined by characterization of the dose–response curve. For bioequivalence determination, pharmacodynamic parameters including the total area under the acute pharmacodynamic effect–time curve, peak pharmacodynamic effect, and time for peak pharmacodynamic effect are obtained from the pharmacodynamic effect–time curve. The onset time and duration of the pharmacokinetic effect may also be included in the analysis of the data. The use of pharmacodynamic endpoints for the determination of bioavailability and bioequivalence is much more variable than the measurement of plasma or urine drug concentrations.

Clinical observations

Well-controlled clinical trials in humans establish the safety and effectiveness of drug products and may be used to determine bioavailability. However, the clinical trials approach is the least accurate, least sensitive, and least reproducible of the general approaches for determining *in-vivo* bioavailability. The FDA considers this approach only when analytical methods and pharmacodynamic methods are not available to permit use of one of the approaches described above. Comparative clinical studies have been used to establish bioequivalence for topical antifungal drug products (eg, ketoconazole) and for topical acne preparations. For dosage forms intended to deliver the active moiety to the bloodstream for systemic distribution, this approach may be considered acceptable only when analytical methods cannot be developed to permit use of one of the other approaches.

Design of Single Dose Bioequivalence Study and Relevant Statics

The *in-vivo* bioequivalence study requires determination of relative bioavailability after administration of single dose of test and reference formulations by the same route, in equal dose, but at different times. The reference product is generally a previously approved product, usually the innovator's product or some suitable reference standard. The study is performed in fasting, young, healthy, adult male volunteers to assure homogeneity in the population and to spare the patients, elderly or pregnant women from rigors of such a clinical investigation. Homogeneity in the study population permits focus on formulation factors.

Fasting study

- ✓ Bioequivalence studies are usually evaluated by a single-dose, two-period, two-treatment, two-sequence, open-label, randomized crossover design comparing equal doses of the test and reference products in fasted, adult, healthy subjects.
- ✓ This study is required for all immediate-release and modified-release oral dosage forms.

✓ Both male and female subjects may be used in the study.

✓ Blood sampling is performed just before (zero time) the dose and at appropriate intervals after the dose to obtain an adequate description of the plasma drug concentration–time profile.

✓ The subjects should be in the fasting state (overnight fast of at least 10 hours) before drug administration and should continue to fast for up to 4 hours after dosing.

✓ No other medication is normally given to the subject for at least 1 week prior to the study.

✓ In some cases, a parallel design may be more appropriate for certain drug products, containing a drug with a very long elimination half-life.

✓ A replicate design may be used for a drug product containing a drug that has high intersubject variability.

Food intervention study

✓ Co-administration of food with an oral drug product may affect the bioavailability of the drug.

✓ Food intervention or food effect studies are generally conducted using meal conditions that are expected to provide the greatest effects on GI physiology so that systemic drug availability is maximally affected.

✓ The test meal is a high-fat (approximately 50% of total caloric content of the meal) and high-calorie (approximately 800–1000 calories) meal.

✓ A typical test meal is two eggs fried in butter, two strips of bacon, and two slices of toast with butter, 4 ounces of brown potatoes, and 8 ounces of milk.

✓ This test meal derives approximately 150, 250, and 500–600 calories from protein, carbohydrate, and fat, respectively.

✓ For bioequivalence studies, drug bioavailability from both the test and reference products should be affected similarly by food.

✓ The study design uses a single-dose, randomized, two-treatment, and two-period, crossover study comparing equal doses of the test and reference products.

✓ Following an overnight fast of at least 10 hours, subjects are given the recommended meal 30 minutes before dosing.

✓ The meal is consumed over 30 minutes, with administration of the drug product immediately after the meal.

✓ The drug product is given with 240 mL (8 fluid ounces) of water.

✓ No food is allowed for at least 4 hours post dose.

✓ This study is required for all modified-release dosage forms and may be required for immediate-release dosage forms if the bioavailability of the active drug ingredient is known to be affected by food (eg, ibuprofen, naproxen).

✓ For certain extended-release capsules that contain coated beads, the capsule contents are sprinkled over soft foods such as apple sauce, which is taken by the fasted subject and the bioavailability of the drug is then measured.

✓ Bioavailability studies might also examine the affects of other foods and special vehicles such as apple juice.

Table 7.7: Latin-square crossover design for a bioequivalence study of three drug products in six human volunteers

Subject	Drug Product		
	Study Period 1	**Study Period 2**	**Study Period 3**
1	A	B	C
2	B	C	A
3	C	A	B
4	A	C	B
5	C	B	A
6	B	A	C

Crossover designs

Subjects who meet the inclusion and exclusion study criteria and have given informed consent are selected at random. A complete crossover design is usually employed, in which each subject receives the test drug product and the reference product. Examples of **Latin-square crossover designs** for a bioequivalence study in human volunteers, comparing three different drug formulations (A, B, C) or four different drug formulations (A, B, C, D).

The Latin-square design plans the clinical trial so that each subject receives each drug product only once, with adequate time between medications for the elimination of the drug from the body.

In this design, each subject is his own control, and subject-to-subject variation is reduced. Moreover, variation due to sequence, period, and treatment (formulation) are reduced, so that all patients do not receive the same drug product on the same day and in the same order. Possible carryover effects from any particular drug product are minimized by changing the sequence or order in which the drug products are given to the subject. Thus, drug product B may be followed by drug product A, D, or C. After each subject receives a drug product, blood samples are collected at appropriate time intervals so that a valid blood drug level–time curve is obtained. The time intervals should be spaced so that the peak blood concentration, the total area under the curve, and the absorption and elimination phases of the curve may be well described.

Table 7.8: Latin-square crossover design for a bioequivalence study of four drug products in 16 human volunteers

Subject	Drug Product			
	Study Period 1	Study Period 2	Study Period 3	Study Period 4
1	A	B	C	D
2	B	C	D	A

Drug Product				
Subject	Study Period 1	Study Period 2	Study Period 3	Study Period 4
3	C	D	A	B
4	D	A	B	C
5	A	B	D	C
6	B	D	C	A
7	D	C	A	B
8	C	A	B	D
9	A	C	B	D
10	C	B	D	A
11	B	D	A	C
12	D	A	C	B
13	A	C	D	B
14	C	D	B	A
15	D	B	A	C
16	B	A	C	D

Period refers to the time period in which a study is performed. A two-period study is a study that is performed on two different days (time periods) separated by a washout period during which most of the drug is eliminated from the body—generally about 10 elimination half-lives. A sequence refers to the number of different orders in the treatment groups in a study. For example, a two-sequence, two-period study would be designed as follows:

	Period 1	Period 2
Sequence 1	T	R
Sequence 2	R	T

Where R = reference and T = treatment.

Shows a design for three different drug treatment groups given in a three-period study with six different sequences. The order in which the drug treatments are given should not stay the same in order to prevent any bias in the data due to a residual effect from the previous treatment.

Replicated crossover design

Replicated crossover designs are used for the determination of individual bioequivalence, to estimate within-subject variance for both the Test and Reference drug products, and to provide an estimate of the subject-by-formulation interaction variance. Generally, a four-period, two-sequence, two-formulation design is recommended by the FDA.

	Period 1	Period 2	Period 3	Period 4
Sequence 1	T	R	T	R
Sequence 2	R	T	R	T

Where R = reference and T = treatment.

The same reference and the same test are each given twice to the same subject. Other sequences are possible. In this design, Reference-to-Reference and Test-to-Test comparisons may also be made

Evaluation of the data

• Analytical method

The analytical method for measurement of the drug must be validated for accuracy, precision, sensitivity, and specificity. The use of more than one analytical method during a bioequivalence study may not be valid, because different methods may yield different values. Data should be presented in both tabulated and graphic form for evaluation. The plasma drug concentration–time curve for each drug product and each subject should be available.

• Pharmacokinetic evaluation of the data

For single-dose studies, including a fasting study or a food intervention study, the pharmacokinetic analyses include calculation for each subject of the area under the curve to the last quantifiable concentration (AUC_{0-t}) and to infinity ($AUC_{0-\infty}$), T_{max}, and C_{max}. Additionally, the elimination rate constant, k, the elimination half-life, $t_{1/2}$, and other parameters may be estimated. For multiple-dose studies, pharmacokinetic analysis includes calculation for each subject of the steady-state area under the curve, (AUC_{0-t}), T_{max}, C_{min}, C_{max}, and the percent fluctuation [$100 \times (C_{max} - C_{min})/C_{min}$]. Proper statistical evaluation should be performed on the estimated pharmacokinetic parameters.

• Statistical evaluation of the data

Bioequivalence is generally determined using a comparison of population averages of a bioequivalence metric, such as AUC and C_{max}. This approach, termed **average bioequivalence**, involves the calculation of a 90% confidence interval for the ratio of averages (population geometric means) of the bioequivalence metrics for the Test and Reference drug products. To establish bioequivalence, the calculated confidence interval should fall within a prescribed bioequivalence limit, usually, 80–125% for the ratio of the product averages. Standard crossover design studies are used to obtain the data. Another approach proposed by the FDA and others is termed **individual bioequivalence**. Individual bioequivalence requires a replicate crossover design, and estimates within-subject variability for the Test and Reference drug products, as well as subject-by-formulation interaction. Presently, only average bioequivalence estimates are used to establish bioequivalence of generic drug products.

To prove bioequivalence, there must be no statistical difference between the bioavailability of the Test product and the Reference product. Several statistical approaches are used to compare the bioavailability of drug from the test dosage form to the bioavailability of the drug from the reference dosage form. Many statistical approaches (parametric tests) assume that the data are distributed according to a normal distribution or "bell-shaped curve". The distribution of many biological parameters such as C_{max} and AUC has a longer right tail than would be observed in a normal distribution. Moreover, the true distribution of these biological parameters may be difficult to ascertain because of the small number of subjects used in a bioequivalence study. The distribution of data that has been transformed to log values resembles more closely a normal distribution compared to the distribution of non-log-transformed data. Therefore, log transformation of the bioavailability data (eg, C_{max}, AUC) is performed before statistical data evaluation for bioequivalence determination.

(1) Analysis of variance (ANOVA)

An analysis of variance (ANOVA) is a statistical procedure used to test the data for differences within and between treatment and control groups. A bioequivalent product should produce no significant difference in all pharmacokinetic parameters tested. The parameters tested usually include AUC_{0-t}, $AUC_{0-\infty}$, t_{max}, and C_{max} obtained for each treatment or dosage form. Other metrics of bioavailability have also been used to compare the bioequivalence of two or more formulations. The ANOVA may evaluate variability in subjects, treatment groups, study period, formulation, and other variables, depending on the study design. If the variability in the data is large, the difference in means for each pharmacokinetic parameter, such as AUC, may be masked, and the investigator might erroneously conclude that the two drug products are bioequivalent.

A statistical difference between the pharmacokinetic parameters obtained from two or more drug products is considered statistically significant if there is a probability of less than 1 in 20 times or 0.05 probability ($p \leq 0.05$) that these results would have happened on the basis of chance alone. The probability, p, is used to indicate the level of statistical significance. If $p < 0.05$, the differences between the two drug products are not considered statistically significant.

To reduce the possibility of failing to detect small differences between the test products, a power test is performed to calculate the probability that the conclusion of the ANOVA is valid. The power of the test will depend on the sample size, variability of the data, and desired level of significance. Usually the power is set at 0.80 with a $\beta = 0.2$ and a level of significance of 0.05.

The higher the power, the more sensitive the test and the greater the probability that the conclusion of the ANOVA is valid.

(1) Two one-sided tests procedure

The two one-sided tests procedure is also referred to as the **confidence interval approach**. This statistical method is used to demonstrate if the bioavailability of the drug from the Test formulation is too low or high in comparison to that of the Reference product. The objective of the approach is to determine if there are large differences (ie, greater than 20%) between the mean parameters.

The 90% confidence limits are estimated for the sample means. The interval estimate is based on a Student's t distribution of the data. In this test, presently required by the FDA, a 90% confidence interval about the ratio of means of the two drug products must be within $\pm 20\%$ for measurement of the rate and extent of drug bioavailability. For most drugs, up to a 20% difference in AUC or C_{max} between two formulations would have no clinical significance. The lower 90% confidence interval for the ratio of means cannot be less than 0.80, and the upper 90% confidence interval for the ratio of the means cannot be greater than 1.20. When log-transformed data are used, the 90% confidence interval is set at 80–125%. These confidence limits have also been termed the **bioequivalence interval**. The 90% confidence interval is a function of sample size and study variability, including inters- and intersubject variability.

For a single-dose, fasting study, an analysis of variance (ANOVA) is usually performed on the log-transformed AUC and C_{max} values. There should be no statistical differences between the mean AUC and C_{max} parameters for the Test (generic) and Reference drug products. In addition, the 90% confidence intervals about the ratio of the means for AUC and C_{max} values of the Test drug product should not be less than 0.80 (80%) nor greater than 1.25 (125%) of that of the Reference product based on log-transformed data.

Overview of Regulatory Requirements For Conduction of Bioequivalence Studies

1. The **90%** confidence interval of the relative mean AUC of the test to reference formulation should be within **90.0 to 112.0%;** the relevant AUC or AUCs as described in Guidelines A and B are to be determined.

2. The **90%** confidence interval of the relative mean measured C_{max} of the test to reference formulation should be between **80.0 and 125.0%.**

3. These requirements are to be met in both the **fasted and fed states.**

4. These standards should be met on log transformed parameters calculated from the measured data and from data corrected for measured drug content (percent potency of label claim).

5. Steady-state studies are not required for "critical dose drugs" unless warranted by exceptional circumstances. If a steady-state study is required, the **90%** confidence interval of the relative mean measured C_{min} of the test to reference formulation should also be between **80.0 and 125.0%.**

For BE studies, both the test and reference must contain same active ingredient, same dose, similar dosage form and both are given by the same route

1. Single dose or multiple dose study is required.

2. Study is performed in normal healthy volunteers.

3. Volunteers who smoke, who are allergic or who have taken medication within one week of study are excluded.

4. The active ingredient in the test must be within 80 to 125% of reference product.

Note:

❖ Due to the nature of these drugs, it may be necessary to conduct studies in patients rather than in healthy subjects. The variability of the disease states in patients in whom the studies are performed will be an important consideration in deciding the size of cohort which will have to be investigated in order to meet the standards. It is highly recommended that the study group be as homogeneous as possible with respect to predictable sources of variation in drug disposition.

❖ Where a drug is being administered chronically, it may be possible to study bioavailability only during a dose interval at steady-state. The test drug product would be required to replace the reference drug product over a period of at least five half-lives, where feasible, before sampling. Standardization of the study conditions is essential, particularly with respect to the time of day of drug administration and posture of the subject.

❖ Ethical considerations may also dictate that these studies be conducted in parallel groups rather than by a crossover design.

Questions

Essay questions

1. What is bioavailability? Write a note on measurement of bioavailability.

2. What is bioequivalence? Explain single dose bioequivalence study and relevant statics.

3. What are the special concerns in the bioavailability and bioequivalence studies?

Short questions

1. What are the objectives of bioavailability studies?

2. What are the regulatory requirements for conduction of bioequivalence studies?

3. What is the purpose of bioavailability studies?

4. What is the clinical significance of bioequivalence studies?

5. What are the advantages and limitations of randomized, balanced, cross-over study in bioequivalence determination?

6. Define equivalence, chemical equivalence, pharmaceutics equivalence, and therapeutic equivalence.

Chapter—8

BIOAVAILABILITY AND BIOEQUIVALENCE TESTING PROTOCOL

In Vitro Dissolution Studies for Solid Dosage Forms Methods

For an *in vitro* test to be useful, it must predict the *in vivo* behavior to such an extent that *in vivo* bioavailability test need not be performed. Despite attempts to standardize the test performance, the *in vitro* dissolution technique is still by no means a perfect approach. The efforts are mainly aimed at mimicking the environment offered by the biological system.

There are the several factors that must be considered in the design of a dissolution test. They are:

1. Factors relating to the dissolution apparatus such as – the design, the size of the container (several mL to several liters), the shape of the container (round bottom or flat), nature of agitation (stirring, rotating or oscillating methods), speed of agitation, performance precision of the apparatus, etc.

2. Factors relating to the dissolution fluid such as – composition water, 0.1N HCL, phosphate buffer (simulated gastric fluid, simulated intestinal fluid, etc.), viscosity, volume (generally larger than that needed to completely dissolve the drug under test), temperature (generally 37°C) and maintenance of **sink** (drug

concentration in solution maintained constant at a low level) or **nonsink** conditions (gradually increase in the drug concentration in the dissolution medium).

3. Process parameters such as method of introduction of dosage form, sampling techniques, changing the dissolution fluid, etc.

USP method 1 (rotating basket method)

There is the several in vitro drug dissolution methods are as follows:

- A cylindrical vessel, A, made of borosilicate glass or any other suitable transparent material, with a hemispherical bottom and with a nominal capacity of 1000ml.

- A motor with a speed regulator capable of maintaining the speed of rotation of the paddle within 4% of that specified in the individual monograph. The motor is fitted with a stirring element which consists of a basket, D.

- The basket consists of two components. The top part, with a vent, is attached to the shaft C. The lower detachable part of the basket is made of welded-steam cloth, with a wire thickness of 0.254 mm diameter and with 0.381mm square openings, formed into a cylinder. The basket may be plated with a 2.5mm layer of gold for use with acidic media.

- The distance between the inside bottom of the vessel and the basket is maintained at 23 to 27mm during the test.

- A water-bath set to maintain the dissolution medium at 37 ± 0.5°C.

- The dosage form is placed in a dry basket at the beginning of each test.

- In case of non-disintegrating dosage forms this apparatus is superior to apparatus 2 since it constrains the dosage form in steady state fluid flow.

- This apparatus may seem to be inferior for testing of dosage forms, which contains gums due to clogging of the screen matrix.

- In case of floating dosage forms this method performs well.

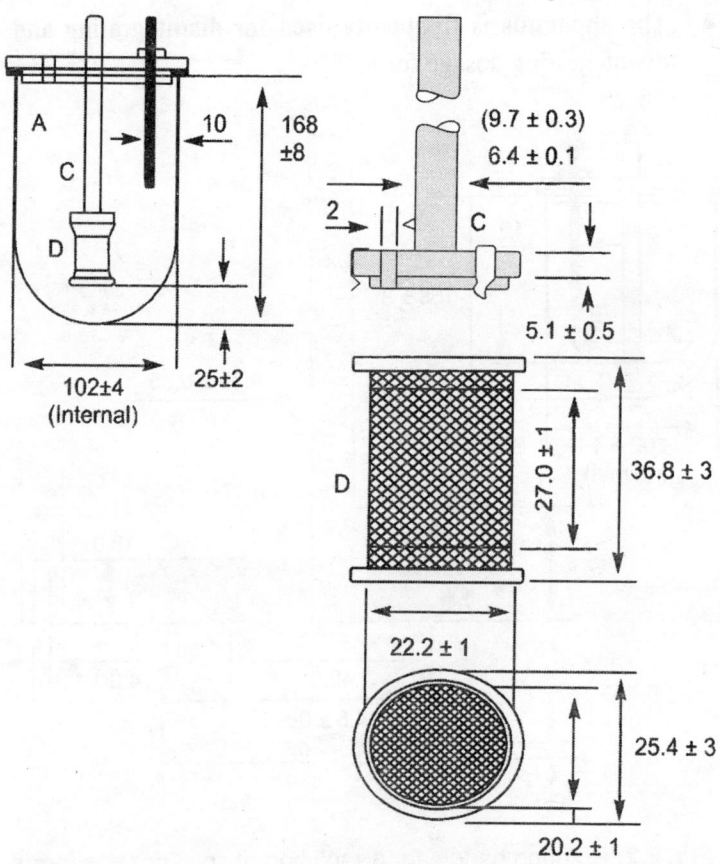

Fig. 8.1: Rotating basket for dissolution of solid dosage forms

USP method 2 (rotating paddle method)

The assembly consists of the following:

- The assembly is the same as in Apparatus 1 except that the motor is fitted with a stirring element which consists of a drive shaft and blade forming a paddle.

- The dosage form is allowed to sink to the bottom of the vessel before rotation of the blade is started.

- The apparatus is frequently used for disintegrating and non-disintegrating dosage forms.

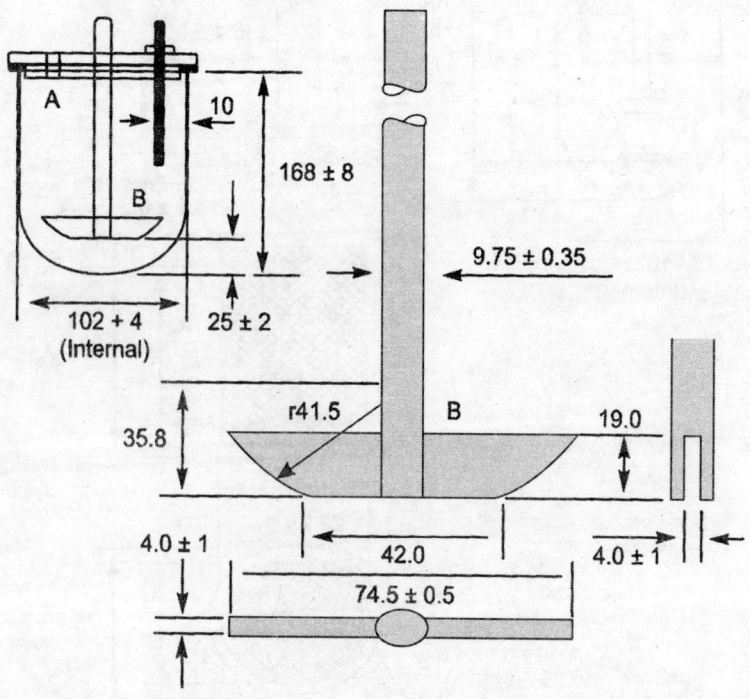

Fig. 8.2: Rotating paddle for dissolution of solid dosage forms.

➤ **Dissolution medium:**

- Use the dissolution medium specified in the individual monograph.

- If the medium is a buffered solution, adjust the solution so that its pH is within 0.05 units.

- The dissolution medium should be deaerated prior to testing.

➤ Method:

- Introduce the stated volume of the dissolution medium, free from dissolved air, into the vessel of the apparatus. Warm the dissolution medium to 37 ± 0.5 °C.

- When Apparatus 1 is used, place the tablet or capsule in a dry basket at the beginning of each test. When Apparatus 2 is used, allow the tablet or capsule to sink to the bottom of the vessel prior to the rotation of the paddle.

- Operate the apparatus at the speed of rotation specified in the individual monograph.

- Within the time interval specified, withdraw a specimen from a zone midway between the surface of the dissolution medium and the top of the rotating blade or basket, and replace the aliquots withdrawn for analysis with equal volumes of fresh dissolution medium at 37°C.

- For each of the tablet or capsule tested, calculate the amount of dissolved active ingredient in solution as a percentage of the stated amount.

- If the results do not conform to the requirements at stage S1 given in the acceptance table, continue testing with additional tablets or capsules through stages S2 and S3.

Table 8.1: Acceptance table

Stage	Number	Tested Acceptance criteria
S1	6	Each unit is not less than D* + 5%
S2	6	Average of 12 units (S1+S2) is equal to or greater than D and no unit is less than D –15%.
S3	12	Average of 24 units (S1+S2+S3) is equal to or greater than D, not more than 2 units are less than D–15% and no unit is less than D–25%

* D is the amount of dissolved active ingredient, expressed as a percentage of the stated amount.

USP method 3 (reciprocating cylinder)

The assembly consists of the following:

- A set of glass reciprocating cylinders.
- A motor and drive assembly to reciprocate the cylinders vertically inside the vessels.
- The vessels are immersed in a suitable water bath maintained at a temp. $37 \pm 0.5°C$.

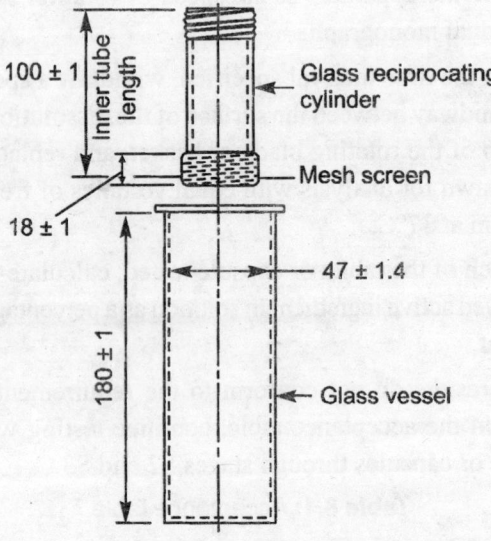

Fig. 8.3: Reciprocating cylinder for dissolution of solid dosage forms

The apparatus consists of 6 rows of outer tubes which contain media (25o ml capacity for each tube), while in each row there are 6 inner tubes containing the product and an additional 7th tube for standard solution to be analyzed.

Advantage of this reciprocating cylinder is that gastrointestinal tract conditions can be easily stimulated, and easy to make time dependent pH changes.

This apparatus is most suitable for dissolution of:

- Non-disintegrating (extended release) or
- Delayed release (enteric coated) dosage forms.

USP method 4 (flow through cell)

The assembly consists of:

- A reservoir and a pump for dissolution medium.
- A flow through cell.
- A water bath that maintains dissolution medium at $37 \pm 0.5°C$.

The pump forces the dissolution medium upwards through the flow through cell. The pump has a delivery range b/w 240 and 960 ml/hr, with the standard flow rates of 4, 8, 16 ml/min.

The **advantage** of this apparatus is its ability to test drugs of low aq. Solubility and ability to change pH conveniently during test.

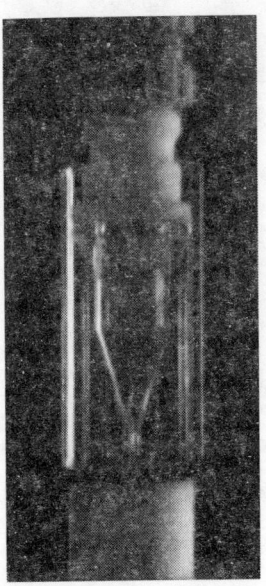

Fig. 8.4: Flow through cell for dissolution of solid dosage forms

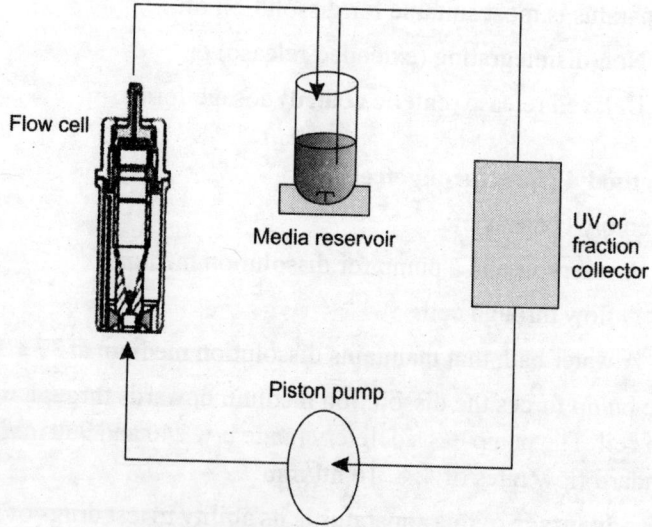

Fig. 8.5: Closed loop configuration

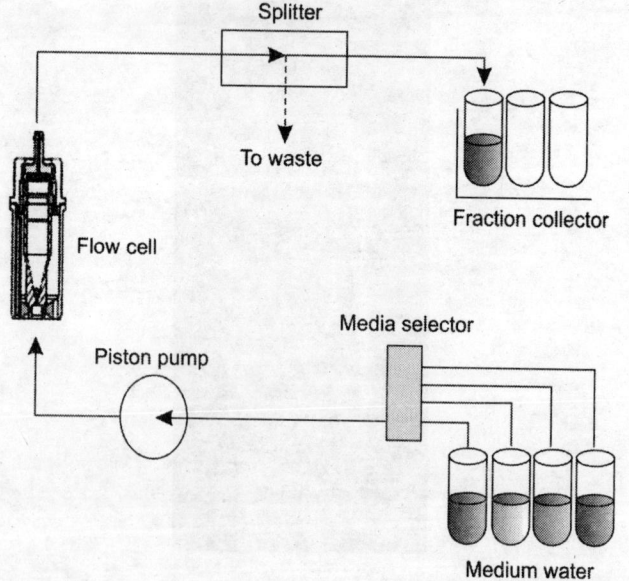

Fig. 8.6: Open loop configuration

USP method 5 (paddle over disk)

The apparatus 2 is used, with the addition of a stainless steel disk assembly for holding the transdermal system at the bottom of the vessel and temperature is maintained at 32 ± 0.5 °C.

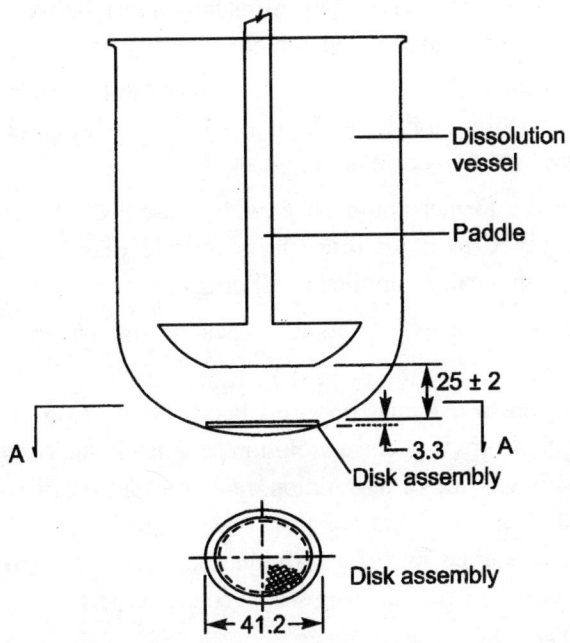

Fig. 8.7: Paddle over disk for dissolution of solid dosage forms

In Vitro – In Vivo Correlation

A simple *in vitro* dissolution test on the drug product will be insufficient to predict its therapeutic efficacy. Convincing correlation between *in vitro* dissolution behavior of a drug and its *in vivo* bioavailability must be experimentally demonstrated to guarantee reproducibility of biologic response.

The two major objectives of developing such a correlation are:

(1) To ensure batch-to-batch consistency in the physiologic performance of a drug product by use of such *in vitro* values.

(2) To serve as a tool in the development of a new dosage form with desired *in vivo* performance.

There are two basic approaches by which a correlation between dissolution testing and bioavailability can be developed:

(1) By establishing a relationship, usually linear, between the *in vitro* dissolution and the *in vivo* bioavailability parameters, and

(2) By using the data from previous bioavailability studies to modify the dissolution methodology in order to arrive at meaningful *in vitro – in vivo* correlation.

Though the former approach is widely used, the latter still holds substance, since to date; there is no single dissolution rate test methodology that can be applied to all drugs.

Some of the often used quantitative linear *in vitro – in vivo* correlations are:

(1) Correlation based on the plasma level data: Here, linear relationships between dissolution parameters such as percent drug dissolved, rate of dissolution, rate constant for dissolution, etc. and parameters obtained from plasma level data such as percent drug absorbed, rate of absorption, C_{max}, t_{max}, K_a etc. are developed; for example, percent drug dissolved versus percent drug absorbed plots.

(2) Correlation based on the urinary excretion data: Here, dissolution parameters are correlated to the amount of drug excreted unchanged in the urine, cumulative amount of drug excreted as a function of time, etc.

(3) Correlation based on the pharmacologic response: An acute pharmacologic effect such as LD_{50} in animals is related to any of the dissolution parameters.

Statistical moment theory can also be used to determine the relationship such as mean dissolution time (*in vitro*) versus mean residence time (*in vivo*).

Though examples of good correlations are many, there are instances when positive correlation is difficult or impossible; for example, in case of corticosteroids, the systemic availability may not depend upon the dissolution characteristics of the drug. Several factors that limit such a correlation include variables pertaining to the drug such as dissolution methodology, physicochemical properties of the drug such as particle size, physiologic variables like presystemic metabolism, etc.

Bioavailability Testing Protocol and Procedures

Introduction

Ensuring uniformity in standards of quality, efficacy and safety of pharmaceutical products is the fundamental responsibility of CDSCO. Reasonable assurance has to be provided that various products, containing same active ingredients, marketed by different licensees, are clinically equivalent and interchangeable.

Accordingly, the bioavailability of an active substance from a pharmaceutical product should be known and reproducible. In most cases, it is cumbersome and unnecessary to assess this by clinical studies. Bioavailability and bioequivalence data is therefore required to be furnished with applications for new drugs, as required under Schedule Y, depending on the type of application being submitted.

Both bioavailability and bioequivalence focus on the release of a drug substance from its dosage form and subsequent absorption into the systemic circulation. For this reason, similar approaches to measuring bioavailability should generally be followed in demonstrating bioequivalence.

Bioavailability can be generally documented by a systemic exposure profile obtained by measuring drug and/or metabolite concentration in the systemic circulation over time. The systemic exposure profile determined during clinical trials in the early drug development can serve as a benchmark for subsequent BE studies.

Bioequivalence studies should be conducted for the comparison of two medicinal products containing the same active substance. The studies should provide an objective means of critically assessing the possibility of alternative use of them. Two products marketed by different licensees, containing same active ingredient(s), must be shown to be therapeutically equivalent to one another in order to be considered interchangeable. Several test methods are available to assess equivalence, including:

i. Comparative bioavailability (bioequivalence) studies, in which the active drug substance or one or more metabolites is measured in an accessible biological fluid such as plasma, blood or urine.

ii. Comparative pharmacodynamic studies in humans.

iii. Comparative clinical trials.

iv. *in-vitro* dissolution tests.

The guidelines describe when bioavailability or bioequivalence studies are necessary and describe requirements for their design, conduct, and evaluation. The possibility of using *in vitro* instead of *in vivo* studies with pharmacokinetic end points is also envisaged.

For classes of products, including many biological such as vaccines, animal sera, and products derived from human blood and plasma, and product manufactured by biotechnology, the concept of interchangeability raises complex which may be addressed by the applicant on the basis of contemporary scientific rationale.

In vivo bioequivalence/bioavailability studies recommended for approval of modified release products should be designed to ensure that:

i. The product meets the modified release label claims

ii. The product does not release the active drug substance at a rate and extent leading to dose dumping.

iii. There is no significant difference between the performance of the modified release product and the reference product, when given in dosage regimes to arrive at the steady state.

iv. There must be a significant difference between the performance of modified release product and the conventional release product when used as reference product.

It is appreciated that pharmacokinetic studies can be conducted during any phase of a clinical trial for New Chemical Entities (NCEs). While these guidelines deal with pharmacokinetic / pharmacodynamic studies vis-à-vis bioavailability or bioequivalence studies for a generic drug, the principles described herein, are applicable for any pharmacokinetic / pharmacodynamic study.

Definitions

• Bioavailability

Bioavailability refers to the relative amount of drug from an administered dosage form which enters the systemic circulation and the rate at which the drug appears in the systemic circulation.

• Bioequivalence

Bioequivalence of a drug product is achieved if its extent and rate of absorption are not statistically significantly different from those of the reference product when administered at the same molar dose.

• Clinical trial

A clinical trial is a systematic study of pharmaceutical products in human subject(s), in order to discover or verify the clinical, pharmacological (including pharmacodynamic / pharmacokinetic), and/or adverse effects, with the object of determining their safety and/or efficacy.

• Good clinical practice (GCP) guidelines:

Good clinical practice guidelines issued by directorate general of health services, ministry of health and family welfare, government of india.

• Modified release dosage forms

Modified-release dosage forms are those for which the drug-release characteristics of time course and/or drug-release location are chosen to accomplish such therapeutic or convenience objectives that are not offered by immediate-(conventional) release dosage forms.

• Pharmaceutical equivalents

Pharmaceutical equivalents are drug products that contain identical amounts of the identical active drug ingredient, i.e., the same salt or ester of the same therapeutic moiety, in identical dosage forms, but not necessarily containing the same inactive ingredients.

● **Pharmaceutical alternatives**

Pharmaceutical alternatives are drug products that contain the identical therapeutic moiety, or its precursor, but not necessarily in the same amount or dosage form or as the same salt or ester.

● **Pharmacodynamic evaluation**

Pharmacodynamic evaluation is measurement of the effect on a pathophysiological process as a function of time, after administration of two different products to serve as a basis for bioequivalence assessment.

● **Pharmacokinetics**

Pharmacokinetics deals with the changes of drug concentration in the drug product and changes of concentration of a drug and/or its metabolite(s) in the human or animal body following administration of the drug product, i.e., the changes of drug concentration in the different body fluids and tissues in the dynamic system of liberation, absorption, distribution, body storage, binding, metabolism, and excretion.

● **Non-linear pharmacokinetics**

Nonlinear kinetics or saturation kinetics refers to a change of one or more of the pharmacokinetic parameters during absorption, distribution, metabolism, and excretion by saturation or overloading of processes due to increased dose sizes.

● **Reference product**

For purpose of these guidelines, the reference product is a pharmaceutical product which is identified by the Licensing Authority as "Designated Reference Product" and contains the same active ingredient(s) as the new drug. The Designated Reference Product will normally be the global innovator's product. An applicant seeking approval to market a generic equivalent must refer to the Designated Reference Product to which all generic versions must be shown to be bioequivalent. For subsequent new drug applications in India the Licensing Authority may, however, approve another Indian product as Designated Reference Product.

● **Supra-bioavailability**

This is a term used when a test product displays an appreciably larger bioavailability than the reference product.

● **Sustained release dosage form**

These are modified release dosage forms where the liberation (drug release) rate constant is smaller than the unrestricted absorption rate constant.

● **Steady state**

Steady state is the state when the plasma concentration of drug at any time point during any dosing interval should be identical to the concentration at the same time during any other dosing interval. The steady state drug concentrations fluctuate (oscillate) between a maximum and a minimum steady state concentration within each of the dosing intervals.

● **Therapeutic equivalents**

Therapeutic equivalents are drug products that contain the same active substance or therapeutic moiety and, clinically show the same efficacy and safety.

Pharmacokinetic terms

● C_{max}

This is the maximum drug concentration achieved in systemic circulation following drug administration.

● C_{min}

This is the minimum drug concentration achieved in systemic circulation following multiple dosing at steady state.

● C_{pd}

This is the pre-dose concentrations determined immediately before a dose is given at steady state.

● T_{max}

It is the time required to achieve maximum drug concentration in systemic circulation.

- **AUC_{0-t}**

Area under the plasma concentration - time curve from 0 h to the last quantifiable concentration to be calculated using the trapezoidal rule

- **$AUC_{0-\infty}$**

Area under the plasma concentration-time curve, from zero to infinity to be calculated as the sum of AUC plus the ratio of the last measurable concentration to the elimination r ate constant.

- **$AUC_{0-\tau}$**

Area under the plasma concentration - time curve over one dosing interval following single dose for modified release products.

- **$AUC_{0-\tau (ss)}$**

Area under the plasma concentration - time curve over one dosing interval in multiple dose study at steady state.

- **K_{el}**

Apparent first-order terminal elimination rate constant calculated from a semi-log plot of the plasma concentration versus time curve.

- **T1/2**

Elimination half life of a drug is the time necessary to reduce the drug concentration in the blood, plasma, or serum to one-half after equilibrium is reached.

Scope of the guidelines

Bioavailability and Bioequivalence studies are required by regulations to ensure therapeutic equivalence between a pharmaceutically equivalent test product and a reference product. Several in vivo and in vitro methods are used to measure product quality.

- **When bioequivalence studies are necessary and types of studies required**
  - ➢ **In vivo studies**

For certain drugs and dosage forms, *in vivo* documentation of equivalence, through either a bioequivalence study, a comparative clinical pharmacodynamic study, or a comparative clinical trial, is regarded as especially important. These include:

a. Oral immediate release drug formulations with systemic action when one or more of the following criteria apply:

    i. Indicated for serious conditions requiring assured therapeutic response;

    ii. Narrow therapeutic window/safety margin; steep dose-response curve;

    iii. Pharmacokinetics complicated by variable or incomplete absorption or absorption window, nonlinear pharmacokinetics, pre-systemic elimination/high first-pass metabolism >70%;

    iv. Unfavourable physicochemical properties, e.g., low solubility, instability, meta-stable modifications, poor permeability, etc.;

    v. Documented evidence for bioavailability problems related to the drug or drugs of similar chemical structure or formulations;

    vi. Where a high ratio of excipients to active ingredients exists.

b. Non-oral and non-parenteral drug formulations designed to act by systemic absorption (such as transdermal patches, suppositories, etc.).

c. Sustained or otherwise modified release drug formulations designed to act by systemic absorption.

d. Fixed-dose combination products with systemic action.

e. Non-solution pharmaceutical products which are for non-systemic use (oral, nasal, ocular, dermal, rectal, vaginal, etc. application) and are intended to act without systemic absorption. In these cases, the bioequivalence concept is not suitable and comparative clinical or pharmacodynamic studies are required to prove equivalence. There is a need for drug concentration measurements in order to assess unintended partial absorption.

Bioequivalence documentation is also needed to establish links between:

i. Early and late clinical trial formulations

ii. Formulations used in clinical trials and stability studies, if different

iii. Clinical trial formulations and to be marketed drug products

iv. Other comparisons, as appropriate

In each comparison, the new formulation or new method of manufacture shall be the test product and the prior formulation (or respective method of manufacture) shall be the reference product.

➤ In vitro studies

In following circumstances equivalence may be assessed by the use of *in vitro* dissolution testing:

a. Drugs for which the applicant provides data to substantiate all of the following:

i. Highest dose strength is soluble in 250 ml of an aqueous media over the pH range of 1-7.5 at 37 °C.

ii. At least 90% of the administered oral dose is absorbed on mass balance determination or in comparison to an intravenous reference dose

iii. Speed of dissolution as demonstrated by more than 80% dissolution within 15 minutes at 37 °C using IP apparatus 1, at 50 rpm or IP apparatus 2, at 100 rpm in a volume of 900 ml or less in each of the following media:

1. 0.1 N hydrochloric acid or artificial gastric juice (without enzymes)

2. A pH 4.5 buffer

3. A pH 6.8 buffer or artificial intestinal juice (without enzymes)

b. Different strengths of the drug manufactured by the same manufacturer, where all of the following criteria are fulfilled:

i. The qualitative composition between the strengths is essentially the same;

ii. The ratio of active ingredients and excipients between the strengths is essentially the same, or, in the case of small strengths, the ratio between the excipients is the same;

iii. The method of manufacture is essentially the same;

iv. An appropriate equivalence study has been performed on at least one of the strengths of the formulation (usually the highest strength unless a lower strength is chosen for reasons of safety); and

v. In case of systemic availability - pharmacokinetics have been shown to be linear over the therapeutic dose range. *In vitro* dissolution testing may also be suitable to confirm unchanged product quality and performance characteristics with minor formulation or manufacturing changes after approval.

➢ When bioequivalence studies are not necessary

In following formulations and circumstances, bioequivalence between a new drug and the reference product may be considered self-evident with no further requirement for documentation:

a. When new drugs are to be administered parenterally (e.g., intravenous, intramuscular, subcutaneous, intrathecal administration etc.) as aqueous solutions and contain the same active substance(s) in the same concentration and the same excipients in comparable concentrations;

b. When the new drug is a solution for oral use, and contains the active substance in the same concentration, and does not contain excipients that is known or suspected to affect gastro-intestinal transit or absorption of the active substance;

c. When the new drug is a gas;

d. When the new drug is a powder for reconstitution as a solution and the solution meets either criterion (a) or criterion (b) above;

e. When the new drug is an otic or ophthalmic or topical product prepared as aqueous solution and contains the same active substance(s) in the same concentration(s) and essentially the same excipients in comparable concentrations;

f. When the new drug is an inhalation product or a nasal spray, tested to be administered with or without essentially the same device as the reference product, prepared as aqueous solutions, and contain the same active substance(s) in the same concentration and essentially the same excipients in comparable concentrations. Special *in vitro* testing is required to document device performance comparison between reference inhalation product and the new drug product.

For (e) and (f) above, the applicant is expected to demonstrate that the excipients in the new drug are essentially the same and in comparable concentrations as those in the reference product. In the event this information about the reference product cannot be provided by the applicant, *in vivo* studies need to be performed.

Design and conduct of studies
- **Pharmacokinetic studies**
- ➢ **Study design**

The basic design of an in-vivo bioavailability study is determined by the following:

i. What is the scientific question(s) to be answered.

ii. The nature of the reference material and the dosage form to be tested.

iii. The availability of analytical methods.

iv. Benefit-risk ratio considerations in regard to testing in humans.

The study should be designed in such a manner that the formulation effect can be distinguished from other effects. Typically, if two formulations are to be compared, a two-period, two-sequence crossover design is the design of choice with the two phases of treatment separated by an adequate washout period which should ideally be equal to or more than five half life's of the moieties to be measured. Alternative study designs include the parallel design for very long half-life substances or the replicate design for substances with highly variable disposition. Single-dose studies generally suffice. However situations as described below may demand a steady-state study design:

i. Dose or time-dependant pharmacokinetics.

ii. Some modified release products (in addition to single dose investigations)

iii. Where problems of sensitivity preclude sufficiently precise plasma concentration measurements after single-dose administration.

iv. If intra-individual variability in the plasma concentration or disposition precludes the possibility of demonstrating bioequivalence in a reasonably sized single-dose study and this variability is reduced at steady state.

➤ **Study population**

1. Selection of the number of subjects

The number of subjects required for a study should be statistically significant and is determined by the following considerations:

i. The error variance associated with the primary characteristic to be studied as estimated from a pilot experiment, from previous studies or from published data.

ii. The significance level desired: usually 0.05

iii. The expected deviation from the reference product compatible with bioequivalence.

iv. The required (discriminatory) power, normally $=80\%$ to detect the maximum allowable difference (usually$\pm$ 20%) in primary characteristics to be studied.

The number of subjects recruited should be sufficient to allow for possible withdrawals or removals (dropouts) from the study. It is acceptable to replace a subject withdrawn/drop out from the study once it has begun provided the substitute follows the same protocol originally intended for the withdrawn subject and he/she is tested under similar environmental and other controlled conditions. However, the minimum number of subjects should not be less than 16 unless justified for ethical reasons. Sequential or add-on studies are acceptable in specific cases e.g. where a large number of subjects are required or where the results of the study do not convey adequate statistical significance. In all cases the final statistical analysis must include data of all subjects or reasons for not including partial data as well as the un-included data must be documented in the final report.

2. Selection criteria for subjects

To minimize intra and inter individual variation subjects should be standardised as much as possible and acceptable. The studies should be normally performed on healthy adult volunteers with the aim to minimize variability and permit detection of differences between the study drugs. Subjects may be males or females; however the choice of gender should be consistent with usage and safety criteria.

Risks to women of childbearing potential should be considered on an individual basis. Women should be required to give assurance that they are neither pregnant, nor likely to become pregnant until after the study. This should be confirmed by a pregnancy test immediately prior to the first and last dose of the study. Women taking contraceptive drugs should normally not be included in the studies. If the drug product is to be used predominantly in the elderly attempt should be made to include as many subjects of 60 years of age or older as possible. If the drug product is intended for use in both sexes attempt should be made to include similar proportions of males and females in the studies. For a drug representing a potential hazard in one group of users, the choice of subjects may be narrowed, e.g., studies on teratogenic drugs should be conducted only on males. For drugs primarily intended for use in only males or only females–volunteers of only respective gender should be included in the studies.

For drugs where the risk of toxicity or side effects is significant, studies may have to be carried out in patients with the concerned disease, but whose disease state is stable. They should be screened for suitability by means of a comprehensive medical examination including clinical laboratory tests, an extensive review of medical history including medication history, use of oral contraceptives, alcohol intake, and smoking, use of drugs of abuse.

Depending on the study drugs therapeutic class and safety profile, special medical investigations may need to be carried out before, during and after the study.

3. Genetic phenotyping

Phenotyping and/or genotyping of subjects should be considered for exploratory bioavailability studies and all studies using parallel group design. It may also be considered in crossover studies (e.g. bioequivalence, dose proportionality, food interaction studies etc.) for safety or pharmacokinetic reasons. If a drug is known to be subject to major genetic polymorphism, studies could be performed in panels of subjects of known phenotype or genotype for the polymorphism in question. While designing a study protocol, adequate care should be taken to consider Pharmacogenomic issues in the context of Indian population.

➤ Study conditions

Standardisation of the study environment, diet, fluid intake, post-dosing postures, exercise, sampling schedules etc. is important in all studies. Compliance to these standardisations should be stated in the protocol and reported at the end of the study, in order to reassure that all variability factors involved, except that of the products being tested, have been minimised. Unless the study design requires, subjects should abstain from smoking, drinking alcohol, coffee, tea, xanthine containing foods and beverages and fruit juices during the study and at least 48 hours before its commencement.

1. Selection of blood sampling points/schedules

The blood-sampling period in single-dose trials of an immediate release product should extend to at least three-elimination half-lives. Sampling should be continued for a sufficient period to ensure that the area extrapolated from the time of the last measured concentration to infinite time is only a small percentage (normally less than 20%) of the total AUC. The use of a truncated AUC is undesirable except in certain circumstances such as in the presence of entero-hepatic recycling where the terminal elimination rate constant cannot be calculated accurately.

There should be at least three sampling points during the absorption phase, three to four at the projected T_{max}, and four points during the elimination phase. The number of points used to calculate the terminal elimination rate constant should be preferably determined by eye from a semi-logarithmic plot. Intervals between successive data/sampling points used to calculate the terminal elimination rate constant should, in general, not be longer than the half-life of the study drug. Where urinary excretion is measured in a single-dose study it is necessary to collect urine for seven or more half-lives.

2. Fasting and fed state considerations

Generally, a single dose study should be conducted after an overnight fast (at least 10 hours), with subsequent fast of 4 hours following dosing. For multiple dose fasting state studies, when an evening dose must be given, two hours of fasting before and after the dose is considered acceptable. However, when it is recommended that the study drug be given with food (as would be in routine clinical practice), or where the dosage form is a modified release product, fed state studies need to be carried out in addition to the fasting state studies. Fed state studies are also required when fasting state studies make assessment of C_{max} and T_{max} difficult.

Studies in the fed state require the consumption of a high-fat breakfast before dosing. Such a breakfast must be designed to provide 950 to 1000 KCals. At least 50% of these calories must come from fat, 15 to 20% from proteins and the rest from carbohydrates. The vast ethnic and cultural variations of the Indian sub-continent preclude the recommendation of any single standard high fat breakfast. Protocol should specify the suitable and appropriate diet. The high fat breakfast must be consumed approximately 15 minutes before dosing.

3. Steady state studies

In following cases – an additional "steady state study" is considered appropriate:

i. Where the drug has a long terminal elimination half-life and blood concentrations after a single dose cannot be followed for a sufficient time.

ii. Where assay sensitivity is inadequate to follow the terminal elimination phase for an adequate period of time.

iii. For drugs, which are so toxic that ethically they should only be administered to patients for whom they are a necessary part of therapy, but where multiple dose therapy is required, e.g. many cytotoxics.

iv. For modified-release products where it is necessary to assess the fluctuation in plasma concentration over a dosage interval at steady state.

v. For those drugs which induce their own metabolism or show large intra-individual variability.

vi. For enteric-coated preparations where the coating is innovative.

vii. For combination products where the ratio of plasma concentration of the individual drugs is important.

viii. For drugs that exhibit non-linear (i.e., dose- or time- dependent) pharmacokinetics.

ix. Where the drug is likely to accumulate in the body. In steady state studies, the dosing schedule should follow the clinically recommended dosage regimen.

➢ **Characteristics to be investigated during bioavailability/ bioequivalence studies**

In most cases evaluations of bioavailability and bioequivalence will be based upon the measured concentrations of the active drug substance(s) in the biological matrix. In some situations, however, the measurements of an active or inactive metabolite may be necessary. These situations include (a) where the concentrations of the drug(s) may be too low to accurately measure in the biological matrix, (b) limitations of the analytical method, (c) unstable drug(s), (d) drug(s) with a very short half-life or (e) in the case of prodrugs. Racemates should be measured using an achiral assay method. Measurement of individual enantiomers in bioequivalence studies is recommended where all of the following criteria are met:

(a) The enantiomers exhibit different pharmacodynamic characteristics.

(b) The enantiomers exhibit different pharmacokinetic characteristics.

(c) Primary efficacy / safety activity resides with the minor enantiomers.

(d) Non-linear absorption is present for at least one of the enantiomers.

The plasma-time concentration curve is mostly used to assess the rate and extent of absorption of the study drug. These include pharmacokinetic parameters such as the C_{max}, T_{max}, AUC_{0-t} and $AUC_{0-\infty}$. For studies in the steady state AUC_{0-t}, C_{max}, C_{min} and degree of fluctuation should be calculated.

➤ **Bioanalytical methodology**

The bioanalytical methods used to determine the drug and/or its metabolites in plasma, serum, blood or urine or any other suitable matrix must be well characterised, standardised, fully validated and documented to yield reliable results that can be satisfactorily interpreted. Although there are various stages in the development and validation of an analytical procedure, the validation of the analytical method can be envisaged to consist of two distinct phases:

1. The pre-study phase which comes before the actual start of the study and involves the validation of the method on biological matrix human plasma samples and spiked plasma samples.

2. The study phase in which the validated bioanalytical method is applied to the actual analysis of samples from bioavailability

and bioequivalence studies mainly to confirm the stability, accuracy and precision.

1. Pre-study phase

The following characteristics of the bioanalytical method must be evaluated and documented to ensure the acceptability of the performance and reliability of analytical results:

i. Stability of the drug/metabolites in the biological matrix: Stability of the drug and/or active metabolites in the biological matrix under the conditions of the experiment (including any period for which samples are stored before analyses) should be established. The stability data should also include the influence of at least three freezing and thawing cycles representative of actual sample handling. The absence of any sorption by the sampling containers and stoppers should also be established.

ii. Specificity/Selectivity: Data should be generated to demonstrate that the assay does not suffer from interference by endogenous compounds, degradation products, other drugs likely to be present in study samples, and metabolites of the drug(s) under study.

iii. Sensitivity: Sensitivity is the capacity of the test procedure to record small variations in concentration. The analytical method chosen should be capable of assaying the drug/metabolites over the expected concentration range. A reliable lowest limit of quantification should be established based on an intra- and inter-day coefficient of variation usually not greater than 20 percent. The limit of detection (the lowest concentration that can be differentiated from background levels) is usually lower than the limit of quantification. Values between limit of quantification and limit of detection should be identified as "Below Quantification Limits."

iv. Precision and accuracy: Precision (the degree of reproducibility of individual assays) should be established by replicate assays on standards, preferably at several concentrations. Accuracy is the degree to which the 'true' value of the concentration of drug is estimated by the assay. Precision and accuracy should normally be documented at three concentrations (low, medium, high) where 'low' is in the vicinity of the lowest concentration to be measured, 'high' is a value in the vicinity of C max and 'medium' is a suitable intermediate value.

Intra-assay precision (within days) in terms of coefficient of variation should be no more than 15%, although no more than 20% may be more realistic at values near the lower limit of quantification. Inter-assay precision (between days) may be higher than 15% but not more than 20%. Accuracy can be assessed in conjunction with precision and is a measure of the extent to which measured concentrations deviate from true or nominal concentrations of analytical standards. In general, an accuracy of ±15% should be attained.

v. Recovery: Documentation of extraction recovery at high, medium and low concentrations is essential since methods with low recovery are, in general, more prone to inconsistency. If recovery is low, alternative methods should be investigated. Recovery of any internal standard used should also be assessed.

vi. Range and linearity: The quantitative relationship between concentration and response should be adequately characterized over the entire range of expected sample concentrations. For linear relationships, a standard curve should be defined by at least five concentrations. If the concentration response function is non-linear, additional points would be necessary to define the non-linear portions of the curve. Extrapolation beyond the standard curve is not acceptable.

vii. Analytical system stability: To assure that the analytical system remains stable over the time course of the assay, the reproducibility of the standard curve should be monitored during the assay. A minimal design would be to run analytical standards at the beginning and at the end of the analytical run.

2. Study phase

In general, with acceptable variability as defined by validation data, the analysis of biological sample can be done by single determination without a need for a duplicate or replicate analysis. The need for duplicate analysis should be assessed on a case-by-case basis. A procedure should be developed that documents the reason for re-analysis. A standard curve should be generated for each analytical run for each analyte and should be used to calculate the concentration of the analyte in the unknown samples assayed with that run. It is important to use a standard curve that will cover the entire range of concentrations in the unknown samples. Estimation of unknowns by extrapolations of standard curves below the lowest standard concentration or above the highest standard concentration is not recommended. Instead, it is suggested that standard curve should be redetermined or sample should be re-assayed after dilution. Quality control sample should be used to accept or reject the run.

3. Quality control samples

Quality control samples are samples with known concentration prepared by spiking drug-free biological fluid with drug. These samples should be prepared in low, medium and high concentration. To avoid possible confusion between quality control samples and standard solutions during the review process, preparation of quality control samples at concentrations different from those used for the calibration is recommended. For stable analytes, quality control samples should be prepared in the fluid of interest at the time of pre-study assay validation or at the time of study sample collection, and stored with the study samples. For less stable analytes, daily or weekly quality control samples may have to be prepared. A quality control sample for each concentration should be assayed on each occasion that study samples are assayed, and the concentration determined by reference to that day's calibration standards. If the concentration values determined for the controls are not within ±15% of the expected concentrations, the batch should be considered for re-analysis.

4. Repeat analysis

In most studies some samples will require re-analysis because of aberrant results due to processing errors, equipment failure or poor chromatography. The reasons for re-analysis of such samples should be stated. The criteria for repeat analyses should be determined prior to running the study and recorded in the protocol / laboratory standard operating procedures.

➤ **Statistical evaluation**

1. Data analysis

The primary concern in bio-equivalence assessment is to limit the consumer's risk i.e., erroneously accepting bioequivalence and also at the same time minimizing the manufacture's risk i.e., erroneously rejecting bioequivalence. This is done by using appropriate statistical methods for data analysis and adequate sample size.

2. Statistical analysis

The statistical procedure should be s specified in the protocol itself. In case of bioequivalence studies the procedures should lead to a decision scheme which is symmetrical with respect to the two formulations (i.e. leading to the same decision whether the new formulation is compared to the reference product or the reference product to the new formulation). The statistical analysis (e.g. ANOVA) should take into account sources of variation that can be reasonably assumed to have an effect on the response. The 90% confidence interval for the ratio of the population means (Test/reference) or two one sided-t tests with the null hypothesis of non-bioequivalence at the 5% significance level for the parameter under consideration are considered for testing bioequivalence. To meet the assumption of normality of data underlying the statistical analysis, the logarithmic transformation should be carried out for the pharmacokinetic parameters C max and AUC before performing statistical analysis. However, it is recommended not to verify the assumptions underlying the statistical analysis before making logarithmic transformation. The analysis of T is desirable if it is clinically relevant. The parameter T max should be analysed using non-parametric methods. In addition to above, summary statistics such as minimum, maximum and ratio should be given.

3. Criteria for bioequivalence

To establish Bioequivalence, the calculated 90% confidence interval for AUC and C max should fall within the bioequivalence range, usually 80-125%. This is equivalent to the rejection of two one sided-t tests with the null hypothesis of non-bioequivalence at 5% level of significance. The non-parametric 90% confidence interval for T max should lie within a clinically acceptable range.

Tighter limits for permissible differences in bioavailability may be required for drugs that have:

   i. A narrow therapeutic index.

  ii. A serious, dose-related toxicity.

 iii. A steep dose/effect curve, or

 iv. A non-linear pharmacokinetics within the therapeutic dose range.

A wider acceptance range may be acceptable if it is based on sound clinical justification. In case of supra-bioavailability, a reformulation followed by a fresh bioequivalence study will be necessary. Otherwise, clinical trial data on new formulation will be required to support the application, especially dosage recommendations. Such formulations are usually not being accepted as therapeutically equivalent to the existing reference product. The name of the new product should preclude confusion with the earlier approved product.

4. Deviations from the study plan

The method of analysis should be defined in the protocol. The protocol should specify methods for handling drop-outs and for identifying biologically implausible outliers. Post hoc exclusion of outliers is not recommended. A scientific explanation should be provided to justify the exclusion of a volunteer from the analysis.

➤ **Special considerations for modified-release drug products**

For the purpose of these guidelines modified release products include:

   i. Delayed release

  ii. Sustained release

iii. Mixed immediate and sustained release

iv. Mixed delayed and sustained release

v. Mixed immediate and delayed release

Generally, these products should:

i. Act as modified-release formulations and meet the label claim

ii. Preclude the possibility of any dose dumping effect

iii. There must be a significant difference between the performance of modified release product and the conventional release product when used as reference product.

iv. Provide a therapeutic performance comparable to the reference immediate-release formulation administered by the same route in multiple doses (of an equivalent daily amount) or to the reference modified-release formulation;

v. Produce consistent pharmacokinetic performance between individual dosage units; and

vi. Produce plasma levels which lie within the therapeutic range (where appropriate) for the proposed dosing intervals at steady state. If all of the above conditions are not met but the applicant considers the formulation to be acceptable, justification to this effect should be provided.

i. Study parameters

Bioavailability data should be obtained for all modified release drug products although the type of studies required and the pharmacokinetic parameters which should be evaluated may differ depending on the active ingredient involved. Factors to be considered include whether or not the formulation represents the first market entry of the drug substance, and the extent of accumulation of the drug after repeated dosing. If the formulation is the first market entry of the drug substance, the product's pharmacokinetic parameters should be determined. If the formulation is a second or subsequent market entry then comparative bioavailability studies using an appropriate reference product should be performed.

ii. Study design

Study design will be single dose or single and multiple dose based on the modified release products that are likely to accumulate or unlikely to accumulate both in the fasted and non-fasting state. If the effect of food on the reference product is not known (or it is known that food affects its absorption), two separate two-way cross-over studies, one in the fasted state and the other in the fed state, may be carried out. If it is known with certainty (e.g. from published data) that the reference product is not affected by food, then a three-way cross-over study may be appropriate with:

  a. The reference product in the fasting state
  b. The test product in the fasted state, and
  c. The test product in the fed state.

iii. Requirements for modified release formulations unlikely to accumulate

This section outlines the requirements for modified release formulations which are used at a dose interval that is not likely to lead to accumulation in the body ($AUC0\text{-}t / AUC0\text{-}\infty = 0.8$). When the modified release product is the first market entry of that type of dosage form, the reference product should normally be the innovator's immediate-release formulation. The comparison should be between a single dose of the modified release formulation and doses of the immediate-release formulation which it is intended to replace. The latter must be administered according to the established dosing regimen. When the modified release product is the second or subsequent entry on the market, comparison should be with the reference modified release product for which bioequivalence is claimed. Studies should be performed with single dose administration in the fasting state as well as following an appropriate meal at a specified time. The following pharmacokinetic parameters should be calculated from plasma (or relevant biological matrix) concentrations of the drug and/or major metabolite(s):$AUC0\text{-}t$, $AUC0\text{-}t$, $AUC0\text{-}\infty$, $Cmax$ (where the comparison is with an existing modified release product), and $k\ el$. The 90% confidence interval calculated using log transformed data for the ratios (Test: Reference) of the geometric mean AUC (for both AUC_{max} and AUC) and generally be within the range 80 to 125% both in the fasting state and following the administration of an appropriate meal at a specified time before taking the drug. The pharmacokinetic parameters should support the claimed dose delivery attributes of the modified-release dosage form.

iv. Requirements for modified release formulations likely to accumulate

This section outlines the requirements for modified release formulations that are used at dose intervals that are likely to lead to accumulation ($AUC0-\tau / AUC0-\infty < 0.8$).

When a modified release product is the first market entry of the modified release type, the reference formulation is normally the innovator's immediate-release formulation. Both a single dose and steady state doses of the modified release formulation should be compared with doses of the immediate-release formulation which it is intended to replace. The immediate-release product should be administered according to the conventional dosing regimen.

Studies should be performed with single dose administration in the fasting state as well as following an appropriate meal. In addition, studies are required at steady state. The following pharmacokinetic parameters should be calculated from single dose studies: $AUC0-t$, $AUC0-t$, $AUC0-\infty$, C max (where the comparison is with an existing modified release product), and k_{el}. The following parameters should be calculated from steady state studies: $AUC_{0-\tau\ (ss)}$, C_{max}, C_{min}, Cpd and degree of fluctuation. When the modified release product is the second or subsequent modified release entry, single dose and steady state comparisons should normally be made with the reference modified release product for which bioequivalence is claimed. The 90% confidence interval for the ratio of geometric means (Test: Reference drug) of AUC (for both AUC_{0-6} and AUC_{0-t}) and C max (where the comparison is with an existing modified release product) determined using log transformed data should generally be within the range 80 to 125% when the products are compared after single dose administration in both the fasting state and the fed state. The 90% confidence interval for the ratio of geometric means (Test: Reference drug) for AUC0-t(ss), C max , and C min determined using log-transformed data should generally be within the range 80 to 125% when the formulations are compared at steady state. The pharmacokinetic parameters should support the claimed attributes of the modified-release dosage form. Pharmacodynamic data may reinforce or clarify interpretation of differences in the plasma concentration data. Where these studies do not show bioequivalence, comparative efficacy and safety data may be required for the new product.

➢ **Pharmacodynamic studies**

Studies in healthy volunteers or patients using pharmacodynamic parameters may be used for establishing equivalence between two pharmaceutical products. These studies may become necessary if quantitative analysis of the drug and/or metabolite(s) in plasma or urine cannot be made with sufficient accuracy and sensitivity. Furthermore, pharmacodynamic studies in humans are required if measurements of drug concentrations cannot be used as surrogate endpoints for the demonstration of efficacy and safety of the particular pharmaceutical product e.g., for topical products without an intended absorption of the drug into the systemic circulation. In case, only pharmacodynamic data is collected and provided, the applicant should outline what other methods were tried and why they were found unsuitable. The following requirements should be recognised when planning, conducting and assessing the results from a pharmacodynamic study:

i. The response measured should be a pharmacological or therapeutic effect which is relevant to the claims of efficacy and/ or safety of the drug.

ii. The methodology adopted for carrying out the study should be validated for precision, accuracy, reproducibility and specificity.

iii. Neither the test nor the reference product should produce a maximal response in the course of the study, since it may be impossible to distinguish differences between formulations given in doses that produce such maximal responses. Investigation of dose-response relationship may become necessary.

iv. The response should be measured quantitatively under double-blind conditions and be recorded in an instrument-produced or instrument-recorded fashion on a repetitive basis to provide a record of pharmacodynamic events which are a substitute for plasma concentrations. If such measurements are not possible, recordings on visual-analog scales may be used. In instances, where data are limited to qualitative (categorized) measurements, appropriate special statistical analyses will be required.

v. Non-responders should be excluded from the study by prior screening. The criteria by which responders *versus* non-responders are identified must be stated in the protocol.

vi. Where an important placebo effect can occur, comparison between products can only be made by a priori consideration of the placebo effect in the study design. This may be achieved by adding a third period/phase with placebo treatment, in the design of the study.

vii. A crossover or parallel study design should be used, as appropriate.

viii. When pharmacodynamic studies are to be carried out on patients, the underlying pathology and natural history of the condition should be considered in the study design. There should be knowledge of the reproducibility of the base-line conditions.

ix. In studies where continuous variables could be recorded, the time course of the intensity of the drug action can be described in the same way as in a study where plasma concentrations are measured. From this, parameters can be derived which describe the area under the effect-time curve, the maximum response and the time when the maximum response occurred.

x. Statistical considerations for the assessments of the outcomes are in principle, the same as in pharmacokinetic studies.

xi. A correction for the potential non-linearity of the relationship between dose and area under the effect-time curve should be made on the basis of the outcome of the dose ranging study. The conventional acceptance range as applicable to pharmacokinetic studies and bioequivalence is not appropriate (too large) in most cases. This range should therefore be defined in the protocol on a case-to-case basis.

➤ Comparative clinical studies

In several instances, the plasma concentration time-profile data may not be suitable to assess equivalence between two formulations. Whereas in some of the cases pharmacodynamic studies can be an appropriate tool for establishing equivalence, in other instances this type of study cannot be performed because of lack of meaningful pharmacodynamic parameters which can be measured and a comparative clinical study has to be performed in order to demonstrate equivalence between two formulations. Comparative clinical studies may also be required to be carried out for certain orally administered drug products when pharmacokinetic and pharmacodynamic studies are not feasible. However, in such cases, the applicant should outline what other methods were tried and why they were found unsuitable. If a clinical study is considered as being undertaken to prove equivalence, the appropriate statistical principles should be applied to demonstrate bioequivalence. The number of patients to be included in the study will depend on the variability of the target parameters and the acceptance range, and is usually much higher than the number of subjects in bioequivalence studies. The following items are important and need to be defined in the protocol in advance:

a. The target parameters which usually represent relevant clinical end-points from which the intensity and the onset, if applicable and relevant, of the response are to be derived.

b. The size of the acceptance range has to be defined case-to-case taking into consideration the specific clinical conditions. These include, among others, the natural course of the disease, the efficacy of available treatments and the chosen target parameter.

In contrast to bioequivalence studies (where a conventional acceptance range is applied) the size of the acceptance range in clinical trials cannot be based on a general consensus on all the therapeutic classes and indications.

c. The presently used statistical method is the confidence interval approach. The main concern is to rule out that the test product is inferior to the reference product by more than the specified amount. Hence, a one-sided confidence interval (for efficacy and/ or safety) may be appropriate. The confidence intervals can be derived from either parametric or nonparametric methods.

d. Where appropriate, a placebo leg should be included in the design.

e. In some cases, it is relevant to include safety end-points in the final comparative assessments.

➢ **In vitro studies**

In certain situations a comparative *in vitro* dissolution study may be sufficient to demonstrate equivalence between two drug products. The test methodology adopted should be in line with the pharmacopoeial requirements unless those requirements are shown to be unsatisfactory. Alternative methods may be acceptable provided they have sufficient discriminatory power. Dissolution studies should generally be carried out under mild agitation conditions at 37±0.5 °C and at physiologically relevant pH. More than one batch of each formulation should be tested. Comparative dissolution profiles, rather than single point dissolution test data, should be generated. The design should include:

i. Individually testing of at least twelve dosage units (e.g., tablets, capsules) of each batch. Mean and individual results should be reported along with their standard deviations or standard errors.

ii. Measuring the percentage of nominal content released at a number of suitably spaced time points to provide a profile for each batch, e.g. at 10, 20 and 30 minutes or as appropriate to achieve virtually complete dissolution.

iii. Determining the dissolution profile in at least three aqueous media covering the pH range of 1.0 to 6.8 or in cases where considered necessary, pH range of 1.0 to 8.0.

iv. Conducting the tests on each batch using the same apparatus and, if possible, on the same or consecutive days.

Comparisons of the dissolution profiles may be made by any of the established model-independent or model-dependent methods.

Documentation

With respect to the conduct of bioequivalence/bioavailability studies following important documents must be maintained:

i. Clinical Data:

    a. All relevant documents as required to be maintained for compliance with GCP Guidelines

ii. Details of the analytical method validation including the following:

    a. System suitability test.

    b. Linearity range

    c. Lowest limit of quantitation

    d. QC sample analysis

    e. Stability sample analysis

    f. Recovery experiment result

iii. Analytical data of volunteer plasma samples which should include the following:

    a. Validation data of analytical methods used

    b. Chromatograms of all volunteers, including any aberrant chromatograms

    c. Inter-day and intra-day variation of assay results

    d. Details including chromatograms of any repeat analysis performed

    e. Calibration status of the instruments

   iv. Raw data

   v. All comments of the chief investigator regarding the data of the study submitted for review.

   vi. A copy of the final report

Study report

The bioequivalence or bioavailability report should give the complete documentation of its protocol, conduct and evaluation. The report should include (as a minimum) the following information:

a. Table of contents

b. Title of the study

c. Names and credentials of responsible investigators

d. Signatures of the principal and other responsible investigators authenticating their respective sections of the report

e. Site of the study and facilities used

f. The period of dates over which the clinical and analytical steps were conducted

g. Names and batch numbers of the products compared

h. A signed declaration that this was identical to that intended for marketing.

i. Results of assays and other pharmaceutical tests (e.g., physical description, dimensions, mean weight, weight uniformity, and comparative dissolution) carried out on the batches of products compared

j. Full protocol for the study including a copy of the ICF and criteria for inclusion/exclusion or withdrawal of subjects

k. Report of protocol deviations, violations

l. Documentary evidence that the study was approved by an independent ethics committee and was carried out in accordance with GCP/GLP.

m. Demographic data of subjects

n. Names and addresses of subjects

o. Details of and justifications for protocol deviations

p. Details of dropout and withdrawals from the study should be fully documented and accounted for

q. Details of analytical methods used, full validation data, quality control data and criteria for accepting or rejecting assay results

r. Representative chromatograms covering the whole concentration range for all, standard and quality control samples as well as specimens analysed

s. Sampling schedules and deviations of the actual times from the scheduled

t. Details of how pharmacokinetic parameters were calculated

u. Documentation related to statistical analysis:

   i. Randomization schedule

   ii. Volunteer wise plasma concentration and time points for test and reference products

   iii. Volunteer wise AUC_{0-t} , $AUC_{0-\infty}$, C_{max} , T , K_{el} , and $t1/2$ for test and reference products

   iv. Logarithmic transformed measures used for BE demonstration

   v. ANOVA for AUC_{0-t}, AUC_{0-t}, C_{max}

   vi. Inter-subject, intra-subject and/or total variability if possible

   vii. Confidence intervals for AUC_{0-t}, $AUC_{0-\infty}$, C_{max}

   (Confidence interval (CI) values should not be rounded off; therefore, to pass a CI range of 80 to 125, the values should be at least 80.00 and not more than 125.00

   viii. Geometric mean, arithmetic mean, ratio of means for AUC_{0-t}, $AUC_{0-\infty}$, C_{max}

   ix. Partial AUC, only if it is used

x. C_{min}, C_{max}, C_{pd}, AUC, degree of fluctuation [(C max – C min)/C av] and swing [(C max – C min)/C min], if steady state studies are employed

Facilities for conducting bioavailability and/or bio-equivalence studies

Legal identity

The organization, conducting the bioequivalence / bioavailability studies, or the parent organization to which it belongs, must be a legally constituted body with appropriate statutory registrations.

Impartiality, confidentiality, independence and integrity:

The organization shall:

a. Have managerial staff with the authority and the resources needed to discharge their duties.

b. Have arrangements to ensure that its personnel are free from any commercial, financial and other pressures which might adversely affect the quality of their work.

c. Be organized in such a way that confidence in its independence of judgment and integrity is maintained at all times.

d. Have documented policies and procedures, where relevant, to ensure the protection of its sponsors' confidential information and proprietary rights.

e. Not engage in any activity that may jeopardize the trust in its independence of judgement and integrity.

f. Have documented policies and procedures for the safety of human rights and the use of human subjects in research consistent with Schedule Y (refer Drugs & Cosmetics Act and Rules) and GCP Guidelines.

g. Have documented policies and procedures for scientific integrity including procedures dealing with and reporting possible scientific misconduct.

Organization and management:

The study site organization must include the following:

a. An Investigator who has the overall responsibility to provide of the human subjects. The Investigator(s) should possess appropriate medical qualifications and relevant experience for conducting pharmacokinetic studies.

b. The site should have identified adequately qualified and trained personnel to perform the following functions:

    i. Clinical Pharmacological Unit (CPU) management

    ii. Analytical laboratory management

    iii. Data handling and interpretation

    iv. Documentation and report preparation

    v. Quality assurance of all operations in the centre

Documented standard operating procedures

The center shall establish and maintain a quality system appropriate to the type, range and volume of its activities. All operations at the site must be conducted as per the authorized and documented standard operating procedures. These documented procedures should be available to the respective personnel for ready reference. The procedures covered must include those that ensure compliance with all aspects of:

a. GCP Guidelines

b. Good laboratory practice guidelines issued by Ministry of Health & Family Welfare

A partial list of procedures for which documented standard operating procedures should be available includes:

a. Maintenance of working standards (pure substances) and respective documentation.

b. Withdrawal, storage and handling of biological samples.

c. Maintenance, calibration and validation of instruments.

d. Managing medical as well as non-medical emergency situations

e. Handling of biological fluids

f. Managing laboratory hazards

g. Disposal procedures for clinical samples and laboratory wastes

h. Documentation of clinical pharmacology unit observations, volunteer data and analytical data

i. Obtaining informed consent from volunteers

j. Volunteer screening and recruitment and management of ineligible volunteers

k. Volunteer recycling (using the same volunteer for more than one study

l. Randomization code management

m. Study subject management at the site (including check-in and check-out procedures)

n. Recording and reporting protocol deviations

o. Recording, reporting and managing scientific misconduct

p. Monitoring and quality assurance

Wherever possible, disposable (sterile, wherever applicable) medical dev ices must be used for making subject interventions. If services of a laboratory or a facility other than those available at the site (whether with in India or outside the country) are to be availed – its/their name(s), address(s) and specific services to be used should be documented.

Clinical pharmacological unit

It must have adequate space and facilities to house at least 16 volunteers. Adequate area must be provided for dining and recreation of volunteers, separate from their sleeping area.

Additional space and facilities should also be provided for the following:

a. Office and administrative functions

b. Sample collection and storage

c. Control sample storage
d. Wet chemical laboratory
e. Instrumental Laboratory
f. Library
g. Documentation archival room
h. Facility for washing, cleaning and Toilets
i. Microbiological laboratory (Optional)
j. Radio Immuno – Assay room (optional)

Maintenance of records of BA/BE studies

All records of in vivo or in vitro tests conducted on any marketed batch of a drug product to assure that the product meets a bioequivalence requirement shall be maintained by the Sponsor for at least 2 years after the expiration date of the batch and submitted to CDSCO on request.

Retention of BA/BE samples

All samples of test and reference drug products used in bioavailability / bioequivalence study should be retained by the organization carrying out the bioavailability / bioequivalence study for a period of three years after the conduct of the study or one year after the expiry of the drug, whichever is earlier. The study sponsor and/or drug manufacturer should provide to the testing facility batches of the test and reference drug products in such a manner that the reserve samples can be selected randomly. This is to ensure that the samples are in fact representative of the batches provided by the study sponsor and/or drug manufacturer and those they are retained in their original containers. Each reserve sample should consist of a quantity sufficient to carry out twice all the in-vitro and in-vivo tests required during bioavailability / bioequivalence study.

The reserve sample should be stored under conditions consistent with product labeling and in an area segregated from the area where testing is conducted and with access limited to authorized personnel.

Special topics

- **Food effect bioavailability studies**

Food effect study is required when there is a possibility to have effect of food on the bioavailability of the drug. Food effect bioavailability studies focus on effects of food on the release of the drug substance from the drug product as well as the absorption of the drug substance. Usually, a single dose crossover study is recommended for BA and BE studies.

- **Long half-life drugs**

For BE determination of an oral product with long half life, a single dose crossover study can be conducted, provided an adequate wash out period is used. If due to longer periods, chances of drop outs as well as intra subject variation are higher with routine cross over designs; parallel group designs can be used. In all cases, blood sampling period should be adequate to describe the plasma concentration time profile. C max and a suitably truncated AUC can be used to characterize peak and total drug exposure, respectively. For drugs, demonstrating high intra-subject variability in distribution and clearance, AUC truncation warrants caution. In such cases, sponsors and/or applicants should consult the regulatory authority.

- **Early exposure**

In general, bioequivalence may be demonstrated by measurements of peak and total exposure for an immediate release product. However, in situations such as rapid onset of an analgesic effect or to avoid an excessive hypotensive action of an antihypertensive, an early exposure measure may be informative on the basis of appropriate clinical efficacy/safety trials and/or pharmacokinetic / pharmacodynamic studies that call for better control of drug absorption into the systemic circulation. In these situations, use of partial AUC is recommended as an early exposure measure. The partial area should be truncated at T values for the reference formulation. At least two quantifiable samples should be collected before the expected peak time to allow adequate estimation of the partial area.

- **Individual and population bioequivalence**

The current practice of evaluating bioequivalence has been termed as average bioequivalence. Whereas in individual bioequivalence, determination of the intra subject variation of drug response is important. By "population bioequivalence" we mean a bioequivalence criterion that requires the distribution of the formulation to be sufficiently similar to that of the reference in some appropriate population. Average bioequivalence is a special case of population bioequivalence.

The average bioequivalence of the two formulations is important in the case of prescribability. However, Individual bioequivalence is required in case of switchability. Assessment of individual bioequivalence is an interesting and exciting alternative to the current practice of evaluating average bioequivalence. The evaluation of individual bioequivalence requires values of intra-subject variability of the test and reference formulations. Hence the assessment of individual bioequivalence is done based on three or four period designs. Replicate study designs provide such information. Up till now, bioequivalence studies are designed to evaluate average bioequivalence. Experience with population and individual bioequivalence studies is limited. Hence no specific recommendation is proposed on this matter. However, for highly variable drugs, individual bioequivalence can be considered.

In Vivo Methods of Evaluation – Statistical Treatment

(See statistical evaluation in bioavailability testing protocol and procedure)

Questions

Essay questions

1. Write a note on bioavailability and bioequivalence protocol and procedure.
2. Explain *in vitro* drug dissolution testing models. What factors should be considered in the design of dissolution testing models?

Short questions

1. What are the objectives and approaches in developing in *vitro–in vivo* correlation?

2. Discuss the various methods of developing quantitative linear in vitro–in vivo correlationships.

3. What are the special considerations for modified release drug product?

4. What are the special facilities for conducting bioavailability and bioequivalence studies?

5. Write a note on statistical treatment.